The Dog

Its Behavior,

Nutrition,

and Health

Linda P. Case

Iowa State University Press / Ames

Linda P. Case teaches companion animal science in the Animal Sciences Department at the University of Illinois at Urbana-Champaign. She owns AutumnGold Dog Training Center and consults for the Iams Company.

Illustrations and cover by Kerry Helms

© 1999 Iowa State University Press

Iowa State University Press
2121 South State Avenue, Ames, Iowa 50014

Orders: 1-800-862-6657
Office: 1-515-292-0140
Fax: 1-515-292-3348
Web site: www.isupress.edu

⊚ Printed on acid-free paper in the United States of America

First edition, 1999

International Standard Book Number: 0-8138-1259-3

Library of Congress Cataloging-in-Publication Data

Case, Linda P.
     The dog: its behavior, nutrition, and health / Linda P. Case.
        P.   cm.
     Includes bibliographical references (p.   ) and index.
     ISBN 0-8138-1259-3
     1. Dogs.   2. Dogs—Behavior.   3. Dogs—Nutrition.   4. Dogs—Health.   I. Title.
SF426.C375   1999
636.7—dc21   98-39307

The last digit is the print number: 9   8   7   6   5   4   3   2   1

To Roxie, Sparks, Gusto, and Nike
who continue
to bring laughter, joy, and love
to our household

And in memory of Fauna
who brought true meaning
to the word "spirit"

And Stepper
whose heart held all
that is good about dogs

Contents

Preface

TODAY, APPROXIMATELY 38 percent of households in the United States own at least one dog—a total of more than 55 million dogs. An 8-billion-dollar pet food industry and the more than 7 billion dollars that pet owners spend on veterinary care each year provide tangible evidence of the increasing importance that dogs have in our society. This devotion is further illustrated by the recent growth of the pet supply industry, which includes pet "super-stores," play-parks, training centers, and dog day care centers in many communities. The bond that owners have with their dogs and the many health benefits that are afforded by this bond have been the topic of numerous research studies in the past 25 years. The dog as a cherished companion and family member is here to stay, and many owners, students, and companion animal professionals are eager to learn more about man's best friend, *Canis familiaris*.

This comprehensive study of the domestic dog is written for people who are either pursuing or are currently engaged in a profession or avocation that involves dogs: dog trainers, breeders, kennel owners, veterinary technicians, veterinarians, and other companion animal professionals. In addition, *The Dog: Its Behavior, Nutrition, and Health* is an essential text for college students who are studying the physiology, care, behavior, and nutrition of companion animals.

The book is divided into four topical sections. Part 1, "Man's Best Friend: The Animal within the Companion," examines the origin of the relationship between humans and dogs and follows the development of the dog from the first stages of domestication through present day. This part also contains basic information about the dog's physiology, structure, reproduction, and genetics. The status of the dog today and the importance of proper pet selection and responsible ownership are discussed in the final chapter of this section.

Part 2, "Behavior: Communicating with Man's Best Friend," examines the developmental behavior of the dog from birth to adulthood. Species-specific behavior patterns are examined, followed by a discussion of breed-specific behaviors. Learning processes and principles of training are the topic of Chapter 9. Basic tenets of learning are first reviewed, followed by an examination of successful training methodologies. Various training principles are compared and contrasted, and practical examples are provided throughout the chapter. The final chapter in this section identifies several common behavior problems and their solutions.

Part 3, "Health and Disease," concerns health maintenance and the prevention and treatment of disease. Infectious and non-infectious diseases and common internal and external parasitic diseases are included. Types of vaccines, procedures for their use, and vaccination schedules are also discussed.

The final chapter in the section reviews emergency care and first aid procedures that are essential skills for all pet care professionals and dog owners.

Part 4, "Nutrition: Feeding for Health and Longevity," provides an overview of the dog's nutrient requirements and examines available pet foods and methods of feeding. Detailed instructions for feeding throughout the dog's life cycle and criteria for the selection of optimal pet foods are included. The final chapter of the book reviews four common medical disorders that can be treated or managed through diet.

A complete list of relevant and up-to-date books and journal articles for further reading is found at the end of the book along with a glossary of terms used in the book and an easy-to-reference index. Terms that appear in the text in boldface generally are defined in the glossary.

This book is intended not only as a helpful resource but also as an enjoyable and interesting exploration of domestic dogs, our relationship with them, and the best methods of caring for them. The knowledge gained can only strengthen the well-established and enduring bond that exists between dogs and their human caretakers in our culture today.

Acknowledgments

THIS BOOK would not have been possible without the help of several friends and colleagues. First and foremost, many thanks go to one of my proofreaders and editors, Jean S. Palas, whose experience as a dog person and professional trainer were invaluable (thanks, Mom!). The illustrations and diagrams are the work of Kerry Helms, whose positive attitude, creativity, and friendship made this project an enjoyable endeavor. Many thanks also go to my department head, Dr. Robert Easter, who has provided continuing support and enthusiasm for the Companion Animal Program. The behavior chapters of this book would not be what they are without the help and ideas of several trainers at my training center, AutumnGold. Pam Wasson's understanding of dogs and her positive approach to training have had a strong influence on the ideas contained in this book. In addition, the continuing help and input of trainers Mary Stuart and Susan Helmink have been invaluable. And last, many thanks to my husband, Mike, who provided support, editing help, and many hours of "dog help" throughout this project.

Part 1   Man's Best Friend: The Animal within the Companion

1 Man and Wolf: The Process of Domestication

TODAY, APPROXIMATELY 38 percent of households in the United States own at least one dog—a total of more than 55 million dogs.[1] Each year, pet owners are spending more than 8 billion dollars on food for their animals, and an equal amount of money is spent on veterinary care. Although recent research studies have shown that pet ownership is good for both our physical and our psychological health, most dog owners have known this for generations. It is undeniable that the dog is a valued and important member of our society. Unlike any other nonhuman species, the dog has become fully integrated into our lives, and it appears that he is here to stay. So what exactly was it that brought man and dog together many years ago? And more importantly, what characteristics of these two very different species enabled them to forge the strong, on-going partnership that is still so important to us today?

The Dog's Phylogeny (Evolutionary History)

The dog, like the cat, is a member of the order Carnivora, which includes a diverse group of animals that are all predatory in nature. Carnivores are so named because of their enlarged carnassial teeth. These include the enlarged upper fourth premolar and the lower first molar on each side of the mouth. These adaptations make the teeth efficient at shearing and tearing prey. All carnivores also have small, sharp incisors for holding prey and, often, elongated canine teeth for stabbing and tearing.

During the time period when dinosaurs dominated the earth, a group of animals called the miacids were evolving. The Miacidae family included a diverse group of predatory mammals, many of whom were small, tree-dwelling animals. This group existed about 62 million years ago and formed the ancestral family for all members of the order Carnivora. The miacids all walked on the palms/soles of their feet (plantigrade), were long-bodied and slim, and were the first animals with carnassial teeth, an indication of their predatory nature.

Over time, the viveravines branched off from the miacids and are now known to be the oldest ancestor of our domestic cat. A second branch that evolved from the miacids was the miacines. Animals in this group were the ancestors of the dog, bear, raccoon, and weasel. They existed about 60 million years ago and eventually gave rise to *Hesperocyon* (meaning western dog), who is designated as the oldest member of the Canidae family. Remains of *Hesperocyon* have been found in South Dakota, Nebraska, Colorado, and Wyoming and are estimated to have existed about 36 to 38 million years ago. Interestingly, current evidence indicates that the Canidae family evolved completely in North America and did not migrate into Eurasia until much later in its development. *Hesperocyon* was a digitigrade mammal, meaning it walked on its toes, and was long-bodied and long-legged, obviously adapted for speed. Its dentition, including the presence of carnassial teeth, and body structure showed it to be an agile predator. By the end of the Oligocene period, about 23 million years ago, *Hesperocyon* had evolved into *Leptocyon*. *Leptocyon* is thought to be the most recent common ancestor of all of today's canids, although there is some controversy over this mammal's eventual fate.[2] Some accounts claim that *Leptocyon* gave rise to *Tomarctus*, who became the wolf's and the domestic dog's primary ancestor. Other records depict *Tomarctus* and *Leptocyon* as two separate branches of *Hesperocyon*. Regardless, it appears that *Leptocyon*, and probably *Tomarctus*, gave rise to the dominant group of canids in North America who were destined to become all of our modern-day canid species.

The Dog's Taxonomy (Present-Day Classification)

Today, the domestic dog is classified as a member of the Canidae family (Table 1.1). This family also includes the wolf, coyote, fox, jackal, and Cape hunting dog. The dog's genus is *Canis*, and its species is *familiaris*. Other members of *Canis* are the coyote (*Canis latrans*), two species of wolf (the gray or timber wolf *Canis lupus* and the red wolf *Canis rufus*), and four species of jackal. The extreme regional variations that are observed in wolves all represent varieties (subspecies) of *Canis lupus*, rather than separate species. Twenty to thirty subspecies have been identified, some of which have become extinct in this century. The genetic plasticity of the wolf as a species is illustrated by the great variation in physical and behavioral attributes in various subspecies. For example, Alaskan timber wolves (*Canis lupus pambasileus*) typically weigh more than 100 pounds at maturity and live in well-organized packs consisting of an average of five to eight adults. In contrast, the small Asian wolf (*Canis lupus pallipes*) weighs only about 45 to 50 pounds and travels alone or in small packs. There is still dispute over whether or not the red wolf (*Canis rufus*) should be classified as a separate species of wolf or as a sub-

---

TABLE 1.1   Taxonomy of the Dog

Phylum	Animalia
Class	Mammalia
Order	Carnivora
Family	Canidae
Genus	*Canis*
Species	*familiaris*

species. Similarly, there are some experts who feel that the dog should actually be classified as a subspecies of wolf (i.e. *Canis lupus familiaris*), rather than as an entirely different species (*Canis familiaris*).[3]

The immediate wild ancestor of *Canis familiaris* has been the subject of much debate. At one time, it was believed that the dog was descended from the interbreeding of wolves, coyotes, jackals, and other wild canids. During the 1940s, the Nobel prizewinning ethologist, Konrad Lorenz, said that some breeds of dogs were descended from the golden jackal, while others, those that he called "lupus" breeds, were directly descended from the wolf.[4] More recently, wolf and dog expert Michael Fox developed a "missing link" theory. He believes that the dog is descended from a now-extinct European dingo-like dog. However, there is little if any fossil evidence of this ancestor.

Current behavioral, **morphological**, and molecular biological (genetic) evidence supports the wolf (*Canis lupus*) as the primary wild ancestor of our present-day dog. There is still speculation concerning which subspecies of wolf the dog is descended from and whether or not other members of the Canidae family were interbred with wolves on different occasions. Most likely the dog was domesticated simultaneously in different areas of the world from several different subspecies of wolf. For example, in Europe and North America the subspecies would have been the large wolf, *Canis lupus lupus,* while in western and southern Asia the smaller Arabian and Indian wolves *Canis lupus arabs* and *Canis lupus pallipes* would have been the dog's progenitors. Other contributors that have been identified are the Japanese wolf (*Canis lupus hodophylax*) and the Chinese wolf (*Canis lupus chanco*). Support for the interbreeding of the dog with other members of the Canidae family lies in the fact that the domestic dog is still capable of interbreeding with wolves, coyotes, and jackals. Both dogs and wolves have 39 pairs of chromosomes, or 78 total. This is also true for the four species of jackal and the coyote.

Important evidence for the dog's close relationship to the wolf lies in the existence of physical and behavioral similarities between the two species. One of the most basic is the social nature of dogs and wolves. Both species establish social groups, commonly called packs. In contrast, jackals are known to live and hunt alone, while coyotes hunt in pairs or at the most, as a threesome. The typical wolf pack consists of closely related individuals who are each independent, yet voluntarily work together to obtain food, raise young, and protect the pack from other predators. For the wolf, this means survival in a harsh environment in which food is scarce and the primary food source is often large ungulates (hoofed mammals). Hunting such large prey would be impossible for one wolf hunting alone. As individuals, both dogs and wolves seek out contact and interactions with con-specifics (other pack members), and social activity is an important part of their daily life. Common examples include the elaborate greeting rituals, play, and exploratory behaviors of both species.

A second important similarity between the domestic dog and the wolf involves methods of communication. Natural selection has resulted in the establishment of complex communication patterns in all species that are required to work cooperatively for survival. In wolves, primary communication patterns involve body postures, facial expressions, and vocalizations. The domestic dog has inherited some of these communication tools in their complete form, differing little from their expression in *Canis lupus*. Other patterns have been modified through domestication, but vestigial portions are still observed. The wolf and the dog exhibit similar postures that signal aggression, dominance, submission, and fear. However, the level of stimulus that is necessary to evoke these expressions, along with their intensity and completeness, has been modified significantly through domestication. The development of different breeds of dogs for specific purposes has further exaggerated or attenuated both physical and behavioral characteristics of the wolf (see Chapter 2).

The Process of Domestication

Domestication of a species occurs when the breeding and containment of large groups of animals is under the control of humans. Over a period of many generations, this results in the development of an animal who is genetically distinct from members of the original species. Although members of domesticated species can often still mate and produce viable offspring with members of the progenitor species, the domestication process involves a change in genetic structure. This can be contrasted to "taming," which refers to simply decreasing the fear of humans in an individual animal. A tame animal is merely a wild animal who has been habituated to its human caretakers. Such an animal easily reverts to the wild state, most often when it reaches sexual maturity. Domestication must be viewed as a process that affects an entire species over many generations and that involves the geographic, reproductive, and behavioral isolation of the selected group from its wild population.

Currently there are two predominant theories that attempt to explain the morphological and behavioral changes that occurred in the wolf as it was domesticated to become the dog. The first and most popular of these develops a model of the dog as a neotenized wolf.[5,6] The term **neoteny** refers to the persistence of infantile characteristics, either physical or behavioral, into adulthood. In essence, the animal remains permanently immature with respect to the characteristic in question. Physical attributes that are commonly observed in neotenized species include decreased body size, altered jaw size and strength, decreased number and size of teeth, a prominent forehead, shortened limbs, and diminished secondary sexual characteristics in males. In predatory species, such as the dog, these physical changes were necessary to allow handling and management of individuals.

Neotenized behavioral characteristics are of equal significance in the domestic dog. An examination of the normal wolf pup demonstrates a number of behavior patterns that have been selected to persist into adulthood in the domesticated dog. Wolf pups are highly curious about their environments and will readily explore and investigate new animals and objects without showing the characteristic wariness of adult wolves. It is only after a certain age that wolf pups begin to show a fearfulness of unfamiliar stimuli. This is called **xenophobia** or **neophobia,** meaning, respectively, fear of the foreign or fear of the new. Xenophobia has survival value for any species that is living in a harsh environment. However, this trait is not desirable in a domesticated animal. Adaptability to new environments is a key characteristic in domesticated species. For example, an adult dog that is fearful of new situations, people, or animals is not well adapted to living and working with man. Therefore, the artificial selection for dogs with a puppylike trust of new stimuli was of distinct advantage. Moreover, once the dog came under the care of humans, there ceased to be any natural selection for xenophobia, since the wolf's normal predators were no longer a threat.

A second important neotenized characteristic that is seen in the dog is the presence of enhanced and easily elicited subordinate behavior patterns. Wolf pups are naturally subordinate to elder members of their pack and are more sociable with animals of other species. However, as pups mature into adult wolves, subordinate behaviors are not as easily elicited, and a collection of dominant behavior patterns develops that are necessary and vital for the adult wolf's integration into the pack. In the domestic dog, both dominant and subordinate behavior patterns are present, but there is an intensification of subordinate behaviors in the adult dog compared to the wolf. Although there are great variations between breeds in both dominant and subordinate behaviors, in general, the display of dominant behaviors has been attenuated. Genetic selection for a naturally subordinate temperament facilitated training and handling of dogs and enhanced their dependency on human caretakers. By keeping the dog rather puppylike in its relationships to others of its pack, the development of agonistic displays and dominance challenges as the animal matured was less likely.

A theory has recently been advanced that challenges the premise that neoteny can explain all of the morphological and behavioral changes that have occurred in the dog. The "mesomorphic remodeling theory" proposes that there are traits present in the domestic dog that are not to be found in either wolf pups or wolf adults.[7,8,9] This theory proposes that the dog may be looked upon more as being arrested at some point during its adolescence or metamorphic period, rather than being strictly neotic. The mesomorphic period refers to a period during which the young animal is rapidly changing into an adult form. In mammals such as the dog this period is typically referred to as the period of adolescence or the juvenile period. The various stages of life that an individual progresses through (i.e., fertilized egg, fetus, neonate, infant, juvenile, and adult) can be viewed as specialized stages during which the animal is behaviorally and morphologically adapted to the environment in which it exists at that time. Behaviors that are present in the infant slowly recede to give way to behaviors that are adaptive for the juvenile and so on. In wolves, the mesomorphic juvenile exhibits some characteristics of the pup, which are decreasing with time; some traits of the adults, which are increasing with time; and some traits that are present only in the juvenile stage.

An interesting and important aspect of the mesomorphic period is that it represents a period of behavioral flexibility or plasticity. Proponents of this model believe that the mesomorphic period represents a period when a multitude of new and different behaviors can evolve and a period when the animal is highly responsive to learning. This theory maintains that a better model to use for the domesticated dog is one in which the dog represents a wolf whose development has been arrested or halted during the highly unstable mesomorphic period. The juvenile period in the wolf is relatively long in duration, and a number of changes occur during this period. It is theorized that selection for arrestment during different points of the juvenile period could be an important source of the wide variation in size, morphology, and behavior seen in different breeds of domestic dog. The hypothesis of metamorphic remodeling is relatively new. It has not yet been thoroughly tested or examined by behaviorists, but it does represent another possible explanation for many of the behaviors and structural differences seen in the domesticated dog.

In the Beginning: Man Meets Dog

The last glaciation period ended approximately 10,000 years ago, and by that time humans and dogs had already forged a strong, enduring partnership. The earliest remains of a domesticated dog that have been found are dated around 12,000 to 14,000 years ago. The earliest archaeological evidence of domestication comes from a grave site that was excavated in northern Israel. The skeleton of a young human boy was found with his hand resting on the skeleton of a 4- to 5-month-old dog.[10] The position of the two skeletons and the structural features of the dog indicate that the relationship between the two was not predatory but affectionate in nature. Recent studies of DNA changes in dogs and wolves have provided evidence that the dog may actually have been domesticated more than 100,000 years ago.[11] However, the reliability of these dating methods is controversial, and this research has not been corroborated.

Most researchers agree that the dog was first domesticated and selectively bred in the context of a forager (hunter-gatherer) society, not an agrarian society. During the Pleistocene period, humans lived in small tribal groups and hunted large ungulates (hoofed mammals) as one of their food sources. Living and hunting as a social group allowed humans to be successful in hunting prey species that were larger or faster than themselves. At that time, another predatory species, the wolf, was also successfully surviving as a social hunter. Most likely, humans and wolves were competing for the same food sources within geographical areas and existed in relatively close proximity to one another.

The first attempts at taming and domesticating the wolf were probably unintentional and occurred in many areas of the world at the same time. Being opportunists, wolves possibly followed human tribes occasionally to scavenge food from their campsites. It is known that humans of the Pleistocene age were in the habit of taking young animals of many species from the wild and raising them in captivity as pets or novelties. Although the young of other carnivores, such as foxes and jackals, also would have been kept and tamed as young animals, the less social nature of these species would not have facilitated a long-term association with humans. The social nature of wolves, on the other hand, may have encouraged humans to keep them in captivity. In general, species that are less social in nature adapt less well to taming and do not remain habituated to humans once they reach adulthood. This trait is responsible for the prevalence of social species in our group of domesticated animals (with the one exception, of course, being the cat).

Once an individual wolf pup was raised and tamed, it could serve several purposes to tribal people, prime of which was as a food source. However, as time went on, humans began to recognize other advantages to keeping this predatory species as a campsite friend. A wolf's alarm bark would have been beneficial in alerting humans to the approach of other tribes or predators as well as a possible deterrent to these intruders. The social nature of the wolf and its ability to hunt cooperatively led to uses of the wolf/dog in the detection, tracking, and killing of game.

During the Mesolithic period, human culture developed the use of weapons for hunting. This allowed greater distances between hunters and prey and opened the need for canine partners to act as trackers and retrievers. As the climate changed and human populations increased, man slowly evolved from hunter-gatherers to inhabitants of settled agrarian communities. Within communities, the need for dogs to act as sentinels to warn of approaching animals or other tribes increased. The age of agriculture and the keeping of domesticated livestock as a food supply resulted in a need for the dog as a guard and herder. As human lifestyles changed, so did the dog's. Intentional breeding was undertaken to develop specific types of dogs for specific jobs. This process was repeated often in many parts of the world, and the dog slowly diversified to numerous body types, coat types, temperaments, and working abilities. The end result was the dog of today—comprising breeds that range in weight from a few pounds to more than 150 pounds and with temperaments as diverse as the differences in size.

From Wolf to Dog: Changes Due to Domestication

The wolf (*Canis lupus*) is one of the most **pleomorphic** species of mammal alive today. This is demonstrated by the physical and behavioral diversity of the many wolf subspecies. Subspecies of wolf vary from the small Arabian desert wolf (*Canis lupus arabs*), weighing only 40 to 50 pounds, to the largest Arctic tundra wolf, which can weigh more than 170 pounds. Many subspecies of wolf have become extinct in the last century, some of which have shown even greater extremes in size and body type. In addition to their physical diversity, the many subspecies of *Canis lupus* also show distinct variations in behavior. For example, while most wolves hunt as packs, the Chinese wolf (*Canis lupus linger*) is a solitary hunter. Howling is a form of communication between wolves within a pack. However, the Asian wolf (*Canis lupus pallipes*) is unusual because it does not howl.

Like the wolf, the dog has 39 pairs of chromosomes, or 78 total. The breeds of dogs we know today have all evolved from this gene pool. As a result, certain attributes, such as overall skeletal structure, capabilities of the special senses, social organization, and communication patterns, are present in all dogs of all breeds. Differences exist, however, in the manner and intensity with which many of these characteristics are expressed. Because of the wolf's vast genetic plasticity, humans were able to select for specific behavior traits and physical attributes as they gradually created the dog from the wolf. Over many generations, certain changes occurred that have made the dog different enough from its wild ancestor to be considered a separate species and classified as *Canis familiaris.*

Several distinct and important physical changes occurred to *Canis lupus* as it was transformed into the dog. Compared to the wolf, the dog has a smaller jaw, and smaller and fewer number of teeth. Even the largest St. Bernard has smaller teeth and less jaw strength than an adult wolf. In most breeds, the shape of the mandible is more curved than that of the wolf, and the angle between the facial region and cranium is greater, resulting in a pronounced **stop.** Other modifications to the mandible include alterations in length to produce the **brachycephalic,** or shortened muzzle, breeds and doliocephalic, or elongated muzzle, breeds. The dog's ears, tail, and coat type became diversified. The pendulous ear of breeds such as the Cocker Spaniel and Beagle are examples of neoteny. While wolf pups ears often fold, all adult wolves have an erect, or prick, ear. In contrast, the erect ear has been retained in many breeds, such as the German Shepherd dog and the Siberian Husky. Entire body size has been reduced in most dogs. Extreme examples are the toy breeds, such as the Papillon and the Italian Greyhound. In others, giantism has resulted in extremely large animals, such as the Great Dane and St. Bernard.

Most domesticated species demonstrate high fertility and early sexual maturity compared to their wild ancestors.[12] This alteration has distinct economic advantages for humans, who have usually been concerned with producing the largest number of animals in the shortest span of time. The wolf has only one estrous cycle per year, usually in the spring. Female dogs, in contrast, are not seasonal breeders and have approximately two estrous cycles per year. The male wolf only produces sperm seasonally, while the male dog is fertile throughout the year. Dogs also reach puberty at an earlier age, attaining sexual maturity at 6 to 9 months. In contrast, wolves do not become sexually active until they are at least 2 years old. Interestingly, the attainment of social maturity in the domestic dog still occurs at a later date, generally about 18 to 24 months. Social maturity is conveyed by the development of strong social bonds, the onset of dominance relationships, and the active defense of territory. If the dog is of a dominant nature, certain types of aggression may arise as well. Domestication appears to have resulted in an uncoupling of sexual maturity and social maturity in the dog's development. While these two changes occur around the same time in wolves (2 years), social maturity occurs substantially later than sexual maturity in the dog. This dichotomy has important significance when dealing with behavioral problems associated with dominance hierarchies in the dog (see chapters 8 and 10).

The physical and behavioral development of wolf and dog puppies also shows important differences. Compared to dogs, wolf pups develop physically much more quickly during the early weeks of life. Important information was gathered in a study that compared growth and development of a group of wolf pups to a group of Alaskan Malamute puppies.[13] Both groups were raised by the same foster wolf mother and socialized to humans. It was found that the wolf pups developed coordination and locomotor skills more rapidly than did the Malamute puppies. For example, at the age of 3 weeks, the wolf pups were capable of climbing out of a whelping pen with 16-inch sides. At the same age, even though they were of comparable size, the Malamutes pups were unable to traverse a 6-inch barrier. At 6 weeks of age, motor performance was again tested in each group. The wolf pups' coordination was almost equivalent to that of small adult dogs. In contrast, the Malamute pups still showed the uncoordinated, rolling gait of a neonate. Interestingly, by 10 weeks of age, these differences had disappeared. When retested for locomotor skills, the wolf pups and the Malamute pups showed similar performances. It is possible that domestication has resulted in decreased selection for early coordination since the survival value of this trait is lessened in a protected environment.

In addition to physical and developmental changes, the wolf has also undergone important behavioral modifications during domestication. The wolf's relationship to his environment changed drastically when humans removed individuals from their natural habitat. The artificial environment into which they were placed did not include most of the selective pressures of the wolf's natural habitat. This alone would result in changes over time, as the wolf no longer needed to evolve in response to changes in the natural environment. As a species, humans then proceeded to insert themselves into the wolf's social structure, the pack. Behavioral changes such as changes in response to thresholds to certain stimuli, increased subordinance and adaptability, and the perpetuation of certain infantile behavior patterns into adulthood are a direct result of these two constraints that were imposed upon the wolf.

Regardless of whether the neoteny theory or the mesomorphic theory is accepted as the primary model for domestication of the dog, it is generally agreed that all domestic dogs exhibit varying degrees of neotenic or juvenile behavior. Whining is a good example. Whining is commonly observed in wolf pups but rarely in adults. The dog, on the other hand, continues to exhibit whining into adulthood and often uses this verbal pattern as an important communication tool with human caretakers. Play behaviors in dogs are a second example. Although adult wolves do exhibit play behaviors, playfulness, in general, is more exaggerated and more easily evoked (i.e. lower response threshold) in dogs than in wolves.

The natural subordinance of puppies and the demonstration of passive and active submission are probably the most important behavioral traits that have been intensified in the domestic dog. The prolonged display of subordinate behavior into adulthood and a decreased tendency toward dominant challenges as sexual and social maturity is achieved are traits that have allowed the dog to bond closely with human caretakers. It has been hypothesized that both the young puppy's need for maternal care and its natural subordinance to adult pack members are neotenized traits.[4] The need for maternal care manifests as an elevated propensity to bond to caretakers, and enhanced subordinance facilitates acceptance of a leader and, subsequently, ease of training.

It appears that the primary socialization period in pups occurs for a longer span of time in dogs than in wolves (see Chapter 7). In canid species, socialization periods represent an age during which social bonds are easily and strongly established. During the early weeks of this period, pups readily approach and investigate novel stimuli such as new sights, smells, and other animals. However, near the end of this period, pups become progressively fearful of new experiences (neophobic). The adaptive significance of this behavior for wolves is that it facilitates appropriate bonding to the dam, litter mates, and other pack members early in life. However, as the pups grow and become more mobile and capable of wandering farther from the den area, the onset of a "fear of the new" has distinct survival value.

Domestic dogs demonstrate primary socialization and develop social bonds most intensely between 5 and 12 weeks of age. Frequent and positive interactions with humans caretakers during this period have been shown to facilitate strong attachment behaviors and training at a later age. In contrast, puppies that are isolated from humans during the period of primary socialization have a greater tendency to become aloof or even timid toward humans. If no interactions occur between puppies and humans prior to 12 to 14 weeks of age, the formation of normal relationships is often severely compromised. By comparison, the wolf pup's primary socialization period appears to be much shorter in duration than that of the dog, and the manifestation of the fear imprint period is much more intense. It has been hypothesized that this early and intense fear imprint period is the cause of the wolf's inability to bond strongly to humans even when raised in captivity.[14] It appears that while the socialization period starts at about the same time in dogs as in wolves, the fear reaction to new animals and situations is delayed in the puppy and is demonstrated far less intensely.

Even when wolf pups are raised in captivity and spend many hours with humans during the period of primary socialization the bond or orientation that wolf pups develop toward humans is still very weak. Although they will passively accept handling by and interactions with human caretakers until about 7 weeks, they begin to show a strong period of fear imprint between 6 and 8 weeks of age. Throughout their development, if the pups have access to a foster mother or to another adult wolf, they will demonstrate a strong social preference to the member of their own species rather than to the human caretaker. This is in strong contrast to developmental behavior in puppies. The study cited previously reported that as soon as the Malamute puppies were mobile, they would readily abandon their foster mother upon the approach of a human caretaker.[13] Moreover, by the time of weaning, the dog puppies were demonstrably more independent of their foster mother than were the wolf pups at the same age.

Of special interest is the greeting behavior of wolf pups compared to dog puppies. Wolf puppies typically demonstrate an intense, effusive "greeting frenzy" toward elder pack members. This greeting behavior is characterized by body postures and facial expressions that convey submission. Wolf pups consistently demonstrate this type of greeting toward their dam, sire, and other pack members. In contrast, dog puppies greet other dogs much less intensely and reserve most of their frenzied greeting responses for their human caretakers. This is another example of how domestication has shifted the dog's primary social attachment from his conspecifics to that of another species, the human.

As wolf pups attain physical maturity, they begin to show normal **agonistic** behaviors, which include dominance displays and challenges to other pack members. The purpose of these behaviors is to establish a stable social hierarchy within the pack. There are natural selective pressures against overt intragroup aggression in social species that are predatory in nature. There are several reasons for this. First, any energy that is spent on altercations with other individuals within the pack is energy that could be better spent in the procurement of food through cooperative hunting. Since survival is usually a full-time occupation for wild animals, the wolf pack that spends large amounts of time fighting among themselves would be at a distinct disadvantage. Therefore, there is direct selective pressure to minimize the amount of energy that is expended settling disputes within the pack. Second, social animals that are predators have the capability to inflict severe injury and death to other animals. Aggression between pack members could result in injury or death, given the power of their defense mechanisms. If injured by another pack member during a dispute, the injured animal would not be able to hunt efficiently and may even attract other predators because of the presence of blood and its weakened state. Therefore, to prevent the problems associated with agonistic behavior toward others of the pack, evolution produced a set of highly predictable and ritualized dominance and submissive displays, along with a social order within the pack that defined the respective roles of dominant and subordinate animals of decreasing social rank. These displays allow the resolution of conflict and other types of interactions within the pack to occur without the danger of inflicting injury to pack members.

While the dog has inherited most of these ritualized body postures, facial expressions, and vocalizations, two important and opposing pressures of the domestication process have modified the wolf's behavior patterns. During domestication, the natural selective pressure against aggression between pack members was unintentionally relaxed. This occurred because the evolving "wolf-dog" was now under the care of human caretakers and no longer had the need to rely upon its own skill and fitness to procure food. In other words, the need to stay fit (and avoid fights with other wolves) was not as important, since fitness was no longer strongly connected to survival. Moreover, the selective pressure for survival of an entire pack was no longer present. As they became domesticated, dogs were incorporated into the human pack and no longer needed to function as a working unit with other dogs. At the same time, in some areas of the world, dogs were selectively bred for guarding behavior and protectiveness. This selective pressure increased the intensity of aggressive responses and decreased the level of stimulus needed to trigger the agonistic behavior. The end result of these pressures was actually an increase in interdog aggression. The repercussions of this can be seen in some of the highly aggressive breeds of dogs that exist today (see Chapter 2). In direct contrast, a second selective force was at work during domestication. The selection for infantile behaviors, including a more naturally subordinate animal, functioned to decrease aggressive behaviors. The final result of these pressures was the creation of a dog who is naturally more subordinate and less dominant than wolves. However, when aggressive behaviors toward other dogs (or humans) are displayed, they may be of higher intensity, and it may take a lower stimulus level to elicit them.

A final important behavioral change that has occurred during domestication is the alteration of normal predatory behavior. The wolf is a predatory animal that hunts cooperatively with a group to kill prey much larger than itself. The complete sequence of predatory behavior includes finding, stalking, chasing, catching, killing, dissecting, and ingesting prey. This sequence of activity is both diminished in intensity in the dog and is terminated before its end (i.e. killing and dissection of prey are absent or severely diminished in most breeds). In addition, certain parts of the predatory sequence have been exaggerated and others suppressed in the development of certain breeds for certain functions (see Chapter 2).

Conclusions

Human association with *Canis lupus* began more than 10,000 years ago and resulted in morphological, developmental, and behavioral changes. These changes eventually produced *Canis familiaris*—the dog as we know it today. Once the dog was domesticated, selective breeding in different areas of the world, in widely different climates, and for a variety of functions resulted in the development of distinct breeds. An examination of the history of selective breeding and the development of different breeds provides valuable information about individual pets that live with us today.

Cited References

1. Arkow, P. **A new look at overpopulation.** Anthrozoos, 3:202-205. (1994)

2. Wayne, R.K. **Phylogenetic relationships of canids to other carnivores.** In: *Miller's Anatomy of the Dog,* third edition, (H.E. Evans, editor), W.B. Saunders Company, Philadelphia, Pennsylvania, pp. 15-21. (1993)

3. Fox, M.W. *The Dog: Its Domestication and Behavior,* Garland STPM Press, New York, New York. (1978)

4. Lorenz, Konrad. *Man Meets Dog,* first printed in 1953. Kodansha International, New York, New York. (1994)

5. Schenkel, R. **Submission: its features and functions in the wolf and dog.** American Zoologist, 7:319-330. (1967)

6. Kretchmer, K.R. and Fox, M.W. **Effects of domestication on animal behaviour.** Veterinary Record, 96:102-108. (1975)

7. Coppinger, R.P. and Schnieder, R. **Evolution of working dog behavior.** In: *The Domestic Dog: Its Evolution, Behavior and Interactions with People* (J.A. Serpell, editor), Cambridge University Press, Cambridge, United Kingdom. (1995)

8. Coppinger, R.P. and Smith, C.K. **A model for understanding the evolution of mammalian behavior.** In: *Current Mammalogy*, Volume 2 (H. Genoways, editor), Plenum Press, New York, New York, pp. 33-74. (1989)

9. Coppinger, R.P. and Feinstein, M. **Why dogs bark.** Smithsonian Magazine, January, pp. 119-129. (1991)

10. Davis, S.J. and Valls, F.R. **Evidence for domestication of the dog 12,000 years ago in the natufian of Israel.** Nature, 276:608-610. (1978)

11. Vila, C., Savolainen, P., Maldonado, J.E., Amorim, I.R., Rice, J.E., Honeycutt, R.L., Crandall, K.A., Lundeburg, J., and Wayne, R.K. **Multiple and ancient origins of the domestic dog.** Science, 276:1687-1689. (1997)

12. Zeuner, F.E. *A History of Domesticated Animals.* Harper and Row, New York, New York. (1963)

13. Frank, H. and Frank, M.G. **On the effects of domestication on canine social development and behavior.** Applied Animal Ethology, 8:507-525. (1982)

14. Fox, M.W. *Behaviour of Wolves, Dogs and Related Canids.* Harper and Row, New York, New York. (1971)

2 Selective Breeding: The Creation of the Working Dog

IN THE PREVIOUS CHAPTER, the history of human association with the dog and its resultant domestication were reviewed. Current evidence indicates that the dog was originally domesticated, in different parts of the world, for its ability to aid in hunting and in guarding homesteads. As human populations increased and man spread across the world, changes in the climate and habitats in which humans lived started to place different demands on their canine companions and working partners. Different types of dogs evolved to work in different environments and in a variety of capacities. It is estimated that selective breeding of dogs for specific functions and appearance has occurred for about 3,000 to 5,000 years. As early as 2900 B.C., dogs resembling today's greyhound were frequently depicted on paintings and pottery in Egypt and western Asia. Selective breeding of dogs for working abilities flourished during the Middle Ages, but many of the extreme alterations in form and function of the dog have occurred only within the past 150 to 200 years.

The Process of Selective Breeding

The term "selective breeding" refers to discriminative selection of dogs for breeding based on the presence of desired structural or behavioral characteristics. In practical terms, this involves positively selecting for certain traits while ignoring others. For example, the mastiff breeds, which were the original fighting and guarding dogs, were selected for a dominant and protective nature. Males and females that showed the desired temperament were chosen as breeding stock. Those that did not were not bred. Over time, a breed type evolved that included individuals that exhibited very high levels of dominance (and aggression) and reacted to lower intensities of stimuli. In contrast, herding dogs were required to follow, or chase, livestock and move animals into or out of areas of confinement. Herding behaviors represent modified predatory behavior, and those animals that showed a very strong chase instinct were selected for breeding. Dogs that followed the chasing behavior with a predatory bite, however, were not chosen. Over many generations, selective breeding for this type of work resulted in dogs that would readily chase their charges but would curtail the predatory response short of the killing bite.

It is important when discussing dogs to distinguish between the development of breeds and the existence of subspecies. A subspecies occurs when a distinctive subpopulation evolves that is separated geographically and differs

morphologically from the original population. For example, the dingo, the feral dog of Australia, is considered to be a subspecies of the domestic dog. The dingo was introduced to Australia by humans but eventually became fully established as a feral (semiwild) population. The dingo was geographically separated from other domestic dogs for many generations and is now classified as the subspecies *Canis familiaris dingo.* The New Guinea singing dog (*Canis familiaris hallstomi*) has a similar history. Conversely, breeds of dogs comprise groups of animals that have been artificially selected to possess a uniform heritable appearance. Although breeds can differ significantly in appearance and temperament, natural selection is not the cause of their development. Rather, a breed is the direct result of artificial selection by humans. Moreover, unlike subspecies, breeds are not necessarily restricted to a particular geographic area. While earlier classifications of the dog identified five breed types as subspecies of *Canis familiaris,* that classification scheme has since been rescinded.[1,2] Currently, all breeds of dog are considered to be members of the single species *Canis familiaris.*

Early Breeds: The Romans and Their Dogs

Although archaeological and hieroglyphic evidence show that distinctive breeds existed 3,000 to 5,000 years ago, the ancient Romans were the first culture to breed dogs systematically and to record the functions for which they used each type of dog. Written records that are dated during the fifth century B.C. describe dogs that were used for herding, sport, war, arena-fighting, scent hunting, and sight hunting. Those of wealth and power also kept smaller "house" dogs, which probably represent the first true companion animals. Five early types of dogs have been designated as the mastiffs, wolflike (spitz) dogs, greyhounds, pointers, and sheepdogs. The mastiff breeds were developed primarily in the area of Tibet and were later used in battle by the Babylonians, Assyrians, Persians, and Greeks. The wolflike breeds were similar to the spitz that we know today and are believed to be the ancestors of the Siberian Husky, Keeshond, and other arctic breeds. The Greyhound is believed to be one of the oldest breeds, developed in Egypt and identified from drawings on Mesopotamian pottery. The pointer types appear to have been developed from Greyhounds for the purpose of hunting small game, and most of the sheepdogs probably originated in Europe.

The majority of purebred dog breeds that we see today have their origins as some type of working animal. An understanding of this heritage provides insight into an individual dog's temperament and behavior. For example, even though the Shetland Sheepdog who resides with her family in a small suburban home has never seen a live sheep, she still has inherited many characteristics that define a working sheepdog. For this reason, she may enjoy chasing the family cat around the living room or stalking the kids as they play, hoping to herd them into some semblance of a cohesive group.

Darwin's Influence

The Middle Ages was the great era for the proliferation of dog breeds in western Europe, spanning the thirteenth to the fifteenth centuries A.D. This was the time of feudalism and the establishment of the aristocracy, for whom hunting was of great importance as a symbol of power and status. Different dogs were developed to hunt different species of game and were named accordingly. Some common breeds included the Deerhound, Wolfhound, Boarhound, Otterhound, and Bloodhound. Interestingly, although selective breeding by humans caused many variants in type and working ability of dogs during this time period, it was not until the 1800s, when Charles Darwin published his theories of natural selection and the evolution of species that early "breeders" began to have an understanding of artificial selection. The concepts of line breeding and crossbreeding subsequently grew out of an enhanced understanding of genetics and inheritance (see Chapter 4). Prior to that time, dogs were bred according to their ability to work, but careful attention to "lineage" was not of concern and there were no breed standards to which dogs were expected to conform. As a result, the individuals within each breed of dog were much more variable in appearance than we are accustomed to seeing today.

Advent of Organized Dog Shows

The creation of competitive dog shows and the subsequent development of breed standards added constraints other than working ability to breeding programs and goals. The first competitive dog show was held in Great Britain in 1859 in Newcastle and was for Pointers and Setters only. The British Kennel Club was established in 1873 to standardize dog shows and dog breeds. In addition to describing working ability, the breed standards that were accepted by the Kennel Club required rigid conformity in size, color, body shape, and movement. Breeders and owners who had previously been concerned primarily with the dog's working ability now began to focus on physical characteristics such as size, coat type and color, and body shape.

Like domestication, purposeful selective breeding of dogs has resulted in a variety of changes. The decreased size and changes to structure that occurred during domestication have been exaggerated in many breeds. Changes in coat color, markings, length, and texture are seen. The range of colors that wolves exhibit is large, varying from almost completely black to white with lemon or cream markings. The domestic dog shows these same variations, with additional colors that are not seen in wild wolves. Some examples include the deep red of the Irish Setter, the steel gray of the Weimaraner, and the chocolate brown of the Irish Water Spaniel. Color markings are also a direct result of breed development. Certainly no one will argue that the distinctive spots of the Dalmatian or the points on the legs of the Doberman Pinscher occur in nature.

An examination of the early history of selective breeding indicates that most breeds of dogs can be categorized into one of eight primary types of working dogs: spitz breeds, mastiff breeds, sight hounds, scent hounds, terriers, gundogs, herding breeds, and livestock guarding breeds. In addition, there are a number of "toy," or miniature, breeds that generally do not have a working dog origin but were developed primarily as companions.

Spitz Breeds

At one time, the spitz-type dogs were classified as a subspecies of the dog, *Canis familiaris palustris*.[1] They are now considered to be a group of dog breeds rather than a separate subspecies. Although it traditionally has been stated that the spitz breeds are more closely related to their wolf progenitors than other breeds of dogs, recent evidence using genetic and biochemical methods have shown that these breeds are no more closely related to the wolf than are other breeds of dogs.[3] In fact, there is less **mitochondrial** DNA difference between dogs and wolves than there is between different ethnic groups of human beings (who are all considered to be a single species). These data indicate that the dog is correctly classified within the genus *Canis* and lends further evidence to the wolf as the dog's primary wild ancestor.

Archaeological evidence shows that dogs of the spitz type were distributed throughout the world. Along with the sight hounds, they are believed to represent some of the oldest breeds of dogs. Spitz breeds are characterized by their short-bodied, stocky builds and thick double coats. Many were originally developed to work in cold environments where they were used as draft dogs to pull sleds or carts. Examples of these breed types include the sled dog breeds such as the Siberian Husky, Alaskan Malamute, and Samoyed. The Chow Chow and the Norwegian Elkhound are also considered to be spitz-type dogs (Figure 2.1).

FIGURE 2.1   Spitz breeds

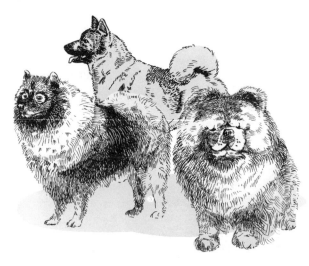

Norwegian Elkhound: The Norwegian Elkhound is a true example of the northern spitz-type group of dogs. The Elkhound's heritage lies with the Vikings of Norway. Ancient fossil remains have been found in Norway that closely resemble this breed as we know it today. The Elkhound was first used to hunt a wide range of animals, including rabbits, bears, and elks. Later they accompanied Viking raiders on their ships. Elkhounds have also been kept as guarding and herding dogs. Small, compact, and agile, they are medium-sized and have the thick double coat of the spitz breeds. The Elkhound is a fairly independent breed, known for its tenacity as a hunter and guarder.

Siberian Husky: The Siberian Husky was developed by the nomadic Chukchi, an Inuit tribe of Siberia. The Husky was needed to pull sleds, herd reindeer, and guard homesteads. The breed was isolated in Siberia for hundreds of years, until fur traders brought it to North America in the early 1900s. As legend has it, the Siberian Husky first won fame when a team carried supplies of diphtheria antitoxin across the state of Alaska to inhabitants of the town of Nome. Huskies are hardy dogs, and their thick double coat makes them capable of withstanding the harsh weather conditions of their native land. Like all dogs bred to pull sleds, they have a high level of energy coupled with a strong desire to pull. A distinctive characteristic of the Siberian Husky is its propensity to howl rather than bark.

Chow Chow: The Chow Chow was developed in Mongolia approximately 4,000 years ago and was later introduced into China. At various points in time the Chow Chow has also been referred to as the tartar dog, the dog of barbarians, and the Chinese spitz. In China, the breed was used principally as a guarding and hunting dog for emperors and the ruling classes. In addition, it served as a source of food and fur. Most people identify the Chow Chow with its very dense double coat and distinctive teddy-bear appearance. However, because of its guarding background, the Chow Chow is considered to be a dominant dog with a tendency to show territorial aggression. Like many breeds from China, it is also characterized as being somewhat independent.

Mastiff Breeds

The Mastiff is considered to be one of the true foundation breeds of dog, as it was a progenitor of many other breeds. Dogs of this type include some of the heaviest and largest breeds. Most were first developed as dogs of war, guardians, and as hunters of large game. Depictions of Mastiffs are found in Egyptian monuments that are dated as early as 3000 B.C. The Romans later developed fighting and war breeds from these dogs. It is known that Julius Caesar had Mastiffs with his troops when he invaded Great Britain but found upon arriving that the natives of that area also had their own Mastiff breeds. It is speculated that Phoenician traders or invading Angles and Saxons had originally introduced the dogs to that area. In addition to being used as a war dog, the Mastiff was used for dog-fighting and bull-baiting. The banning of these activities during the nineteenth century led to a decline in the popularity of the breed in Great Britain and other areas. Examples of modern breeds that are descended from the early Mastiff types are the Mastiff, St. Bernard, and Boxer (Figure 2.2).

Mastiff: The best adjective that describes the Mastiff is massive. It is a heavy-boned dog, standing about 30 inches or more at the shoulder, with a broad, heavy head and short muzzle. The breed declined in numbers during the second World War, and certain kennel lines were lost. However, careful breeding in the United States reestablished the breed, and today it enjoys increased popularity. Although Mastiffs are generally regarded as even-tempered dogs, they retain the ability to guard and protect. They require adequate space but can make faithful, gentle family pets.

St. Bernard: The first known ancestor of the St. Bernard was the heavy Asian "molosser" dog that accompanied Roman armies during the third century A.D. Crossbreeding this dog with the great Pyrenees and Tibetan Mastiff produced a dog that could both guard and herd. Other names for the St. Bernard have been the Alpine Mastiff, the Barryhund, and the Sacred Dog. In the 1700s the St. Bernard was first used as a rescue dog and was given its name from the hospice of the great Saint Bernard Pass. The monks of this hospice bred dogs to serve as guides and rescue dogs for travelers who were traversing the perilous Alpine pass between Switzerland and Italy. The most famous St. Bernard in recorded history was a dog named Barry who, as legend has it, was responsible for saving more than 40 lives.

Boxer: While the St. Bernard is a Swiss derivative of the Mastiff line, the Boxer represents the German variety. Two German dogs of the Mastiff type

FIGURE 2.2   Mastiff breeds

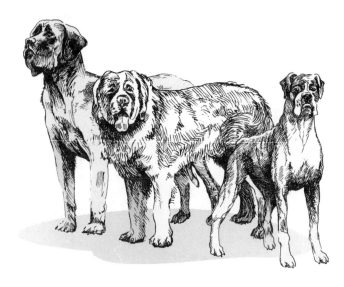

are this breed's primary ancestors: the Bullenbeiszer and the Barenbeiszer. Both of these dogs were originally used for bull-baiting and hunting. Interbreeding with the bulldog led to the creation of the Boxer during the mid-1800s and is responsible for the Boxer's slightly **brachycephalic** head type. The Boxer is an affectionate family dog but does retain the protective instinct of his Mastiff heritage. The breed is somewhat smaller than most Mastiff breeds but is still known for its agility and strength.

Sight Hound Breeds

The hound breeds can be divided into two distinct types: the sight hounds (also referred to as gaze hounds) and the scent hounds. Hounds were the earliest hunting dogs used by man and were important in providing the speed and talent for following game that humans did not possess. Both types of hounds were developed to hunt nonfeathered game, either by sighting and chasing down the quarry (sight hounds) or by following the ground scent of the game (scent hounds).

The ancient Egyptians and Sumerians required dogs that were fast enough to hunt game on the open plains. These cultures were responsible for the early development of the sight hound breeds. Sight hounds are tall and slender and are built for speed. They were developed to chase their quarry using their sense of vision rather than their sense of smell and would overtake and kill game while the hunter followed behind. These dogs are long-legged, deep chested, and slender. Examples of modern-day sight hound breeds include the Greyhound, Saluki, Afghan Hound, and Whippet.

FIGURE 2.3   Sight hounds

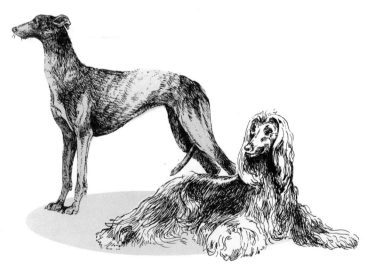

Greyhound: The Greyhound is one of the foundation breeds from which many sight hound breeds are descended. The Greyhound has its origins in the Middle East and was developed to hunt small game such as rabbit and hare. There are depictions of dogs that look like Greyhounds on Egyptian tombs dated 2900 B.C. Phoenician trading ships were responsible for the Greyhound's introduction into Europe. Because of its beautiful appearance and hunting ability, the breed quickly became popular with nobility. Greyhounds were first brought to the Americas by Spanish explorers in the sixteenth century. During the early twentieth century, Greyhound racing was introduced as a gambling sport. Unfortunately, the proliferation of this sport has led to overbreeding and a large surplus of unwanted dogs that were unsuccessful as racing animals. Although they are a coursing breed and, therefore, have a strong chase instinct, the Greyhound is a very gentle, loving dog and can make a wonderful pet. Today, there are numerous nonprofit groups that rescue unwanted Greyhounds from the racing industry and make them available to good homes.

Saluki: Like other sight hound breeds, the Saluki has its origins in the Middle East. The breed can be traced back to Sumer and is named after the ancient Arabian city of Saluk. It has also been called the Gazelle Hound, Arabian Hound, and Persian Greyhound and appears to be closely related to the Afghan Hound. The Saluki was used by various nomadic tribes and as a result quickly spread from the Caspian Sea to the Sahara Desert. Because of the breed's great speed, the Saluki was used to hunt gazelles as well as foxes, hares, and jackals. Today, there are two varieties of Saluki: the feathered and the smooth-haired. The feathered Saluki has light feathering on the backs of its legs and thighs. The Saluki has the characteristic deep-chested, long-legged body type of all of the sight hound breeds.

Afghan Hound: The Afghan Hound is probably one of the most elegant of the sight hound breeds. Also known as the Kabul Dog, this ancient breed is depicted in Afghan drawings dated at more than 4,000 years old. The breed was developed in the Middle East and spread along the trade routes to Afghanistan. It was used to hunt large game such as antelope, gazelles, wolves, and snow leopards. Today, the Afghan Hound is known as a fairly aloof dog, whose major distinction as a sight hound breed is probably its very long, silky coat. This long coat was developed as protection against the bitter cold of the mountain regions of Afghanistan.

Whippet: The Whippet was developed in Victorian times in northeast England by crossing small racing Greyhounds with local terriers. They were used for the sport of "rag racing" in which the small dogs raced toward their owners who were waving a piece of cloth. The Whippet is one of the smallest sight hounds but is considered to be one of the fastest as well. It has been shown to even outpace the Greyhound over short distances. The Whippet makes an excellent house pet and is known for its gentle, loving, sensitive nature. Even though it stands only about 18 to 20 inches at the shoulder, the Whippet still has the characteristic long legs and deep chest of the other sight hound breeds.

Scent Hound Breeds

In addition to developing the sight hounds, the Egyptians and ancient Sumerians are responsible for developing a group of dogs that used their superior sense of smell to locate and track quarry. These breeds are collectively referred to as the scent hounds. During the Middle Ages these breeds were further refined by the landed gentry of Europe. While some breeds were developed to kill their quarry, others were expected to corner the prey and then "give tongue," or bay, to alert the hunter. Stamina and an acute sense of smell are the most important characteristics of these dogs. Compared to the sight hounds, the scent hounds follow game much more slowly and, therefore, possess both a good nose and a build that promotes stamina. Structurally, scent hounds are characterized by strong, sturdy legs; heavy bones; and long heads with pendulous ears. Examples of these breeds include the Bloodhound, Basset Hound, Beagle, and Otter Hound (Figure 2.4).

Bloodhound: The Bloodhound is believed to be the oldest scent hound breed. Its origins are traced back to the eighth century in Belgium. At that time, the breed that was to become the Bloodhound was known as St. Hubert's Dog and was a favorite of French kings. By the twelfth century, the breed was popular as a hunting dog, and kennels often were established at monasteries. Its scenting abilities are promoted as being the keenest of all scent hounds, and the breed often is used today as a search and rescue dog.

FIGURE 2.4   Scent hounds

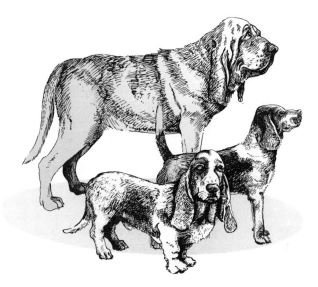

The Bloodhound is also the largest of the scent hound breeds but is still renowned for its gentle, affectionate temperament.

Basset Hound: The Basset Hound was a relative latecomer to the scent dog group. It was developed during the late sixteenth century in France as a hunting companion to hunters who were traveling on foot. Its name is a derivative of the French word "bas" meaning "low," which certainly is descriptive of the Basset's short legs and long body. The Basset's short stature and heavy build are important for providing the breed with its strength and stamina. Like all of the scent hounds, the Basset is tenacious when following a scent but is generally a very gentle-natured dog. This breed is also known for its very distinctive, low bell-like bark that is issued whenever a scent is detected and followed.

Beagle: The Beagle is the smallest of the scent hounds. This breed was developed as a pack-hunting hound. Although its exact origins are unknown, a Beagle-like dog was used by the ancient Egyptians who hunted with a group of dogs in a pack. During the middle of the eleventh century, the Beagle was brought to England where it became a popular hunting dog of the land-owning aristocrats. Like all scent hounds, the Beagle has a strong desire to follow a trail and is known to become selectively deaf when engaged in this occupation. Because of their gentle nature and small size, Beagles can make excellent house pets.

Otterhound: As its name implies, the Otterhound was bred for hunting otters. It is a unique hound in that records indicate crosses of large hounds with several types of terriers were used to develop a dog with a shaggy and rather wiry coat. The Otterhound is known for its persistence as a hunting dog, both on land and in the water, where its webbed feet assist its swimming ability. In recent years, the Otterhound has lost popularity in Europe and Britain but has increased in popularity in the United States. The Otterhound is known as a loyal and very affectionate breed, and can make an effective guard dog.

Terrier Breeds

The word "terrier" is derived from the Latin work *terra,* meaning earth. This aptly describes the nature of the terrier's work. The original purpose for most of these dogs was to dig underground (called "going to earth" or "going to ground") and hunt ground-dwelling quarry such as badger, fox, and various rodents. Terriers can be divided into two main types: long-legged and short-legged. Short-legged terriers were bred to work in rocky dens where little space was available. Their structure allows them to push dirt to the side as they dig. Many also have long bodies to facilitate entering underground dens. The long-legged terriers were developed to hunt larger game such as woodchucks and badgers. They generally have narrow front assemblies and straight legs and work to throw soil between their hind legs as they dig.

Terriers represent some of the most recently developed breeds of dog. Most originated in the United Kingdom and have only been selectively bred for several hundred years. The Miniature Schnauzer and the Dachshund are the only two terrier breeds that were developed outside of Great Britain; both originated in Germany. (Although the American Kennel Club classifies the dachshund as a hound, its original function was as a terrier breed.) All of these dogs were developed to find land-dwelling game. Some were required to bark or worry the quarry until it could be dug out by the hunter; others were expected to kill the quarry upon finding it. Small terriers were bred to hunt animals that were considered vermin, such as rats and mice. Examples of these breeds include the Manchester, Cairn, Border, and Norfolk terriers. Larger terriers, such as the Fox Terrier, Airedale Terrier, and Bedlington Terrier were used to hunt larger game, usually above ground. All of the terrier breeds are known for their resilience and high pain tolerance, necessary requirements for their work. Most possess a wiry, harsh coat that is well adapted to protecting them while working in brush or digging into the ground (Figure 2.5).

Airedale Terrier: The Airedale Terrier is the largest and the youngest breed of terrier. It was developed only about 100 years ago in Yorkshire, England, by crossing a breed called the Black and Tan with the Otterhound. The Black and Tan is also known to be the ancestor of the Irish, Fox, and Welsh terriers. Airedales were first used to hunt fox, badgers, weasels, and other small game. During World War I, they were enlisted as sentries and messengers, and afterward were used for a short period as police dogs. Its Otterhound heritage makes the Airedale an unusually good swimmer and provides this breed with its renowned ability to scent. A smaller version of the Airedale Terrier is the Welsh Terrier, which exhibits the same body type and coat markings as the Airedale but is considerably smaller.

FIGURE 2.5   Terriers

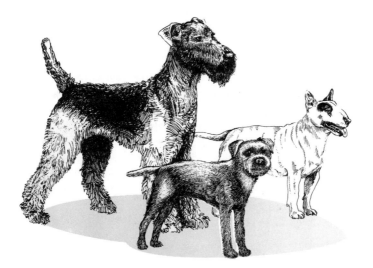

Border Terrier: The Border Terrier is an example of the short, stocky body type that was developed to go to ground after small game. Other terriers with similar body types include the Cairn Terrier, Norwich Terrier, West Highland White Terrier, and Scottish Terrier. The Border Terrier gets its name from the region in which it was originally bred: the rugged, remote countryside between Scotland and England. Border Terriers were originally used to hunt fox but have a history of hunting a variety of small game. The Border Terrier is known for its affectionate, good-natured temperament and its tendency to be a bit more accepting of other dogs than many of the other terrier breeds. Today, Border Terriers enjoy a high degree of popularity in the United States as family pets.

Bull Terrier and related breeds: During the eighteenth century, Bulldogs in England were crossed with various terrier breeds to produce fighting dogs that were used in bull-baiting and dog-fighting. In the mid-1800s the Bull Terrier was refined and all-white dogs became popular. As a result, the Bull Terrier became known as an all-white breed until the early 1900s. However, in the 1920s breeders recognized that deafness was associated with the white coat, so color was gradually reintroduced into the breed. Today, in the United States, colored and white Bull Terriers are shown separately at dog shows, although they are recognized as the same breed. Because it was originally bred as a fighting dog, the Bull Terrier has a tendency to be aggressive toward other dogs. However, if raised properly, these dogs can make good pets in appropriate homes.

The Bull Terrier is related to two breeds that are similar in appearance: the Staffordshire Bull Terrier and the American Staffordshire Terrier. Like the Bull Terrier, the Staffordshire Bull Terrier was originally bred for bull- and bear-fighting but is smaller and has shorter legs than the Bull Terrier. The Staffordshire Bull Terrier crossed the Atlantic in the mid-1800s. Breeding in America gave rise to a slightly larger, heavier-boned version of the breed. This new breed was recognized as the American Staffordshire Terrier in 1972 and is currently cross-registered with the United Kennel Club as the American Pit Bull Terrier.

Gundogs

With the invention of firearms, it was no longer necessary for dogs to follow a scent, chase, and pull down game. Rather, hunters now required a dog that could find game, indicate it, and flush it upon command so the hunter could shoot it. As the range of firearms improved, dogs were developed that would also find and retrieve shot game from long distances. Therefore, the development of firearms was accompanied by a resurgence of selective dog breeding as breeds were created to fill this new working niche. Several types of gundogs resulted. These include the pointers and setters, the spaniels, and the retrievers (Figure 2.6).

Pointers and Setters: This group of breeds was selected to travel ahead of the hunter (who was often on horseback), and locate and indicate game. Pointers communicate the presence of game by standing still and staring toward the hidden animal, sometimes lifting a front leg in a characteristic "point." Setters, on the other hand, indicate by crouching low to the ground (i.e. setting) in response to the presence of game.

The pointer or pointer-type dogs are considered to be the oldest of the gundogs and were developed by English gentry during the 1600s. Early pointers worked in pairs and traveled ahead of the hunter to find and indicate game using their classic pointing stance. Originally, these dogs were used along with Greyhounds. The pointers located the game and froze in their point, then the Greyhounds moved in to flush and chase. The original pointer was the Spanish Pointer, which was a rather slow, houndlike dog. This breed was crossed with Greyhounds to improve speed and with English Foxhounds to improve scenting ability. The result is the English Pointer, a medium-size dog that tracks and points game but does not usually retrieve. Another variety of pointer, developed in Germany, is the German Short-Haired Pointer. This dog was developed by crossing the German Hound with the Spanish Pointer. The German Wire-Haired Pointer is similar in body type to the English Pointer but is slightly heavier in build and sports a longer, wiry coat.

The setter breeds can be traced back to the English Setter, which was also developed during the sixteenth century. The setters aid hunters by locating game using both scent and eyesight, then responding by crouching or sitting. Classically, the dog should wait until the hunter approaches and directs the dog to either hold its position or flush the game. When the setters were first developed, they often were crossed with various types of spaniels. As a result, the early versions of setters and spaniels looked quite similar in appearance.

FIGURE 2.6   Gundogs

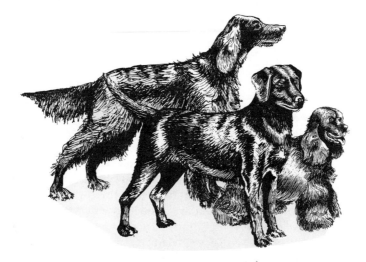

The English Setter as we know it today was first bred by Sir Edward Laverack and was known as the Laverack Setter for a period of time. Two other popular setters are the Gordon and the Irish setters. The Gordon, originally called the Black and Tan, is the largest and strongest of the setter breeds and was developed in Scotland by the Duke of Gordon. The Irish Setter was probably bred in both Ireland and England during the 1800s. The breed originally sported a red and white coat and was a popular all-purpose hunting dog. All of the setter breeds are known for their high-spirited, friendly temperaments. Because the setters that are bred today are quite a bit larger than the dogs that were originally developed for hunting, they require a great deal of exercise and space to live.

Spaniels: The spaniels are known as the "all-purpose" hunting breeds. They were developed to find and indicate game, flush it upon command, and, in some cases, retrieve the prey after it had been shot. When first developed, the spaniels were divided into two types of dogs: water spaniels and land spaniels. Examples include the English Cocker, American Cocker, English Springer, and Brittany spaniels. The English Cocker Spaniel derives its name from a bird called the wood cock, a popular game bird in Wales and southwest England. This breed was introduced into America in the 1880s, where it quickly became popular as a house pet. Breeders in the United States slowly changed the breed by decreasing its size and selecting for a longer, denser coat. Eventually, it became recognized as a separate breed, the American Cocker Spaniel. Today, the American Cocker is one of the most popular companion animals in the United States. The English Springer Spaniel is one of the larger spaniel breeds. It was known as the Norfolk Springer in its early days because the Duke of Norfolk was one of the first to keep a kennel of these dogs. English Springers find, stalk, then "spring" quarry by flushing it from its hiding place. They often were hunted along with falcons. The Brittany is a spaniel breed that was developed in France and is considered to be a bit setterlike in its appearance and working ability. This breed has a natural ability to point and is an excellent retriever. Because of its relatively small size and friendly temperament, the Brittany is increasing in popularity in the United States.

Retrievers: The retrieving breeds are the third type of gundog. These dogs were developed as specialists in finding and retrieving shot game. Many of these breeds were used as water dogs to retrieve ducks and geese. Present-day retrievers include the Golden and Labrador retrievers, the Flat-Coated Retriever, and the Chesapeake Bay Retriever. The Golden Retriever is currently one of the most popular breeds of dog in the United States. This breed has its origins in Scotland, where they were developed on the estate of Lord Tweedmouth. Because his estate was located on the River Tweed, the very distinctive golden-colored dog was first called the Tweed Water Spaniel. Crossbreeding with Flat-Coated Retrievers and Irish Setters resulted in an increased body size and a longer coat. By the end of the nineteenth century, the breed was referred to as the Yellow or Golden Retriever and had gained great popularity as a hunting companion in Britain and the United States. Because of its gentle nature, trainability, and playfulness, this breed makes an excellent family pet.

Despite its name, the Labrador Retriever originated in Newfoundland, not in Labrador. In Newfoundland, these dogs aided fisherman by jumping into the icy waters and retrieving fishing nets. The fishermen of Newfoundland traveled to west England in the nineteenth century and brought their dogs with them. The breed quickly became popular as a gundog and was crossed with other retrieving breeds. Three colors of Labrador Retriever exist: black, yellow, and chocolate. The breed is known for its hardiness and drive as a hunting dog, as well as its gentle, even-tempered nature. Like the Golden Retriever, the Labrador currently enjoys great popularity as a companion and family pet.

Three other retrievers are the Flat-Coated Retriever, the Chesapeake Bay Retriever, and the Curly-Coated Retriever. The Flat-Coated is an all-black, long-coated dog. The Chesapeake Bay Retriever has its origins in the United States during the early nineteenth century and is considered to be one of the strongest retrieving breeds. The Curly-Coated Retriever is probably the least common of the retrieving breeds. It is distinctive for its tightly curled black or brown coat and its hardy working ability.

Livestock-herding Breeds

At the time that the dog was beginning its association with man, humans were slowly evolving from a nomadic lifestyle to a more agrarian lifestyle. Along with these changes came the practice of keeping livestock. Some of the first prey species to be domesticated were goats and sheep, followed closely by cattle. With the arrival of domestic livestock came two new professions for the dog. One group of dogs was bred to control herds and to move livestock from place to place, while another group was developed to guard and protect livestock from wild predators. Both of these types of dogs were originally developed to work in similar habitats (grasslands) and to respond to similar stimuli (livestock). However, the responsibility of a livestock-herding dog is to move the herd from place to place; a livestock-guarding dog lives in the midst of its charges and warns off predators.

The breeds of herding dogs that have been developed vary greatly in appearance, size, and method of working. The Border Collie is known for its agility and ability to work sheep using direct eye contact. In contrast, the small Corgi was developed as a cattle dog to move herds by nipping at the heels of the animals (hence the commonly used term "heelers"). Almost every nation has its own breed of livestock-herding dog. Scotland has the Collie, Hungary has the Pulik, and Wales has the Corgi. Commonly recognized herding breeds in the United States today include the German Shepherd Dog, the Collie, and the Corgi (Figure 2.7).

German Shepherd Dog: This breed, also known as the Alsatian, was developed in Germany from three types of sheep-herding dogs. During the 1800s the German Shepherd Dog was the most popular sheep-herding dog in use.

However, near the end of that century, sheep ranching diminished drastically in Germany and the breed came close to extinction. In 1899, a man by the name of Rittmeister von Stephanitz founded a parent club for the breed in Augsburg, Germany, with the goal of maintaining its working heritage and encouraging new uses for the breed. The German Shepherd Dog was used in World War I for protection and police work. After the war, service men brought the breed to England and the United States, where it quickly gained popularity. The German Shepherd Dog was one of the first breeds to be used as a guide for the sight-impaired and has been used extensively in police work. Although it still retains the ability to herd livestock, the breed is no longer used exclusively for that function.

Collie: The Collie has a long history as a herding dog in Scotland and England. There is evidence that a breed resembling the Collie was established as early as the late 1300s. The name "Collie" may have come from two sources. It may be a derivative of the word "collis," meaning Scottish Highlands. There is also a local breed of black sheep called the Colley that the Collie dog was used to herd (i.e. colley dog). In the mid-1800s Queen Victoria took an interest in the breed and added Collies to the royal kennels at Windsor. This greatly increased their popularity, and by the late 1800s the Collie was commonly seen in both Great Britain and the United States. The Collie continues to enjoy popularity as a family pet today and is still occasionally kept as a working dog.

Welsh Corgi (Pembroke and Cardigan): The two breeds of Welsh Corgis are named for the Welsh word *Corrci,* meaning dwarf dog. The Pembroke Welsh Corgi is tailless and is the more popular of the two breeds. Its lineage can be dated back as far as the 1100s. The Cardigan (with a tail) is a somewhat

FIGURE 2.7   Livestock-herding breeds

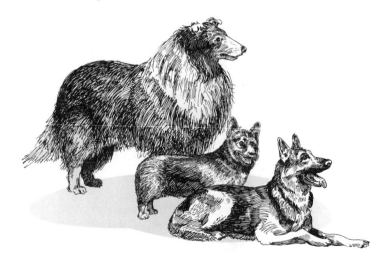

longer bodied, heavier-boned dog. Both Corgis were developed as cattle-herding dogs. Their short stature and agile movement allow them to dart around the legs of the cattle and nip at their heels.

Livestock-guarding Breeds

The livestock-guarding breeds were developed to protect livestock from natural predators, without a need to herd. These dogs are highly attentive, trustworthy, and protective. They must also be large enough to present a deterrent to predator species. Examples are the Komondor, the Kuvasz, and the Great Pyrenees (Figure 2.8).

Komondor and Kuvasz: These two breeds are similar in appearance and were both developed in Hungary. The Komondor is a relatively old guarding breed and can be traced back to about the ninth century A.D. It is distinctive for its naturally cording coat. Left ungroomed, this coat develops into long mats or "cords." This coat is very protective against adverse weather conditions and against attacks by predators. The word Kuvasz is derived from a Turkish word that means "armed guard of the nobility." This breed originated in Tibet and was further refined in Turkey. Both the Kuvasz and the Komondor have enjoyed increased popularity in recent years in central and western United States as herd-guarding dogs.

Great Pyrenees: The Great Pyrenees is a very large, powerful breed and was first developed to protect sheep in the Pyrenees from attacks by wolves and bears. They are descended from the Mastiff breeds and eventually became popular during the fifteenth century as guard dogs. Interestingly, selective

FIGURE 2.8   Livestock-guarding breeds

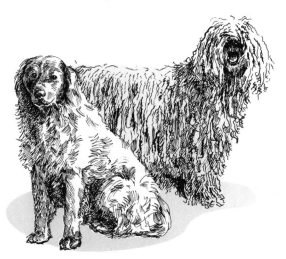

breeding within the last century has caused a decrease in the Pyrenees' protective nature, and this breed is now known for its very gentle, affectionate temperament. The breed is still used as a herd-guarding dog in some areas of the United States and other parts of the world.

Toy Breeds

The toy breeds are probably the first animals to be kept by humans strictly for companionship. Although some of these dogs represent larger breeds that were reduced in size to become companions, others evolved originally as very small breeds of dog. There are records of "dwarf" dogs dating back to the time of early domestication. Modern toy breeds include the Chihuahua, Pomeranian, and the Maltese (Figure 2.9).

Chihuahua: The Chihuahua, standing only about 7 to 10 inches at the shoulder, is believed to be the smallest breed in the history of dogs. The breed has a speculative history. As long ago as the ninth century, the Tolteck Indians of Mexico kept a breed of dogs that was very small and long-coated, called the Techichi. The Chihuahua is believed to have originated from crossing the Techichi with a small hairless breed of dog from Asia. Today, the smooth-coated Chihuahua is more common than the long-coated variety, and the Chihuahua is a popular pet in the United States.

Pomeranian: The Pomeranian is almost certainly a miniaturization of the spitz breeds such as the Keeshond, Norwegian Elkhound, and Samoyed. The breed was originally quite a bit larger and was white in color. It was used in the Pomeranian region (near the border of Poland and Germany) to herd sheep. During the middle of the nineteenth century, Queen Victoria became interested in the breed and actively promoted their popularity in Europe. Increasing popularity resulted in a miniaturization of the breed along with the selection for other colors.

FIGURE 2.9   Toy breeds

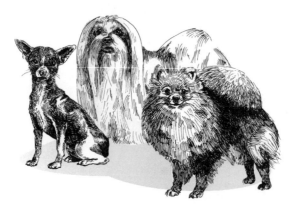

Maltese: The Maltese is one of the oldest breeds of dogs. There are ancient statues depicting a Maltese-like dog in Egyptian tombs of the thirteenth century B.C. The Maltese first arrived in Great Britain with the Roman legions during the first century B.C. It is one of the smallest toy breeds and is known for its long and silky white coat. Those interested in keeping the Maltese as a pet soon learn that this coat requires a great deal of grooming and care.

Dog Breed Registry Organizations

It is currently estimated that there are between 370 and 400 breeds of purebred dogs worldwide. However, since selective breeding has a long history, it is recognized that many breeds that were developed became extinct when their particular function was no longer needed or when another breed was developed to take its place. It is estimated that there have been well over 1,000 different breeds of dogs throughout the history of the dog's domestication.

Beginning in the nineteenth century, dog breeders became interested in standardizing breeds and in keeping records of lineages. During the early 1800s working dog shows (specifically, hound shows) were held in communities throughout Great Britain. However, no standardized regulations were available and no governing body existed to oversee these events. The first kennel club was formed in 1873 in Great Britain as a regulatory body for dog shows. The first kennel club show was held in London in June of 1873 and included 975 entries. Today, as an example of how this sport has grown, the Crufts, which is the most prestigious dog show in England, attracts more than 16,000 entries each year.

The American Kennel Club (AKC) was established in 1884. The original goal of this organization was to set up a uniform code of rules and regulations to be used at dog shows and sporting events. The AKC is set up as a "club of clubs." This means that AKC membership is available to various types of dog clubs, not to individual dog owners, breeders, or exhibitors. The voting power of each member club is appropriated through elected delegates, who meet regularly and are responsible for electing the board of directors. The AKC was established as an organization for amateurs. Therefore, professional judges, trainers, and handlers are not eligible to be delegates.

Another purpose of the AKC is to maintain the stud book. A stud book refers to a record of any animal breeding program. The first dog that was registered in the American Kennel Club Stud Book was named "Adonis." He was an English Setter and was registered in 1878. When the AKC was first established, the stud book contained all purebred dogs that had been registered. However, in the 1940s a decision was made to include only those animals that had been used for breeding one or more times, since these were the only animals that were contributing to the breed's propagation. Today, publication in the Stud Book Register means that the dog has been used for breeding.

The American Kennel Club currently divides its recognized breeds into seven groups: Sporting Dogs, Hounds, Working Dogs, Terriers, Toys, Herding Dogs, and Non-Sporting Dogs. These divisions are based loosely on modern uses for the breeds. Breeds within each of these groups have established breed standards that are maintained by the AKC. Each national parent specialty club (i.e. breed club) writes their breed's standard. This is essentially a description of the ideal dog of that breed, a standard against which dogs are to be judged in the conformation ring. AKC publishes and regularly updates *The Complete Dog Book,* which includes all of the standards for all of the breeds recognized by their registry. Currently, the AKC recognizes more than 130 different purebred breeds of dogs.[4]

Another breed registry organization in the United States is the United Kennel Club (UKC). The UKC was founded in 1898 with the mission of promoting and maintaining the working qualities of purebred dogs. Most of the breeds that are recognized by the UKC are either sporting or hound breeds. For example, UKC registers six different breeds of coonhound: the Black and Tan, Redbone, English, Plott, Bluetick, and Treeing Walker. The UKC also recognizes many breeds that are considered to be unusual or rare. Unlike the AKC, the UKC will provide a "limited privilege" registration to mixed breed dogs, which allows these dogs to be shown in performance events such as agility and obedience trials.

Conclusions

Currently, the AKC recognizes more than 130 purebred breeds of dog, and the UKC lists more than 90 separate breeds. In addition, there are numerous "rare" breeds that are recognized by other registry organizations around the world. Add to this the great assortment of mixed-breed or "random-bred" dogs, and it is obvious that there is an enormous variety of sizes, appearances, coat types, and, most importantly, temperaments to choose from when selecting a dog. However, even with these differences, the dog's overall structure, movement, and use of its special senses are consistent across all breeds and breed types. These basic attributes are examined in Chapter 3.

Cited References

1. Zeuner, F.E. *A History of Domesticated Animals.* Harper and Row, New York, New York. (1963)

2. Clutton-Brock, J. **Dog.** In: *Evolution of Domesticated Animals,* (I.L. Mason, editor), Longman Press, London, United Kingdom, pp. 198-211. (1984)

3. Coppinger, R.P. and Schnieder, R. **Evolution of working dogs.** In: *The Domestic Dog: Its Evolution, Behavior and Interactions with People* (J.A. Serpell, editor), Cambridge University Press, Cambridge, United Kingdom, pp. 21-47. (1995)

4. American Kennel Club. *The Complete Dog Book.* Howell Book House, Inc., New York, New York. (1995)

3 The Dog's Body: Structure, Movement, and Special Senses

AN EXAMINATION of the dog's structure, movement, and special senses must be viewed in light of the original way in which the dog earned its living. The domestic dog's ancestors evolved as group-living, land-dwelling mammalian predators. Although selective breeding has resulted in extreme changes in the size and body proportion of many dogs, the basic skeleton, capabilities of the senses, and principles that govern movement are still consistent in all dogs. In general, the dog is built for speed, with eyes adapted to both detecting the presence of prey and following movement, a sense of smell developed to follow game trails, and ears designed to quickly locate prey and predators.

The Dog's Structure

The skeleton of the dog supports body, provides leverage for locomotion, and protects the internal soft organs (Figures 3.1 and 3.2). For example, the skull protects the brain, the rib cage protects the lungs, and the vertebrae protect the spinal cord. The minerals that make up the skeleton are also important as

FIGURE 3.1   Major bones of the dog

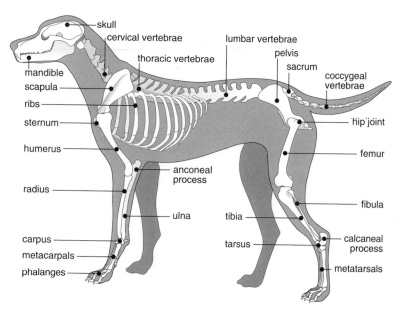

reservoirs that maintain normal levels of essential minerals in body fluids. The average dog skeleton contains a total of 319 bones.

Skull: Some of the greatest differences between breeds of dogs occur in the skull, ranging from the elongated **dolichocephalic** type to the **brachycephalic** type (Figure 3.3). The dolichocephalic head has a narrow skull base and an elongated muzzle. Breeds with this type of head include the Greyhound, Borzoi, and Collie. This head type is designed for speed and is almost always accompanied by a relatively long neck. Together, the narrow skull and long muzzle allow the dog to shift its center of gravity far forward while running, contributing to better balance and greater speed. The **mesaticephalic** structure refers to a moderate head shape with a medium ratio of skull base width to muzzle length. The slightly wider base and relatively shorter muzzle provide additional strength to the jaw. This head type is commonly seen in breeds that were developed to carry, such as the Spaniels and Retrievers. The brachycephalic head type is characterized by an extremely broad skull base and short muzzle. The short compact muzzle confers great jaw strength. This type of head was first seen in breeds that were developed to fight and bite, such as Bulldogs and Boxers. Interestingly, this type of head also occurs in certain toy breeds and may represent a form of **neoteny**. Compared to adults, puppies have a larger, rounder head in proportion to body size. Some breeds, such as the Pug, Pekinese, and Maltese have a brachycephalic head type that resembles the domed skull shape of young puppies. It is theorized that this neotenized look was appealing to the early breeders of toys.[1,2]

FIGURE 3.2   External anatomical terms of the dog

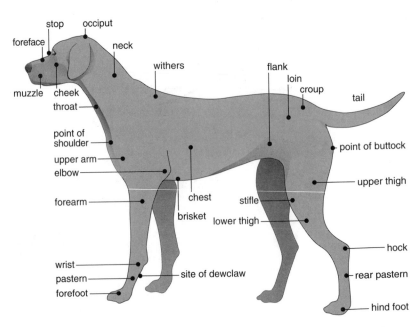

Dentition: The dog has two sets of teeth during its lifetime. The first, deciduous teeth, begin to erupt in the puppy at about 21 days of age. This set totals 28 teeth, which are fully erupted by 5 to 6 weeks of age. The permanent teeth begin to replace the deciduous teeth around 4 months of age and are completely erupted by 6 months of age. There are 42 permanent teeth, representing the general pattern that is seen in most carnivores (Table 3.1). Dogs have three pairs of incisors and a pair of elongated canine teeth on each of the upper and lower jaws. The canine teeth interlock in the closed jaw, with the lower canines located directly in front of the upper canines. The dog also has a pair of carnassial teeth on each side of the jaw. These are represented by the last premolar on the top jaw and the first molar on the bottom jaw. Parts of these teeth are laterally flattened to act as shears for tearing. The dog has a larger number of molars than some of the other carnivores, such as the cat. Molars are adapted for crushing and grinding and indicate the dog's more omnivorous dietary habits.

Neck: The neck is composed of the seven cervical vertebrae (Figure 3.1). The first vertebra, located closest to the head, is called the atlas and provides vertical movement to the head. The neck provides support and movement to the head and the cervical vertebrae, and is an important area for muscle attachment. The many muscles of the neck are involved in the movement of the front assembly. One of the most important of these, the brachicephalicus muscle, extends from an attachment on the head to an attachment on the shoulder blade and works to move the shoulders. The neck also provides bal-

FIGURE 3.3   Skull of the dog: Three types (*from top to bottom*) dolichocephalic, mesaticephalic, brachycephalic

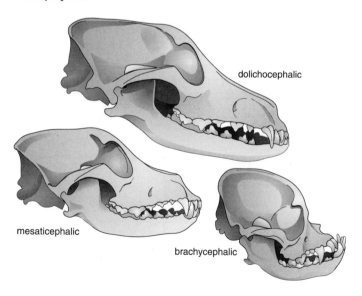

ance to the front assembly and is involved in shifting the dog's center of gravity forward when it is moving. In general, the head and neck are usually related to each other in length. Dogs with a short (or broken) face usually have a short neck, while dolichocephalic heads often have long necks.

Back: Although the term "back" often is used to describe an area extending from the withers all the way to the base of the tail, the actual back only consists of the 13 thoracic vertebrae (Figure 3.1). In most breeds of dogs, the back should be relatively straight, without a noticeable arch. A straight back better absorbs the power that is generated by the hindquarters when the animal is moving. Therefore, the back should be straight and parallel to the ground when the dog is standing stationary.

Loin: The loin consists of the seven lumbar vertebrae (Figures 3.1 and 3.2) and extends from the end of the rib cage to the front of the croup or pelvic girdle. The loin may also be called the lumbar region. This area of the back is important for the attachment of the muscles that contribute to the drive of the hind limbs. The loin also absorbs the concussion of the front end as it lands during movement. Because this section of the body has little support from the front or rear, it acts as a bridge between the two ends of the body. Most breed standards require a slightly arched loin, but this arch is due to muscles in that region, rather than to the shape of the lumbar vertebrae.

Croup: The croup extends from the last lumbar vertebra in the loin to the first tail (coccygeal) vertebra. The vertebrae in this area are fused to form a continuous plate of bone called the sacrum. The croup angle is determined by the horizontal slope of the sacrum and the first two tail vertebrae. The slope of the croup follows the slope of the pelvis bone and is important in determining the tail set. The dog's tail is positioned at the base of the croup.

Tail: The tail is made up of the coccygeal (also called caudal) vertebrae. Although the average number of caudal vertebrae in dogs is 20, the number

TABLE 3.1	Dentition of the Dog			
	Incisors	Canines	Premolars	Molars
Upper	6	2	8	4
Lower	6	2	8	6
TOTAL	12	4	16	10

Eruption of permanent teeth:
Incisors   2 to 5 months
Canines   5 to 6 months
Premolars 4 to 6 months
Molars   5 to 7 months

may vary from six to 23, depending on the breed. Many different types of tails are seen amongst the different dog breeds. These variations are all mutations of the normal straight tail that is seen in the wolf. Although it is banned in many countries and the American Veterinary Medical Association has issued a statement opposing the practice, tail docking is still commonly practiced on several breeds of dogs in the United States.[3] Tail carriage has relevance to behavior and is an indication of a dog's emotional state (see Chapter 8).

Forequarter (shoulder) assembly: The forequarters of the dog refer to the withers, scapula, and length of the humerus. The withers is an area measured from the first to the ninth thoracic vertebrae and includes the highest point of the scapula. The height of a dog is measured at the highest point of the withers. Unlike the hindquarters, which are attached to the body through a ball-and-socket joint, the forequarters are attached to the dog's body only by muscle. The shoulder blade (scapula) slides within limits, back and forth, parallel with the rib cage. If the muscle attachments of the forequarters are inadequate, undesirable movement off of this plane occurs.

Shoulder angulation is the angle that is formed by the slope of the shoulder blade with a line drawn parallel to the ground. The desired conformation of the shoulder is long and sloping, with the scapula forming an angle of approximately 45 to 55 degrees. This is referred to as a shoulder assembly that is "well laid back." This conformation confers optimal forward movement of the front assembly legs because it is associated with maximal extension of the front legs. This results in a long, level stride with minimal upward movement (Figure 3.4). Adequate length to the scapula also provides a large area for muscle attachment and allows proper head carriage and good forward reach of the neck. A shoulder that has an angle of greater than 45 to 55 degrees is called an upright or steep shoulder. This is a fairly common fault in dogs and

FIGURE 3.4   Shoulder assembly: Proper angulation vs. steep shoulders

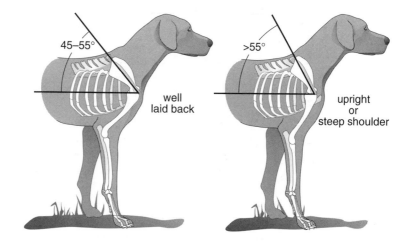

is undesirable because it contributes to a short stride, pounding, and inefficient movement (Figure 3.4).

Shoulder joint: The shoulder joint consists of a modified ball and socket. The lower end of the scapula has a slight indentation called the glenoid cavity into which the articular head of the humerus rests. Although, technically, the shoulder joint can move in all directions (like other ball-and-socket joints), the shape of the glenoid cavity coupled with the connective tissue attachments along the bone limit movement to a forward and backward plane parallel to the body.

Forearm: The radius and ulna are the two bones of the forearm (Figures 3.1 and 3.2). The radius articulates proximally with the humerus to form the elbow joint and distally with the carpus to form the wrist joint (carpus). Although a separate bone, the ulna is closely attached to the radius by muscle. It forms the anconeal process at its proximal end and the coronoid process at its distal end. The proper structure for most breeds of dogs is one in which the forearms are straight, parallel to each other, and positioned vertically to the ground when the dog is standing naturally. This is referred to as a straight front (Figure 3.5).

Carpus: The carpus in the dog is synonymous with the wrist joint in humans. This joint is comprised of seven short carpal bones and their associated **sesamoid** bones, arranged in two rows. The joint is formed by the proximal ends of the carpal bones and the distal end of the forearm (radius and ulna).

FIGURE 3.5   Front types (*from left*): Out at the elbow and too wide, straight, chippendale, too narrow and east-west feet

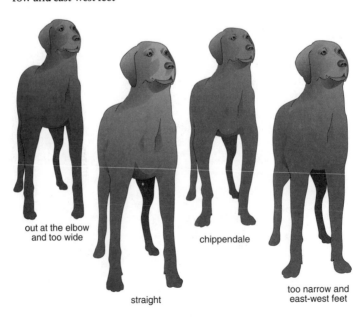

out at the elbow
and too wide

chippendale

straight

too narrow and
east-west feet

Pastern: The pastern is the lower end of the forearm and is made up of several small bones called the metacarpal bones. During movement, the pastern acts as a shock absorber for the dog, absorbing the concussion of each step. For most breeds, the pasterns should not be steep (upright), but should have a slight but definite angle in relation to the bones of the forearm. This angle supplies a certain amount of give and, as a result, gradually diminishes the shock of each step. Straight pasterns are less efficient as shock absorbers and, therefore, pass the impact of footfall directly to the shoulder. The terrier breeds are the only group of dogs that have naturally straight, upright pasterns.

Hindquarter assembly: The dog's hindquarters supply most of its propelling power and consist of the pelvis, femur, tibia and fibula, tarsus (hock), metatarsals, and their associated joints. An examination of the dog's hindquarters from the rear is useful in determining proper structure. For most breeds of dogs, desirable structure is depicted by a straight vertical line through the bones from the pelvis through the upper and lower thigh, the point of the hock, and down to the rear pastern and foot (Figure 3.6). From the side view, both the pelvic angle and the angle of the stifle joint should be evaluated with respect to the dog's breed standard.

Pelvis and its slope: The pelvis, also referred to as the hip bone, is composed of four distinct bones (Figure 3.7). These are the ilium, ischium, pubis and acetabular bones. When puppies are born, these bones are not fully developed. They continue to develop during the first 3 months of life and fuse together to form the butterfly shape of the pelvis at about 12 weeks of age. The socket that forms to hold the end of the femur is called the acetabulum. The acetabulum is an important bone because it bears the weight of the hind

FIGURE 3.6   Rear structure *(from left):* Wide or bandy, correct or straight, cow-hocked

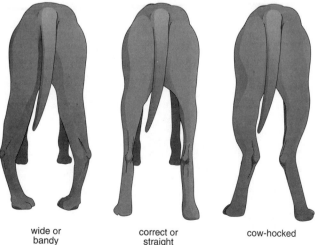

wide or bandy   correct or straight   cow-hocked

end of the dog and absorbs the thrust of rear movement. The three fused sacral vertebrae (the sacrum) are attached to the body of the pelvis by a ligament of dense connective tissue called the sacro-tuberal ligament. The horizontal slope of the pelvis is a factor in determining both rear angulation and movement. In general, an angle of about 30 degrees horizontally is desirable and provides good backward reach to the rear legs as they move. When discussing this angle, it is important to note that the upper thigh (femur) is limited in backward motion. The maximum angle that the femur can make with a properly set pelvis is about 150 degrees. A pelvic slope that is greater than 30 degrees (i.e. a steeper pelvis) will limit this angle and, subsequently, will limit the dog's backward reach (Figure 3.8).

Hip joint: The proximal end of the femur is shaped into a head that fits into the acetabulum of the pelvis to form the hip joint, a ball-and-socket joint. The **teres ligament** attaches the head of the femur to the inner surface of the acetabulum. However, the muscle mass that surrounds the hip joint is primarily responsible for holding the femoral head firmly within the acetabulum in an animal with correct hip structure.

Stifle joint: The angle formed by the femur and the lower thigh bone (tibia/fibula) is called the stifle, or stifle joint. The **trochlea** of the distal end of the femur forms an indentation into which the patella (kneecap) sits. The patella is a sesamoid bone. Sesamoid bones are found within muscles or tendons and function to provide leverage and assist passage of the soft tissue over another area of bone. The stifle joint is stabilized by two important ligaments: the anterior and posterior cruciate ligaments.

Hock joint: The hock joint is formed by the articulation of the lower thigh (tibia/fibula) and the tarsal bones. The tibia is the larger, stronger bone and is

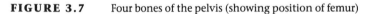

FIGURE 3.7   Four bones of the pelvis (showing position of femur)

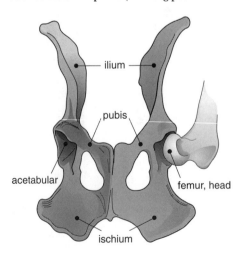

located medially to the fibula. The narrow fibula is a completely separate bone in the dog, but it is closely connected to the tibia, so the two bones work together as the lower thigh. The point of the hock is composed of a bone called the calcaneal process or *os calcis*. This protruding bone is the largest and longest of the seven tarsal bones and corresponds to the heel of the human foot. Another important tarsal bone is the **talus**, or tibial tarsal bone, which directly articulates with the tibia and fibula to form the hock joint. The calcaneus is closely associated with the talus, and this entire area is important for muscle attachment to the point of the hock. The central tarsal bone is found between the proximal and distal rows of tarsals. This is also called the scaphoid bone and is more prone to fracture in dogs that are used for tracking or pulling. The angle of the hock, the length of the calcaneal process, and the height of the hock measured from the ground are all important in determining the type of rear movement that a dog has. For most breeds of dogs, a well-angulated or "bent" hock is desirable for proper movement, but this may vary considerably depending on the original purpose of the breed.

Metatarsus (rear pastern): The rear pastern is comprised of the five metatarsal bones. The length of these bones determines the height of the hock and length of the lower hind limb. In general, high hocks (long metatarsals) correspond with fast movement, and low hocks (short metatarsals) are seen in breeds that were originally developed for endurance.

Feet: Like many mammals that are built for speed, the dog walks on its toes, or phalanges (**digigrade**). The bones of the forepaw and hind foot are quite similar and can be discussed together. The dog has five phalanges, four that are fully functional and weight-bearing, and one that is vestigial. Each phalange is divided into three parts: the proximal, middle, and distal phalanx.

FIGURE 3.8   Pelvic angle and backward reach

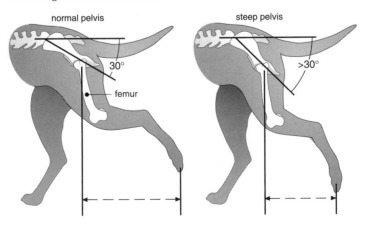

Each is also associated with two sesamoid bones located at the joint with the metacarpal bones. In the front paw, the vestigial phalange forms the dewclaw. Although all dogs are born with this toe, many breeders and veterinarians remove it when the puppies are only a few days old. In the rear, although all dogs have some form of this vestigial phalange, the digit is so reduced in size that it is not apparent in the majority of dogs. Some breed standards specifically describe the presence of a rear dewclaw, however. The shape of a dog's foot is related to the function for which the breed was originally developed. The term "cat foot" refers to a foot that is round and compact with very short distal portions. This type of foot is designed for endurance. In contrast, a "hare foot" has a long digital portion, producing an elongated foot designed for speed. Many sporting breeds have feet that are webbed, with excess skin between the toes. These feet are usually large in size and are well adapted for endurance while swimming.

Balance: A dog's overall conformation is a reflection both of its underlying skeleton and its overlying musculature. The term "balance" refers to the proportion of the dog's various parts to one another; for example, the head to the neck, the depth of chest to length of legs, the overall length of the body to its height, and a front assembly that is balanced with the hindquarter assembly in terms of angulation and strength. A well-balanced animal will have a front end that moves easily in concert with the back end, is able to absorb the power and drive of the back end, and does not interfere with the movement of the hind legs or feet.

The Dog's Movement

The dog evolved as a group-living predator, specializing in both speed and endurance while moving. Selective breeding has resulted in great variations in movement among breeds, but all dogs, regardless of body type, are subject to the same principles that govern movement. The extremes that are seen in today's dogs are evidenced by comparing two of the greatest canine athletes, the racing Greyhound and the racing sled dog. Greyhounds can achieve up to 45 miles per hour for distances of less than a mile, but lack the ability to run for long distances. Racing sled dogs in contrast, run up to 100 miles per day at a pace of 7 to 12 miles per hour while traversing trails such as the 1,100 mile-long Iditarod course.

In all dogs (and all animals, for that matter), movement can be looked upon as simply a series of controlled falls. An understanding of the dog's center of gravity helps to illustrate this. The term "center of gravity" refers to an imaginary point in an object or animal about which all forces are equal (i.e. a balance point). In humans, the body's center of gravity is located at about hip level, toward the center of the body. In the majority of dogs, it is located just behind the shoulders, about one-third of the way up the body. This varies slightly with the length and weight of the head and neck, length of the legs, and weight and structure of the dog's torso.

When the center of gravity is moved out of position without changing the base beneath it, movement results. For example, when a human runner begins to jog, the body leans forward, shifting the center of gravity forward in an arc and ahead of its base of support (the body's trunk and legs). The runner's legs then move to keep the body from falling to the ground, bringing the support of the legs under the center of gravity. In all movement (human and dog), the center of gravity transcribes an arc with the low point at the starting position, moving upward and downward in a cycle with each stride. This upward movement requires muscular effort but does not contribute to forward movement. Therefore, the flatter this arc is, the less energy that is wasted in upward movement.

Walking, trotting and other gaits of the dog are nothing more than upsetting balance then changing position to bring it back under control (i.e. a series of "controlled falls"). In dogs, the center of gravity is positioned closer to the front of the body than to the back. The forequarter assembly is the hardest-working part of the dog and is responsible for supporting more than half of the dog's weight. This is necessary so the hindquarters can be comparatively free to deliver forward drive. As a result, the forequarters also absorb most of the concussion of each step.

Moving efficiently: The goal of proper movement in all animals is to move efficiently (i.e. movement in which the least expenditure of energy occurs for maximal motion in the desired direction). In the dog, efficiency results from moving the center of gravity in as straight a line or arc as possible, while minimizing movement up and down and from side to side (lateral displacement).

One criteria that is used to evaluate movement in dogs is the rise and fall of the withers while trotting. The movement of the dog's withers provides a rough indication of the movement of its center of gravity. Because movement upward does not contribute to forward locomotion but uses energy, the most efficient movement would be that in which the center of gravity moved forward in a straight line, parallel to the ground. However, some lift is necessary for propulsion forward, so the arc of movement, as evidenced by the bob of the withers, should be as flat as possible. When viewed from the side, while the dog is trotting, the withers should show minimal vertical movement. If the withers are bobbing up and down, it is an indication of poor conformation and inefficient movement. Most commonly, bobbing withers are a sign of a steep shoulder set. While evaluating movement from the side, good leg extension is important, without a high-stepping action or pounding as the legs land. Similarly, rear extension should be maximized and the hocks should be fully extended at the end of the swing.

Lateral displacement must also be considered when evaluating movement. When a dog is standing naturally, the four legs support the body at four corners to create a rectangular base. Because the dog's weight is not distributed evenly over this base, its center of gravity, as mentioned previously, is located toward the forward portion of the body. When the dog's legs move forward on alternating sides during locomotion, the center of gravity not only moves forward and vertically but also from left to right. This occurs because the hind legs are not traveling in the same plane, and the thrust forward as they move shifts the center of gravity to the side. The shift of the center of gravity from side to side during movement is called lateral displacement and accounts for the characteristic roll seen in some dogs as they trot. Dogs that are built with a wide base (i.e. short, stocky dogs) naturally show more pronounced lateral displacement than dogs with a narrow base. For example, it is expected that a Bulldog will show more rolling motion while moving than the narrow-based Greyhound.

Although it is a natural consequence of having four legs, lateral displacement represents wasted energy and decreased efficiency of movement. Dogs minimize lateral displacement, within the limits imposed by their structure, by attempting to single-track. Single-tracking involves the dog bringing its feet as close together as possible beneath the vertical center of gravity as it moves. This compensates for lateral displacement by applying the power forward directly over the line of locomotion. Dogs moving at a trot will increase the tendency to single-track as speed increases. Although this inward bend of the leg appears to begin at the elbow when viewed from the front, it actually originates at the shoulder joint. As the dog trots toward or away from the evaluator, its legs should remain in a straight conformation but will bend slightly inward as they attempt to come together beneath the body. The degree to which a dog is capable of actually single-tracking is dependent on overall body conformation and speed when moving.

Gaits of the dog: The term "gait" refers to a given sequence of leg movements that are repeated cyclically. The most common gaits of the dog are the walk, trot, pace, single-suspension gallop and double-suspension gallop. The walk is the slowest and the least tiring gait of the dog. It is a four-beat gait in which three legs are in support of the body at all times. For this reason, the walk is the least tiring of all of the dog's gaits. The trot is a two-beat gait in which diagonal front and rear legs move together as a pair. With the exception of the flying trot, which has a period of suspension, two legs are supporting the body at all times. The right front and left rear first move forward, followed by the left front and right rear. The pace is a two-beat, lateral gait in which the front and hind feet on the same side of the body move together as a pair. Thus, the dog's weight is alternately supported by the right side of the body and the left side of the body. Because of this, the pace results in a rolling motion of the body, exaggerating lateral displacement. In general, most dogs will trot before they will pace. However, many will switch to pacing if they are fatigued or if their structure causes leg interference. The gallop is the fastest gait of the dog. It is a four-beat gait, characterized by extreme shoulder and foreleg extension, followed by movement of the hind legs far forward under the body to provide the propulsive stroke. Most large, heavy dogs demonstrate a single-suspension gallop when they are running. The sight hound breeds, and several other light-boned breeds that are built for speed, run with a double-suspension gallop. The term suspension refers to a short period during which the dog is actually airborne, with no feet touching the ground. In a single-suspension gallop, the dog is airborne one time during a single cycle of the gait. This occurs twice in the double-suspension gallop. During the gallop, both the front and the rear of the dog contribute to forward propulsion. In fact, the front assembly is important for supplying the upward thrust of movement that allows suspension during the gallop.

The Dog's Special Senses

Just as the body structure and movement of *Canis familiaris* are specifically adapted for the niche that this species has filled in the past, so are its special senses. The special senses determine how the dog perceives and responds to the world. Humans have highly developed visual capabilities, so we tend to perceive the environment using vision as our primary sense. In contrast, the dog relies most heavily upon its sense of smell (olfactory) and hearing (auditory) and comparatively has a less well-developed sense of vision. These differences are important when developing an understanding of how a dog perceives, reacts, and learns about its environment.

Vision: Because the wolf is a predator that hunts primarily at twilight (crepuscular), the dog's sense of vision is specialized for maximal efficiency under low light conditions. The retina contains two primary types of light receptors: rods and cones. Rods are specialized for low-intensity light and are the predominant type of receptor found in the dog's retina. Measurements comparing the dog's vision to that of humans have shown that the dog's absolute threshold for the detection of light is about threefold lower than that of humans.[4] This means that the dog is three times as capable of detecting low intensities of light than humans. In contrast, cones are essential for the detection of high-intensity light and are responsible for the perception of color. The dog possesses a much lower density of cones than rods in the retina and has a much lower concentration of these receptors compared to concentrations found in the human eye. Because of this difference, it is often said that dogs are "color-blind." However, recent studies have shown that under bright light, dogs are capable of detecting some color, specifically wavelengths of light within the blue and yellow portion of the light spectrum.[5] However, they are incapable of distinguishing reds and oranges because they have few or none of the cones that are sensitive at the red/orange wavelength. Dogs, therefore, are referred to as being dichromatic. They are capable of detecting two pure colors, blue and green, along with combinations of these two colors.

In addition to the higher concentration of rods, the dog has a second adaptation that aids in dim light vision. The tapetum is a unique anatomical feature of the dog's eye and is composed of a layer of reflective cells that are located immediately behind the retina. This area functions to reflect scattered light back onto the photoreceptive cells of the retina. It is estimated that the tapetum increases the dog eye's light-gathering capability by about 40 percent. The tapetum is responsible for the "red eyes" that are seen when a light is shown straight into the dog's eyes or when pictures are taken with a flash camera.

Like other mammals (with the exception of humans), the dog has an additional membrane located between the eyelid and the eyeball. This is called the third eyelid and is located in the lower inner corner of the eyelid. The third eyelid has several functions. It provides additional protection to the eye, contributes to tear secretion, and helps to restore the tear film over the eye when the dog blinks. In a normal, healthy dog, this lid should not be prominent, but certain eye disorders will cause inflammation of the third eyelid, resulting in **prolapse**.

The dog's visual acuity is adapted to its original role as a predatory species. The dog has excellent dim light vision that is very sensitive to movement. Because of the placement of their eyes on the skull, most dogs also have good lateral vision. The farther to the side of the head that the eyes are placed, the greater the field of vision (Figure 3.9). As a predatory animal, the dog needs a wide field of vision to locate prey. In general, brachycephalic breeds, with frontally placed eyes, have a smaller field of vision, about 200 degrees, compared to the dolichocephalic breeds, which have a field of vision of about 270 degrees. Humans, by comparison, have a range of about 100 degrees. While an increased field of vision is advantageous for detecting moving objects in the environment, it is accompanied by decreased binocular vision. This deficit contributes to the dog's lesser ability to focus on objects that are at close range or to judge distance. Similarly, the dog's eyes are not capable of discriminating fine degrees of form or pattern (poor resolution). This occurs because of the relatively flat shape of its eye, the low concentration of cones in the retina, and the presence of the light-scattering tapetum.

Olfactory (scent): Olfaction is the dog's primary special sense. As a result, odors play an enormous role in the behavior of all dogs. It is often said that a good way to appreciate the importance of scent to the dog is to imagine that the dog perceives its world through "nose pictures." By comparison, humans are woefully inadequate in scenting ability. For example, the dog has approximately 220 million scent receptors in its nose. Humans have about 5 million.

FIGURE 3.9   Differences in field of vision *(from left):* 200° brachycephalic breeds, 270° dolichocephalic breeds

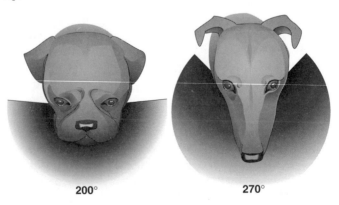

200°

270°

brachycephalic breeds

dolichocephalic breeds

In addition, the olfactory epithelium, the layer of cells that line the passages of the nose, has a surface area in dogs between 18 and 150 centimeters^2, compared to 3 to 4 centimeters^2 in humans.[6]

The dog has several mechanisms that aid in maximizing scenting ability. Most important is the use of sniffing. The sniff is actually a disruption of the normal breathing pattern. This allows the molecules that impart odor to remain within the nasal passages for longer periods of time. Sniffing consists of a series of rapid, short inhalations and exhalations. Air is forced into a space above the subethmoidal shelf, a bony structure that functions to trap inhaled air. The sniffed air rests within this nasal pocket without being inhaled farther into the lungs or being immediately exhaled, as it would during a normal breathing cycle. This allows increased time for the inhaled air and the scent molecules that it carries to interact with scent receptors.

The dog also has a unique scent organ called the vomeronasal organ. The vomeronasal organ (called Jacobson's organ in some species) is comprised of a pair of fluid-filled sacs lined with receptor cells. It is located above the roof of the dog's mouth, just behind the upper incisors. This organ provides a chemical sense in addition to olfaction and is believed to be important for the reception of pheromones (body scents). If this theory is true, the vomeronasal organ is probably involved in normal sexual behavior of the dog and in the dog's ability to identify and recognize other animals and people.

The dog's olfactory acuity is demonstrated most dramatically in its ability to detect, discriminate, and follow scent trails. Controlled tests have shown that dogs trained to indicate a particular scent are capable of detecting extremely minute concentrations. For example, tracking dogs are capable of detecting butyric acid (a volatile fatty acid found in human sweat) at a concentration as low as 10^{-12} Molar.[7] By comparison, this is up to one million-fold greater than the sensitivity of the human nose. Other experiments have demonstrated the dog's excellent discriminatory abilities. A classic study with human subjects showed that trained dogs reliably discriminated between members of a single family, siblings, and identical twins.[8] A final olfactory talent of the dog is its ability to distinguish between the component sources of a smell. When dogs that are trained to detect a particular odor are presented with complex odors that contain the compound, they are still able to detect its presence.

Auditory (hearing): Like olfaction, the dog's ability to hear is also well developed. Most people are aware that dogs are capable of detecting sounds at much higher frequencies than humans. While humans can hear up to 20,000 cycles per second, dogs can detect sounds up to 40,000 cycles per second. In other mammals, such as rodents, the ability to hear very high frequencies often is associated with communication by ultrasound. However, there is no evidence indicating that the dog is capable of producing this type of communication signal. It is more probable that this capability has aided the dog in capturing small prey that use high frequency sounds to communicate. Most dogs have mobile ears, which can pivot to locate sounds. The structure of the dog's ears also enables them to hear over a great distance, about four times farther than humans are capable of hearing.

Touch: As in other mammals, the sense of touch is the earliest developed sense in the newborn dog. Young puppies are responsive to changes in temperature and actively seek out both warmth and tactile comfort. The importance of touch persists throughout the dog's life. Being a social species, the dog uses touch as an essential communication tool in interactions with other dogs and with humans. Some of the first studies of the human/animal bond showed that gentle touch and petting cause a reduction in a dog's heart rate and blood pressure (decreased sympathetic nervous arousal).[9] Humans show this same response to positive interactions with dogs.

Dogs also use touch as a means of investigating and learning about their environment. In most carnivores, an area of the body that is highly sensitive to touch is the muzzle. This is also true for the dog. The nose pad and the skin at the base of the vibrissae (whiskers) are particularly well endowed with sensory nerves. The vibrissae are stiff and do not collapse on contact with surfaces. Although their exact function is not known, it is believed that they provide information to the dog about the location of the head in relation to its immediate surroundings.

Taste: Along with touch, taste is the only other special sense that is fully developed in the dog at birth. As in other mammals, the dog's sense of taste is confined to the mouth, the palate, and the epiglottis. In humans, the sense of flavor is a result of both smell and taste, and it is reasonable to assume that this is true in the dog as well. However, based on the total number of taste receptors in the mouth, dogs' sense of taste appears to be less refined than humans. While humans have about 9,000 taste buds on the tongue, dogs have only about 1,700. In the dog, the most abundant taste buds are those that respond to sugars. This accounts for the fact that most dogs enjoy sweet foods. Interestingly, however, the most potent compounds that trigger the receptors in these taste buds are a certain group of amino acids. The omnivorous nature of the dog is possibly reflected in the ability to detect sugars and other sweet-tasting substances that may be present in some plant materials, such as fruits and some vegetables. The second most abundant group of taste receptors in the dog are the acid receptors. These respond to compounds such as phosphoric acid, carboxylic acids, nucleotide triphosphate, histidine, and several specific amino acids. These are all compounds that are found in meat and meat products.

Recognizing the Normal Dog

As a species, the dog comes endowed with certain physiological constants that can be used by pet owners and companion animal professionals to evaluate health and vitality. These basic indicators of health can be used to establish a normal baseline for a pet by which to measure changes and as an initial evaluation when determining the presence of disease or injury (Table 3.2).

Skin and coat: A dog's skin and coat are good indicators of overall health. The dog's coat forms a physical barrier between the external environment and the skin. Selective breeding has resulted in great variations in coat color, length, and texture. However, a simple way of categorizing coat types is using length (short, medium, or long) and texture (varying degrees of coarseness or fineness). Regardless of the type or length of coat (and regardless of what some breeders or owners insist), all dogs shed their coat. The major differences between breeds relates to the presence or absence of a dense undercoat and the rate at which the hairs grow, mature, and eventually fall out. The amount of shedding that an individual dog shows is also dependent on age, nutritional status, physiological status, housing conditions, and season of the year. Photoperiod has a strong influence on hair growth and shedding in dogs. As day length shortens, the rate of growth decreases and hairs complete their entire growth cycle in a longer time period. As a result, shedding decreases, and the dog develops its "winter" coat. As day length increases, rate of hair growth increases and shedding occurs at a faster rate (i.e. the dog loses its winter coat). When dogs are kept indoors under artificial light, however, shedding often occurs throughout the year, and dogs never develop a heavy winter coat.

The skin of the dog is an important mechanical and biochemical protector for the dog's body. It is also an important sensory structure, conveying information about touch, pressure, pain, and environmental temperature. The skin is composed of the epidermis and the dermis. The epidermis is the uppermost layer and consists of an **avascular** layer of epithelial cells. It is firmly attached to the underlying dermis layer that is made up of connective tissue, blood vessels, and nerve fibers. The sebaceous glands of the skin produce sebum, an oily substance that functions to protect the skin. Although the skin is important in dissipating the body's heat, dogs have a minimal number of sudoriferous (sweat) glands in their skin, so perspiration from the skin is not an effective mechanism of heat loss for the dog. A healthy animal will have clean, pliable skin that is free from dirt, sores, excessive oil, and dryness.

TABLE 3.2   Vital Statistics for Healthy Dogs

Skin and Coat	Normal shine, growth, and shedding pattern for breed or breed type; skin that is pliable, clean, and free of lesions
Mucous Membranes	Light pink in color (if unpigmented); normal CRT (~ 1 second)
Food Intake and Body Weight	Normal and consistent appetite; maintenance of ideal (lean) body weight
Body Temperature	100 to 102.5 degrees F (average 101.5)
Pulse (Resting)	60 to 140 beats/minute
Respiration Rate	10 to 30 inhalations/minute

Mucous membranes: Mucous membranes are the lubricating membranes that line all body openings, such as the mouth, nostrils, eyelids, anus, and reproductive tract. Checking the color and capillary refill time of the mucous membranes can be used as an indicator of a change in either the amount or the composition of blood that is flowing to the extremities. The membranes inside the eyelids, called the conjunctivae, and those inside the mouth are good locations to examine for normal membrane color. Normal mucous membranes should be pale pink in color (if not pigmented) and have normal capillary refill time (CRT). The presence of blood vessels close to the surface of these tissues imparts the light pink color (provided the membrane does not contain dark pigment). Pale mucous membranes are a sign of decreased red blood cells (anemia), blood loss, or reduced blood flow. Some problems that may cause pale membranes include bleeding, destruction or lack of production of red blood cells, heart disease, or circulation collapse (shock). Jaundiced, or yellow-tinged, mucous membranes are a result of an accumulation of bilirubin. Bilirubin is a waste product that is produced when hemoglobin is **catabolized** by the liver. When the liver is incapable of metabolizing hemoglobin normally, or if there is an increased rate of red blood cell destruction, bilirubin accumulates in the body and jaundice occurs. Bright red mucous membranes are seen in the early stages of heat stroke. However, if the red color is confined only to the conjunctiva, it may indicate topical irritation to the eye or an eye infection. Mucous membranes that are cyanotic (bluish or purple in color) indicate a lack of oxygenation of the blood. This can be caused by blocked airways, certain types of heart problems, and some types of poisons.

The dog's CRT is a second way of evaluating blood flow to the extremities. It can be quickly measured by lifting the upper lip and pressing a thumb firmly against the gum area above the upper teeth for 6 to 8 seconds. After releasing, the number of seconds that the blanched area takes to return to normal color is recorded. Normal CRT is about 1 second and indicates normal blood circulation. If the CRT is 2 seconds or longer, this is an indication of decreased blood circulation. Most commonly, CRT is used as a rough indicator of the presence of circulatory collapse in injured or ill animals.

Food intake and body weight: Daily food intake and body weight are important indicators of health in dogs. In American dogs, the condition of obesity contributes to more health problems than underweight conditions. Currently, obesity is the leading nutritional malady seen in American cats and dogs (see Chapter 19). This problem is caused by a combination of overfeeding and underexercising. Long-term effects of obesity include a decrease in exercise tolerance and increased incidence of chronic diseases such as diabetes, heart disease, and degenerative joint disease. Maintaining proper body weight throughout a dog's life contributes to longevity and the prevention of chronic diseases. Growing puppies and adult dogs should be fed an amount of food that supports ideal body condition. A dog that is at ideal body weight will have a lean body condition. The ribs should be barely visible and can be easily felt upon palpation. An overweight animal's ribs will not be visible and an overlying layer of fat can be felt. When viewed from above, the dog should have an hourglass appearance, with a slight indentation in the loin area. The loss of a waist (i.e. indentation behind the ribs) indicates excess weight. Providing regular vigorous exercise contributes to both energy expenditure and to the maintenance of lean body tissue.

Monitoring food intake is also important because, in many cases, one of the first signs of illness will be decreased food intake or **anorexia**. Decreased intake at one or two meals is not usually cause for concern, but a sudden drop in food intake or a sudden loss of weight may be signs of disease or illness.

Body temperature: The normal body temperature of the dog is between 100 and 102.5 degrees Fahrenheit (F), with an average of 101.5 degrees F. The major means that the dog uses to rid itself of body heat is by increased respiration (panting) through the mouth and nasal passages. Although most water would appear to be lost from the tongue and oral cavity, in reality, the nasal cavities expend more heat for the dog than the oral cavity. As its body temperature rises, the dog will first breathe exclusively through the nose, but as it has the need to rid itself of heat continues, it will inhale through the nose and exhale (pant) through the open mouth. Unlike the human, the dog does not have sweat glands in the skin, so it does not perspire through the skin over most of the body. However, it does have eccrine sweat glands located between the toes of the feet, which function to remove body heat through perspiration. These are the only sweat glands used for heat loss by the dog. The dog's body temperature should be taken using a rectal thermometer, preferably one that is designed and sold for companion animals.

Elevated body temperature occurs when the dog is unable to get rid of body heat at a rate equal to the rate at which it is gained. This can be a result of either an internal (metabolic) cause or an external (environmental) cause. A fever is a metabolic cause of elevated body temperature caused by a change in the body's thermoregulatory mechanisms. The temperature "set-point" in the brain is temporarily increased so that the body works to maintain a higher than normal body temperature. As a result, dogs with a fever will try to conserve heat by seeking warm areas or sleeping in a curled position. In general, a moderate fever is not dangerous to the dog and represents a defense mechanism used by the body to fight infection or disease. An elevated body temperature of up to about 105 degrees F can be tolerated by the dog. However, if a fever should rise to 106 degrees or greater, or if fever persists for more than one day, measures should be taken to bring the body's temperature down.

High environmental temperature and humidity or excessive muscular work can cause hyperthermia. In this case, the dog is observed making efforts to rid itself of the excess body heat through panting and seeking a cool environment. Early signs include bright red mucous membranes and elevated body temperature. Dogs experiencing heat stroke can develop a body temperature as high as 110 degrees F. Heat exhaustion and heat stroke should always be treated as a medical emergency, and veterinary care should be sought immediately (see Chapter 15).

Pulse: Pulse is the local, rhythmic expansion of an artery that corresponds to each contraction of the left ventricle of the heart. An animal's pulse is an indicator of the ability of the heart to pump blood through the body. Normal pulse rates vary greatly, depending on the age, size, fitness, and physiological state of the dog. A normal range of resting pulse rate is 60 to 140 beats per minute in alert, resting dogs. The pulse rate of small dogs is usually at the high end of this scale, while large and giant breeds will have slower pulse rates. Puppies have slightly higher pulse rates compared to adult dogs of the same size. Debilitating diseases often cause a weak, slow pulse, while the presence of a fever is associated with an increased pulse rate. A dog's pulse can be taken by either directly palpating the heart or by feeling it in the femoral artery of the back leg. Gently pressing on the lower chest wall immediately behind the dog's shoulder (in the lower third of the chest cavity) can be used to directly feel the dog's heart beat. The femoral artery is found crossing the femur about halfway down the bone. Gently pressing with two or three fingers on this artery provides a good measure of the dog's pulse (Figure 3.10). A normal resting pulse should be strong, easily felt, and have an even rhythm.

Respiration rate: Respiration rate refers to the number of inhalations or exhalations per minute and is an important indicator of the functioning of the respiratory system. This can easily be monitored by counting the number of inhalations or exhalations when watching the movement of the rib cage. The normal range of respiration rates for dogs is 10 to 30 breaths per minute, with an average of 20.

Conclusions

Although the dog has been domesticated for more than 12,000 years, and selective breeding has resulted in many variations in size, appearance, and tem-

FIGURE 3.10   Measuring the dog's pulse at the femoral artery

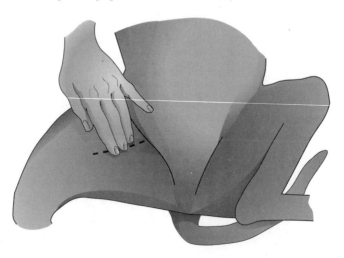

perament, all dogs enter the world with the same basic skeletal structure, special senses, and manner of moving and perceiving the world. Some of these basic physiological constants can be used by companion animal professionals to monitor the health and well-being of dogs. In the following chapter, the manner in which dogs reproduce and, specifically, the uniqueness of this species' reproductive physiology and cycles will be examined in detail.

Cited References

1. Ritvo, H. **The emergence of modern pet-keeping.** In: *Animals and People Sharing the World,* (A.R. Rowan, editor), University Press of New England, Hanover, New Hampshire, pp. 13-31. (1988)

2. Fox, M.W. **Origin and history of the dog.** In: *Understanding Your Dog,* Coward, McCann, and Geoghegan, New York, New York, pp. 1-17. (1974)

3. American Veterinary Medical Association. **AVMA position paper (1994): tail docking and ear cropping.** American Veterinary Medical Association. (1994)

4. Bradshaw, J. **Behavioural biology of the dog and cat.** In: *The Waltham Book of Dog and Cat Behaviour* (Thorne, C., editor), Pergamon Press, Oxford, England, pp. 35-48. (1992)

5. Neitz, J., Geist, T., and Jacobs, J.H. **Color vision in the dog.** Visual Neuroscience, 3:119-125. (1989)

6. Dodd, G.H. and Squirrel, D.J. **Structure and mechanism in the mammalian olfactory system.** Symposia of the Zoological Society of London, 45:35-36. (1980)

7. Moulton, D.G., Ashton, E.H., and Eayrs, J.T. **Studies in olfactory acuity. 4. Relative detectability of n-aliphatic acids by the dog.** Animal Behaviour, 8:117-128. (1960)

8. Kaimus, H. **The discrimination by the nose of the dog of individual human odours and in particular of the odours of twins.** Animal Behaviour, 3:25-31. (1955)

9. Katcher, A.H. and Friedmann, E. **Potential health value of pet ownership.** Compendium on Continuing Education for the Practicing Veterinarian, 2:117-122. (1980)

4   Reproduction and Breeding Management

THE DOG HAS INHERITED the major components of the wolf's reproductive physiology and breeding cycle, with several important behavioral and physiological changes that occurred during the domestication process. Both dogs and wolves are seasonally monestrous, meaning that they have only a single group of follicles mature and release ova during each cycle or "season." However, while the estrous cycle of the wolf is affected by the amount of daylight, selective breeding in the dog has resulted in disconnecting the breeding cycle from seasonal changes in daylight length. Dogs also attain sexual maturity at an earlier age than wolves and are considered to be less sexually selective. Wolves attain sexual maturity around 2 years of age, but female dogs (bitches) become sexually mature between 6 and 16 months, depending on size and breed. Male dogs generally reach sexual maturity around 10 months of age. This chapter examines the dog's reproductive anatomy, reproductive cycle, mating, pregnancy, whelping, and neonatal care.

Reproductive Anatomy of the Bitch

The bitch's anatomy is designed to enable the female to produce litters containing several offspring. The major organs of the reproductive tract of the bitch include the ovaries, oviducts, uterus, vagina, vulva, and the secondary sex organs, or the mammary glands (Figure 4.1). The ovaries are relatively small, lima-bean shaped organs, located **caudally** to the kidneys. They function to produce ova (eggs) and certain reproductive hormones. The oviducts are small, thin tubes connecting the ovaries to the uterus and function to transport the ova from the ovaries to the uterus. In the dog, as in many mammals, the ova mature and are fertilized while moving through the oviducts. Following ovulation and release into the oviducts, the ova spend approximately two days moving through the oviducts to the uterus. The oviducts enter the uterus at the upper end of each horn. Depending on the time of breeding and the rate that the ova mature, fertilization usually takes place near the end of the oviducts (closest to the uterus). The uterus is a muscular, hollow, Y-shaped organ, consisting of two long horns, a short body, neck, and cervix. The cervix is an oval-shaped fibrous/muscular structure that serves as the channel from the uterus to the vagina. The vagina, commonly referred to as the "birth canal" is a long, narrow muscular/membranous canal that extends from the cervix to the vulva. The vagina is lined with stratified, squamous epithelial cells. These cells change in shape and structure during the bitch's estrous cycle. These changes can be used as a method for detecting ovulation in the bitch. The vulva comprises the external genitalia of the bitch, including the **clitoris** and the external folds of the **labia**. The secondary sex organs of the female are the mammary glands. Female dogs have between four and six pairs, located in two parallel rows along the ventral abdomen. Milk is delivered to puppies through the teats (nipples). Prior to puberty, there is little development of these glands. The production of estrogen during the first proestrus stimulates the development of the duct system within the gland and specialization of milk-producing cells. Secretory cells within the gland develop fully during pregnancy and produce milk during lactation.

Reproductive Anatomy of the Male

The reproductive system of the male dog consists of the paired testes (testicles), scrotum, duct system, prostate gland, and penis (Figure 4.2). The testes function to produce sperm (spermatogenesis) and are the major site of testosterone synthesis. In the dog, sperm production occurs throughout the year, without the seasonal fluctuations that are seen in wolves and many other mammals. The testes are divided into lobules, each of which contains long, tightly coiled seminiferous tubules.

Cells lining the seminiferous tubules, the germinal cells, are responsible for spermatogenesis (production of spermatozoa). Sperm are in various stages of production and maturation at different places along the seminiferous tubules, and a complete cycle of spermatogenesis takes 62 days. The Leydig cells, located between the tubules, produce testosterone. This hormone is

FIGURE 4.1   Reproductive organs of the bitch

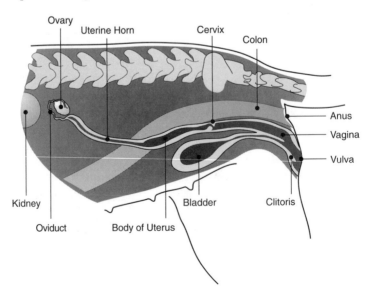

necessary for normal spermatogenesis, development of secondary sexual characteristics, and sexual performance in the male. The seminiferous tubules eventually straighten and empty into collecting ductules that merge to form the epididymis, where sperm maturation takes place. Sperm spend approximately 10 to 14 days traveling the length of the epididymis. Each epididymis empties into the vas deferens (also called the ductus deferens), which eventually empties into the urethra. The prostate is the only accessory sex gland in the dog. It surrounds the urethra where it joins the urinary bladder and produces a watery secretion that is ejaculated after the sperm-containing portion of the semen. The urethra is a hollow tube running through the penis from its origin at the neck of the bladder. It serves to transport urine and, during mating, to transport the sperm-containing semen during ejaculation.

The penis of the dog has several unique characteristics. Within the glans (free portion of the penis), there is a small bone, called the os penis. This bone gives the penis support during the early stages of mating. At one end of the os penis is a penile swelling called the bulbus glandis. This area enlarges to a spherical shape during coitus (mating) and is responsible for the "coital tie" in dogs. This tie prohibits the male and female from separating immediately following intercourse and ejaculation, and generally lasts between 5 and 80 minutes.

There are several important hormones of reproduction in the male dog. The pituitary gland secretes luteinizing hormone (LH) and follicle-stimulating hormone (FSH) in both male and female dogs. In males, these hormones stimulate the production of spermatozoa and hormones by the testes. Specif-

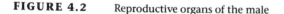

FIGURE 4.2   Reproductive organs of the male

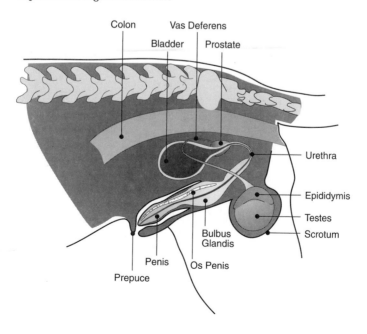

ically, FSH initiates spermatogenesis and the production of **androgens**; LH stimulates the secretion of testosterone. Testosterone is produced by the Leydig cells located in the connective tissue surrounding the seminiferous tubules. Testosterone is important for the development and maintenance of male sex characteristics; it stimulates male sexual behavior and spermatogenesis, and maintains the reproductive tract.

The Female Estrous Cycle

The dog's estrous cycle has several stages. These are anestrus, proestrus, estrus, and diestrus (Figure 4.3). The "heat" or "season" is actually only one stage (the estrus stage) of the entire estrous cycle. It is during the estrus stage that ovulation takes place and the bitch is receptive to breeding by a male. Ovulation is the process of releasing mature ova from the ovaries into the oviduct so that fertilization with a sperm cell can occur. Like many mammals, the dog is a spontaneous ovulator. This means that ova are released from the ovaries at periodic intervals in response to changing hormone levels in the body. This can be contrasted to animals that are induced ovulators (such as the cat) that require both hormonal preparation of the reproductive tract and the stimulation of mating to trigger ovulation. The ova in the ovaries develop within follicles, which are fluid-filled sacs composed of specialized cells. Follicular development leads to ovulation and is under hormonal control. Following the release of ova into the oviducts, the follicular cells at the ovulation sites proliferate, change in structure and function, and form a corpus luteum. The corpus luteum is a transient hormone-producing gland present during the diestrus stage of the estrous cycle.

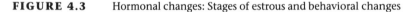

FIGURE 4.3   Hormonal changes: Stages of estrous and behavioral changes

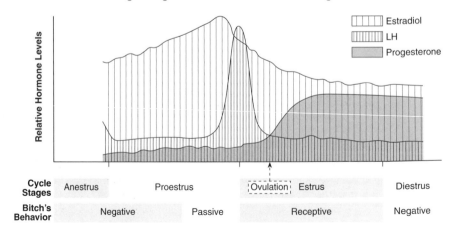

Anestrus: Anestrus is considered to be a period of reproductive quiescence or rest. In a nonpregnant female, it begins at the end of diestrus and ends at the start of proestrus. In a female that has gone through a pregnancy, anestrus begins after whelping. The duration of anestrus varies considerably in females. Factors such as age, state of health, living conditions, and breed will affect this period. A range of 2 to 10 months is seen, with an average anestrus period of 5 1/2 months. An anestrus period of 5 1/2 months results in an estrous cycle that lasts about 8 months.

Proestrus: The start of proestrus is typically defined as the day on which a blood-tinged vaginal discharge first appears. This is accompanied by enlargement and swelling of the vulva. At the beginning of proestrus, the vulva is **turgid**. If mating were attempted during proestrus, intromission (insertion of the penis) would be impossible or very difficult. However, as proestrus proceeds, the vulva becomes softened and more pliable, eliminating this impediment to mating. The bloody discharge that is seen during proestrus is due to the loss of red blood cells by **diapedesis** (leaking) of vessels lining the uterus into the lumen of the uterus. During this stage, the reproductive tract is largely under the influence of estrogen that is produced by the developing follicles. As proestrus proceeds, females often act playful and may even tease males but will not allow mounting or mating by male dogs. Late in proestrus, the bitch often becomes increasingly passive about the male's approach. The length of proestrus usually varies between 6 and 11 days, with an average of 9 days.

Several hormonal changes occur during this period. The hormones FSH and LH from the pituitary gland act upon the ovaries to stimulate growth and development of follicles (Figure 4.3). The follicles are the primary site of estrogen synthesis in the female's body. Estrogen is responsible for the behavioral changes seen during proestrus, as well as the preparation of the uterus and vagina for mating and pregnancy. Estrogen concentrations increase steadily as the follicles develop and prepare for ovulation. Proestrus ends with the onset of estrus, which is characterized by the female allowing a male dog to mount and breed.

Estrus: The estrus period is characterized by sexual receptivity in the bitch. These behavioral changes occur in response to a decline in circulating estrogen level and an increase in circulating progesterone concentration (Figure 4.3). Estrus technically begins on the first day that the female will stand for mounting and ends when the female no longer accepts the male. Behavioral changes in the female include allowing or even initiating interactions with the male, crouching and elevating the rear quarters toward the male when he approaches or attempts to mount, deviating the tail to one side, and tensing of the rear legs to support the weight of the male during mating. The vaginal discharge that is seen during estrus usually has progressed to a straw-colored or only slightly pink color. The vaginal secretions now also contain **pheromones,** which make the bitch very attractive to male dogs. The average duration of estrus is about 5 to 9 days, but this stage can last from just a few days to almost 3 weeks.

Hormonal influences during estrus include a decline in estrogen and an increase in progesterone. The change in estrogen concentration stimulates the release of FSH and LH from the pituitary gland, which in turn causes ovulation. Ovulation and mating take place during the estrus period. Ovulation occurs 24 to 72 hours after the LH surge from the pituitary gland (Figure 4.3). The number of eggs released varies somewhat depending on the age and breed of the female. In general, smaller breeds produce fewer eggs (and hence have smaller litter sizes) than larger breeds. Small breeds generally ovulate between 2 and 10 ova per cycle; the large breeds may release between 5 and 20. All of the ova are released within 24 to 48 hours and are at similar stages of development. This ensures that if fertilization takes place, the fetuses will all be close to the same age.

At the time of ovulation, the ova are still immature and do not complete meiosis until approximately 24 hours after ovulation. Capacitation is the process of maturation by which the ova become capable of being fertilized by sperm. This process takes 2 to 3 days. Once mature, the ova are viable and capable of being fertilized for a period of 12 to 72 hours. Fertilization takes place in the distal portion of the oviduct. Following ovulation, the ruptured follicles of the ovaries convert to corpora lutea and begin increasing their production of progesterone. The corpus luteum is a transient hormone-producing gland that develops at the site of the ruptured follicles on the surface of the ovaries. It is this organ that is responsible for rising progesterone levels during estrus (Figure 4.3).

Diestrus: Diestrus is the 2-month period following estrus when the reproductive organs of the female are under the hormonal influence of progesterone produced by the corpora lutea. It begins with the cessation of sexual receptivity by the bitch and lasts until the corpora lutea regress. This period is equivalent to the period of gestation, if the female has been bred and is pregnant. In a pregnant bitch, diestrus ends abruptly at the time of **parturition**, approximately 65 days after fertilization. In a nonpregnant bitch, the luteal phase wanes more slowly as the corpora lutea regress and ovaries return to the anestrus state.

The dog is somewhat unusual in that its diestrus period lasts the same amount of time in pregnant and nonpregnant females. In the pregnant animal, the corpora lutea are responsible for secreting progesterone and other hormones that are important for the maintenance of pregnancy. Progesterone is responsible for completing the preparation of the uterus for pregnancy and maintaining it in a quiescent state throughout pregnancy. In most species, the corpora lutea will regress and the female will return to anestrus earlier if pregnancy has not occurred. In the female dog, however, the corpora lutea are maintained and remain functional for the same period of time whether or not the female is pregnant. While pregnant bitches have slightly higher progesterone concentrations than nonpregnant bitches during diestrus, individual variation between females precludes the measurement of progesterone as a tool for pregnancy detection. Physiologically, this means that the female dog's genital organs experience a complete breeding cycle, whether or not the bitch has been bred and becomes pregnant. The hormonal changes that are experienced and the resultant changes in behavior and in the reproductive organs are the same in the nonpregnant and the pregnant state.

This is an important difference because it means that all nonpregnant, healthy bitches become pseudo pregnant during diestrus because all females have functioning corpora lutea despite a lack of pregnancy. Behaviorally, the pseudo-pregnant state during diestrus varies greatly in females. While some females show no outward signs, others may demonstrate an increased appetite, decreased activity level, and increases in maternal behavior. Some bitches will even lactate near the end of diestrus. During diestrus, the vulva gradually decreases in size, eventually returning to normal (anestrus) appearance. Following diestrus, the bitch eventually returns to anestrus stage, and the cycle begins again.

Detection of Ovulation in the Bitch

Ovulation occurs during the estrus stage of the estrous cycle. When a female is going to be bred, an estimation of the time of ovulation is essential for successful breeding. Although behavioral cues are helpful in providing a general time frame, breeders are usually interested in precisely identifying the time of ovulation. Most bitches will accept the approach of males and will stand to be bred several days prior to ovulation. If behavioral cues alone are being used to determine breeding dates, the bitch should be bred on the first day of acceptance of the male, then 2 and 4 days later. While this method is successful in some cases, it is not highly accurate. Other methods of determining ovulation (and, therefore, breeding dates) include vaginal exfoliation cytology and sequential measurement of serum progesterone levels.

Vaginal exfoliation cytology is the most commonly used diagnostic tool for the detection of ovulation in female dogs.[1] Because estrogen directly affects the thickness and cellular morphology of the vaginal epithelium, vaginal cytology provides a rough estimation of the bitch's estrogen status. As a result, changes in cells lining the vagina are an excellent aid in distinguishing between the stages of proestrus, estrus, and diestrus (Figure 4.4). During anestrus, the vaginal lining is only a few cell layers thick and is composed of small cuboidal cells. As the reproductive tract becomes influenced by rising estrogen levels during proestrus, this layer greatly increases in thickness, and the cells develop into stratified squamous epithelium. These cells are large and flat and serve as a protective barrier for the vagina. As proestrus proceeds, the thickening of the epithelial layer pushes the cells lining the lumen farther away from their blood supply. This avascular state causes characteristic cellular changes, and eventually cellular death and **exfoliation** (sloughing of the cell).

A vaginal smear can be obtained quickly and painlessly from the bitch by a veterinarian or experienced breeder. The smear will contain exfoliated epithelial cells. The size and shape of these cells provide information about the stage of the female's reproductive cycle. Parabasal cells are the least mature epithelial cells and are seen only during anestrus, early in proestrus, and again in diestrus. Intermediate cells represent a transitional stage between parabasal cells and fully mature superficial cells. In the early stages of proestrus, these cells are small and round, but become more angular as proestrus proceeds (Figure 4.4). The final, fully mature cells are called superficial, or cornified, cells. These are seen during most of the estrus period and contain large amounts of keratin. Keratin is a structural protein that confers strength to protective cells. Fully cornified cells are flat and irregular in shape, with angular sides. A nucleus is either not present or barely visible in the cell. During proestrus, neutrophils (a type of white blood cell) are also seen in the smear. The number of these cells diminishes later in proestrus and in estrus.

The progression of epithelial cells from the parabasal cells of early proestrus to the fully cornified cells of estrus can be used to estimate the time of ovulation. A series of vaginal smears should be obtained over a period of 4 to 10 days, starting at the beginning or middle of proestrus. At the beginning of proestrus, almost all of the cells in the smear are parabasal cells, with some intermediate cells. As proestrus progresses, the number of fully (100 percent) cornified cells gradually increases until these cells make up almost 100 percent of the epithelial cells observed in the smear. This will stay constant for a period of 10 to 14 days, after which a sharp decline occurs. On the day that the female ovulates, the cells have been fully cornified for an average of 6 days. Therefore, the use of a series of slides is essential for identifying the first day that smears are fully cornified. Because ova require 2 to 3 days for capacitation, the bitch should first be bred 4 to 5 days after the day that fully cornified cells reach 100 percent. She can then be bred every day or every other day

FIGURE 4.4   Vaginal exfoliation cytology: Changes during estrous cycle

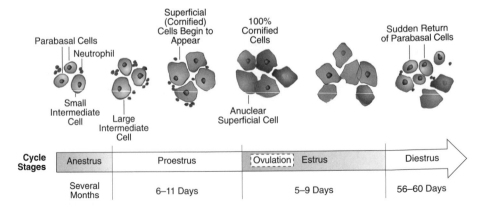

for 3 or 4 consecutive matings. This span will ensure that viable sperm are present when ovulation takes place.

Progesterone levels in the blood provide a second method for detecting ovulation. During the final days of proestrus, declining estrogen levels and increasing progesterone concentration result in the LH surge from the pituitary gland, which induces ovulation. The LH peak is the most reliable indicator of ovulation. Because rising progesterone levels are highly correlated with the LH peak, progesterone concentration in the serum can be used to estimate time of ovulation. Ovulation occurs 2 days after the LH peak. Ova then take an additional 2 to 3 days to mature and are viable for approximately 12 to 72 hours. Therefore, the most highly fertile period is 4 to 7 days after the LH peak.

As with vaginal cytology, progesterone concentrations are most valuable when a sequence of measurements is made. Test kits are available through veterinarians. Blood samples should be collected and tested during proestrus and estrus. Baseline progesterone concentration is between 0 and 1 nanogram/milliliter.[2,3] This increases to greater than 1.0 ng/ml at the onset of estrus. As the corpora lutea predominate during the final stages of estrus and diestrus, progesterone concentration increases slowly and reaches 15 to 60 ng/ml during the first 2 to 3 weeks of diestrus. A series of blood tests is used to determine the day upon which the serum progesterone level first begins to rise. This day is considered to coincide with the LH peak. The first breeding should take place 2 days later and be repeated every other day for several matings.

A less reliable method of detecting ovulation in the bitch is counting days from the first day of proestrus. In general, ovulation occurs around the 10th to 14th day after the onset of proestrus. However, this is extremely variable in dogs and is subject to human error since the onset of proestrus is not always obvious or accurately observed by owners. It also is often suggested that breeding should begin when the vaginal discharge changes in color from pink or red to a translucent yellow or a clear color. This is also not a reliable method because many females have a red-tinged discharge throughout both proestrus and estrus. Similarly, a change in the size and turgidity of the vulva is not a reliable method to use to determine breeding dates in female dogs.

Breeding Management

Before a decision to breed is made, several important factors must be considered. Because of the pet overpopulation problem our country is currently facing, it is imperative that any decision to breed a dog be made with the welfare and health of the puppies and the availability of good homes in mind (see Chapter 6).

Once a decision has been made to breed, the health of the animal must be thoroughly evaluated. Written records should be kept. For bitches, these should include information concerning previous estrus periods (i.e. length of proestrus, estrus, and diestrus; signs of pseudo pregnancy; occurrence of any abnormal cycles); previous breeding dates and the outcomes; vaginal cytology information; and a complete health record. The health record should include vaccination dates, information about the dog's physical condition, and presence of diseases or structural abnormalities. Clearances for any hereditary disorders common to the dog's breed (for example canine hip dysplasia or cataracts) also should be included in the file. A canine brucellosis test should be conducted before breeding. Although canine brucellosis is not a common disease, its presence in a breeding kennel can be devastating (see page 75). Finally, prior to breeding, the female should be given a complete physical examination, including an examination of her reproductive tract. The breeding record for a male dog should contain the same health information as the female's records. Records of semen viability should also be kept. In the dog, sperm with an average of 75 percent or progressive motility is considered normal.

The bitch is usually brought to the male for breeding. Courtship behavior is initiated by the male dog, and the female either will respond positively or will reject the male by showing avoidance or aggression. Courtship behavior in the male includes intense sniffing of the female's face, flank, and urogenital area; licking of the vulva; and chasing or playing behaviors. If the female stands for mounting, the male will mount and clasp the flanks of the female with his forelegs. In the dog, the os penis allows intromission to occur prior to the development of an erection. An erection develops immediately after intromission and is accompanied by rapid stepping movements of the male's hind legs. The enlargement of the bulbus glandis occurs at this time and is eventually responsible for the coital tie. The first portion of the dog's ejaculate contains only sperm-free prostatic fluid and is ejaculated within 1 minute of intromission. Following the development of an erection, the male will dismount by placing both front feet to one side and lifting one hind leg over the female's back so that they are "locked" or "tied" together tail to tail. The enlarged bulbus glandis of the male prevents withdrawal of the penis from the female's vagina during the tie. The sperm-rich portion of the semen is ejaculated during the first 1 to 5 minutes of the tie. Internal ties normally last between 5 and 60 minutes. The female and male should be allowed to separate naturally, once the bulbus glandis has reduced in size sufficiently.

Gestation

Fertilization: The viable life of ova in the female reproductive tract is approximately 12 to 72 hours. On the average, fertilization occurs around the 7th day of estrus. Sperm from a natural mating will reach the ova in the oviduct of the bitch within 30 seconds of ejaculation and have a viable life within the female reproductive tract of up to 7 days. This allows fertilization to take place several days after breeding if the ova are not yet mature on the day of breeding. Fertilization and early fetal development occur in the oviducts, and the developing embryos move into the uterus 6 to 10 days after conception. Implantation within the uterine wall occurs 17 to 21 days after fertilization. The fetuses will usually be evenly spaced throughout the two uterine horns. In general, larger breeds of dogs produce larger litters. Toy breeds may have as few as 1 to 3 puppies; the large breeds average between 7 and 12 puppies per litter.

Detection of pregnancy: Unlike many other mammals (horses and humans), there are no significant specific hormonal changes that occur in pregnant bitches that distinguish them from nonpregnant bitches. During diestrus, pregnant and nonpregnant females both have functioning corpora lutea and, therefore, have similar serum progesterone concentrations. As a result, there is currently no reliable blood test that can be used to detect pregnancy in the female dog. However, there are several indirect methods that can be used, often in concert, to detect pregnancy.

Palpation of the bitch's abdomen for the presence of uterine swellings at individual **placental** sites is a relatively simple method. This is reliable if conducted by an experienced veterinarian, technician, or breeder, and if it is performed at the correct time during gestation. Individual fetuses are usually palpable between 20 and 30 days of gestation, counting from the day of the first breeding. The fetuses appear as oval- to round-shaped swellings and will be distinctly separated from one another within the uterine horns. As an example, the fetal swelling of a 40-pound dog will be approximately 2 inches in length. Palpation becomes less reliable after about day 30 of gestation because the uterus then becomes diffusely enlarged and separations between fetuses are difficult to detect.

Ultrasound is a second method for pregnancy detection and can recognize fetal forms within the uterus relatively early, around day 16 to 20 of gestation. Visualization of functioning hearts can be seen as early as day 25. The ability to detect and monitor heartbeats and placental circulation is an added benefit of ultrasound diagnostics. However, limiting factors of ultrasound are that the required equipment can be expensive and not all veterinarians have the capability of providing ultrasound diagnostics to their clients.

Radiographs are a reliable tool for detecting pregnancy and determining number of fetuses. However, in order to identify a fetus radiographically, there must be a certain level of fetal skeletal development. Between days 21 and 42 of gestation, a radiograph may indicate enlarged, fluid-filled uterine horns, but there is not sufficient skeletal development to make a definitive diagnosis. By day 42 to 52, fetal skeletons can be detected. Because radiographs are not reliably diagnostic until the latter portion of gestation, they are not usually used for pregnancy diagnosis but rather for determination of the number of fetuses present. Veterinarians may also suggest radiographs if there is concern for **dystocia** (whelping problems).

There are several secondary signs of pregnancy that can be used as supportive evidence but are not conclusive. These signs also are often seen in pseudo-pregnant bitches. Provided the female is not being overfed, enlargement of the abdomen occurs fairly late in gestation, around 5 weeks. In females that are at optimal weight at the time of breeding, no weight gain or enlargement of the abdomen should be observed during the first 4 weeks of gestation. The development of mammary tissue can be variable but usually starts around day 35. This is seen as generalized enlargement of the glands and, eventually, hair loss around the teats (nipples). Milk production usually begins about day 58 to 60 of gestation. Also, most pregnant females will show a clear to cloudy vaginal discharge starting around day 32 and continuing until shortly before parturition.

Length of gestation and parturition: Because the timing of ovulation is relatively difficult to identify in the bitch and because most females are bred on multiple days during an estrus period, it is difficult to identify the precise day that fertilization occurs. A range of 56 to 72 days counted from the first day of breeding provides a good estimation of gestation length. Average gestation length is 63 to 65 days. Vaginal exfoliation cytology smears can be used to provide a more exact estimate. This is useful if the female is likely to require a cesarean section. Whelping date is determined to be 56 to 58 days after the first day of diestrus, as determined by vaginal cytology. The size of the litter can significantly affect length of gestation. Large litters tend to have shorter gestation lengths (by 1 to 3 days) than litters with only one to three puppies.

In the dog, parturition (giving birth) is referred to as whelping. Approximately 20 to 30 hours before parturition begins, maternal plasma progesterone concentrations begin to decline. A decrease in the female's body temperature is observed about 12 to 24 hours before whelping. Rectal temperatures usually fall from 101.5 degrees Fahrenheit (F) to 100 degrees F or lower. This change is frequently used by breeders as an indication of impending parturition. The major stimulus for the onset of parturition comes primarily from the fetuses through increased production of glucocorticoids by the adrenal cortex. It appears that the fetal glucocorticoids cause an increased synthesis of estrogen in the placenta, which in turn enhances the synthesis and release of prostaglandin F-2-alpha (PGF-2a) by the placenta and uterus. This locally acting hormone causes regression of the corpus lutea and a subsequent decrease in progesterone. The loss of progesterone's effects on the reproductive tract allows uterine contractions to occur. Estrogen also enhances the action and release of oxytocin, which in turn causes increased PGF-2a production. The hormone **relaxin** is important during parturition, functioning to induce elongation of the interpubic ligament. This allows separation of the pubic bones, necessary for the passage of fetuses through the birth canal.

There are three stages of labor and delivery. Stage 1 is usually unnoticed by the owner because the uterine contractions that occur are not visible externally. During this stage, the cervix relaxes and dilates, and mild contractions begin. The female will usually become restless and nervous, and may shiver or even vomit. Stage I lasts approximately 6 to 12 hours. Stage 2 is characterized by the strong contractions of labor with eventual expulsion of the fetus. Stage 3 begins after expulsion of the fetus and ends with expulsion of the placenta. Therefore, bitches that are whelping more than one puppy alternate between stages 2 and 3 for the duration of whelping. In general, females will deliver their entire litter over a period of several hours. The time between initiation of the strong contractions of stage 2 labor and birth of a puppy is normally 10 to 30 minutes. Active straining of greater than 30 to 60 minutes is a sign of dystocia and a veterinarian should be consulted. Placentas usually are expelled (stage 3) within 5 to 15 minutes after the birth of each puppy.

A quiet area that is draft-free and, preferably, temperature controlled should be provided as a whelping area. The pregnant bitch should be introduced to this area and to the whelping box at least 5 days before her estimated date of parturition. This allows her to become adjusted to the area before the puppies are born. Whelping boxes may have a variety of designs but should be warm and dry, easy to clean, and allow easy access to the mother while preventing the puppies from escaping as they grow. The box should be enclosed on three sides with an entrance cut on the fourth side. The entrance should be approximately 4 to 6 inches off the ground (depending on the height of the female). The bitch should be able to step into it, but the puppies should not be able to climb out. The box should be large enough for the bitch to stretch out in full length on her side and have room to spare. A box that measures 1 1/2 to 2 times the length of the bitch is ideal. A railing or ledge should be placed 3 to 4 inches from the floor around the entire inside periphery of the box. This ledge prevents the bitch from crushing or suffocating a puppy that may get caught between her body and the sides of the box when she is lying down to nurse. The bedding material that is used should provide good traction, be easily cleaned, and be made of a material that will not be easily ingested by the puppies. Examples of appropriate bedding materials include old towels, mattress pads, diapers, or pieces of indoor/outdoor carpeting.

A source of supplemental heat should be placed in the whelping box. During the first week of life, puppies are unable to shiver (a mechanism for producing extra body heat) and are inefficient at regulating their own body temperature. They must rely upon the bitch's body heat and the warmth of their litter mates to maintain normal body temperature. Therefore, during the first few weeks of life, the environmental temperature around the whelping box is vitally important as an aid to keeping the puppies warm. If needed, supplemental heat sources for whelping areas should be placed so that the puppies can move to their own comfort area and escape from the heat source altogether if they become too hot. Appropriate sources of heat include heat lamps and electric or water-filled heating pads.

Care of Newborn Puppies

While the mother provides most of the care of newborn puppies, management of a healthy litter includes providing a proper environment; recognizing the signs of healthy, normal newborns; and identifying signs of trouble or illness. Several vital signs can be monitored as indicators of health (Table 4.1). At birth, puppies are relatively immature. Their eyelids are not yet open, so they cannot see. Their ears are also not yet functioning. When picked up, healthy newborn puppies should have good muscle tone, feel "firm and

TABLE 4.1   Vital Statistics for Neonatal Puppies

	Respiration (breaths/minute)	Heart Rate (beats/minute)	Body Temperature (degrees F)
Newborn (day 1)	8–10	120–150	94–95
First 5 Weeks	15–35	150–220	98–100
Adult Dog	10–30	80–140	100–102.5

plump," and wiggle vigorously. Healthy puppies are also quiet most of the time, crying only when they are hungry or cold. Excessive or prolonged crying is often the first sign of a problem.

Newborns should spend the majority of their time sleeping, and when they are awake, nursing. They do not lie quietly or still when sleeping, but show activated sleep for about 75 percent of their sleeping hours. This is characterized by continual twitching, jerking, stretching, and shifting of position. Activated sleep is important for the development of the neuromuscular system and appears to be the mechanism by which newborn puppies develop muscle tone and begin to develop coordination.

All newborn puppies should show normal neonatal reflexes. The suckling reflex should be seen whenever a puppy's mouth comes into contact with the teat. While some puppies will show this reflex within minutes of birth, all healthy puppies should show a strong suckling reflex within several hours. The rooting reflex is observed when puppies push forward with the head and crawl toward the bitch's side or a hand when it is placed in contact. The puppy will naturally travel in a circular pattern when rooting, and it is believed that this reflex (and its direction) ensures that puppies can find a teat shortly after birth. When the puppy is inverted onto its back, it should immediately be able to flip back over and right itself. All newborn puppies should show reactions to odors, touch, pain, and changes in temperature.

The most important indication of puppy health during the first few days and weeks of life is the demonstration of regular and normal weight gain. After the first day or two, puppies should steadily increase in weight and should double their birth weight by 7 to 10 days. A general rule of thumb to determine normal weight gain during the first 3 to 4 weeks of life is to expect 1 to 1 1/4 grams of gain per day for every pound of expected adult weight. For example, if a puppy is expected to weigh approximately 60 pounds as an adult, it should gain 60 to 75 grams per day for the first 3 to 4 weeks. This is equivalent to 2 to 2.5 ounces of weight gain per day. Puppies should be weighed daily for the first 2 weeks of life, then weekly until weaning.

Most breeders remove puppies' dewclaws when they are between 2 and 5 days of age. The dewclaw is the first toe that is attached to the carpal of the forepaw, but it is a vestigial, functionless appendage. All dogs have dewclaws on the front legs, and a few breeds also have them on the back. When found on the back legs, the dewclaw often lacks an internal bone structure. Front dewclaws almost always have a complete internal bone. Dewclaws usually are removed to prevent injury in active dogs or to prevent ingrowth of the associated nail. When they are removed at this young age, sutures usually are not needed and healing is rapid. However, the puppies' reaction indicates that this procedure is painful, and for this reason, some breeders choose not to remove the dewclaws of their puppies.

The term "weaning" refers to the gradual, permanent decrease in dependency of puppies upon their mother for care. Puppies typically are weaned by breeders when they are between 6 and 8 weeks of age. Seven to 8 weeks has been identified as an ideal time to wean and place puppies into their new homes (see Chapter 7). Nutritional weaning involves a gradual change in diet from bitch's milk to dog food. Puppies can first be introduced to supplemental food when they are 3 to 4 weeks of age. The pet food used to wean the puppies should be the food they will be fed throughout growth. When first introducing puppies to solid food, the mother should be separated from the litter for a few hours to ensure that the puppies are hungry. A soupy "gruel" can be made by mixing dry dog food with warm water and should be offered several times per day in a large shallow bowl. Because the puppies must change their method of obtaining food from suckling to lapping (then chewing), this will at first be a messy process. Gradually, the amount of water added to the dry food can be decreased until the puppies are eating dry food. The length of time the mother is separated from the litter also should be gradually increased (most bitches will initiate these separations voluntarily). By the time the puppies are 6 weeks of age, they should be fed dog food almost exclusively and should be nursing very little. However, it is advisable to continue to allow interactions between the mother and her puppies until 7 to 8 weeks because these interactions are important for normal social development.

Because puppies' gastrointestinal tracts are capable of switching from mother's milk to dog food when they are 4 to 5 weeks of age, it is possible, from a nutritional standpoint, to fully wean them at this age. For behavioral reasons, however, this is not desirable. Primary socialization occurs when puppies are between 5 and 12 weeks of age. The period of 3 to 7 weeks is very important for puppies to learn species-specific behaviors from their mother and through interacting with their litter mates. Weaning prior to 7 weeks deprives them of these important interactions and learning experiences. Most bitches will naturally begin to wean puppies in a gradual manner and should be allowed to discipline puppies as they proceed through the weaning process (see Chapter 7).

Reproductive Problems in the Bitch

Abnormal cycles: Fertility problems in bitches often are caused by either abnormal estrous cycles or hormonal imbalances that may or may not be related directly to reproduction. Silent heats and cycles with abnormal durations are common problems. The term "silent heat" refers to a female that is in estrus but is not exhibiting any behavioral or physical signs. This may occur either because she has little or no vaginal discharge, she keeps herself very clean through self-grooming, or she has had little or no contact with male dogs. Silent heats occur most commonly in young females, and vaginal cytology is often necessary to determine estrus and ovulation.

Some females exhibit very short estrous cycles. On the average, five months is considered to be the minimum length of a complete normal estrous cycle. Bitches that cycle more often than this (every 3 to 4 months) are often infertile. It is believed this is due to an inability of the endometrium to fully regenerate between cycles. **Ovariohysterectomy** (spaying) is usually recommended when a female shows recurrent short estrous cycles. In contrast, a cycle that is longer than 15 months is also considered abnormal. A common cause of this problem is hypothyroidism. Although this disorder is successfully managed, it may have a hereditary basis. Therefore, breeding a female with hypothyroidism is not recommended. Persistent estrus occurs in some females and is caused by the presence of excessive concentrations of estrogen. This may be due to ovarian tumors, follicular cysts, or excess administration of estrogenic compounds. If cysts or tumors are the cause, surgery is necessary to rupture the cysts or remove the ovaries. In most cases, an ovariohysterectomy is performed at the same time. Hypoestronism (low levels of estrogen produced by the ovaries) is caused by the failure of the ovaries to develop to sexual maturity. Estrus does not occur due to low estrogen concentrations. Ovariohysterectomy is recommended. Hyperadrenalcorticism is caused by high levels of adrenal cortical hormones. Almost all females dogs with this disorder will be infertile and will demonstrate prolonged intervals between heats, failure to conceive, or failure to ovulate. Although therapy can be given for the disorder, infertility often is not corrected due to degeneration of the ovaries, and ovariohysterectomy is recommended.

Infectious diseases: Several infectious diseases can affect the female reproductive tract. Vaginitis occurs when pathogenic bacteria invade the vagina and cause infection. Signs include the development of an abnormal discharge that may be bloody, clear, or purulent. The discharge may cause an odor that may attract males as if the female is in estrus. Most cases of vaginitis are successfully treated with antibiotic therapy.

Pyometra is a hormonally mediated infectious disorder that is always associated with diestrus. The disease occurs when the uterus has been under the influence of progesterone and is caused by abnormal bacterial growth in the uterus. Pyometra occurs most commonly in females over the age of 6 years. Clinical signs depend on the state of the cervix at the time of infection. If the cervix is open, a large amount of bloody pus is discharged. If the cervix is closed, pus collects and stays in the uterus, making pyometra much more difficult to diagnose. Other signs of pyometra include refusal to eat, depression, frequent urination, excessive thirst, low-grade fever, and abdominal distension. Because pyometra can lead to **septicemia** and **toxemia,** it should be treated as a medical emergency. Untreated cases are often fatal. Immediate ovariohysterectomy is the recommended treatment. Medical treatment in the form of systemic antibiotic therapy often is not successful and may prolong the disease. Prostaglandin therapy has been successful with the open-type of pyometra.[4] This medication causes strong contractions of the uterus and reduction in circulating progesterone concentrations, and may aid in the relaxation of the cervix.

Canine brucellosis is a disease caused by the bacterium *Brucella canis*. It is distributed worldwide in canine populations, and it is estimated that 1 to 5 percent of the canine population in the United States is infected.[5] There is considerable variation in geographic distribution, partially because *B. canis* is vulnerable to environmental conditions and does not survive well outside of the host animal. In females, the bacterium is found in greatest concentrations in the placenta and in vaginal secretions. Brucellosis is transmitted primarily via the vaginal discharge and mammary secretions of infected bitches and through the semen of males. Many females do not show overt signs of infection. When **bacteremia** is present, signs may include slight enlargement of the lymph nodes, depression, and fatigue. However, these signs often go unnoticed. Reproductive signs in the female include infertility, abortion after 35 days of gestation, litters containing dead puppies, and early embryonic death. Screening for this disease can be conducted with a rapid slide agglutination test that detects the presence of *B. canis* antibodies in the blood. This test has a high negative predictive value, providing 99 percent certainty that the dog is clear of the disease. However, false positives can occur 30 to 50 percent of the time. Therefore, a positive rapid slide agglutination test for canine brucellosis should always be confirmed with a more specific assay.

Two assays that can be used are the tube agglutination test and the agar gel immunodiffusion test. In kennels, the existence of canine brucellosis is very serious, and all positively diagnosed dogs should be removed from the breeding program and the premises. Treatment with antibiotics is successful in controlling bacteremia when present. However, because the *B. canis* organism is capable of being sequestered in the lymph nodes and reproductive tissues, bacteremia often returns after the antibiotic is withdrawn. For this reason, infected individuals should never be used for breeding.

Mastitis is an infection and inflammation of the mammary glands caused by bacterial infection with *Streptococci* sp. The female develops painful, reddened, hard teats and produces abnormal milk that often is blood-tinged. The disease is accompanied by a fever, depression, and anorexia. Puppies should immediately be prevented from nursing from an infected gland because they can become ill from infected milk. Antibiotic therapy is the recommended treatment.

Reproductive Problems in the Male

Infertility: There are numerous causes of infertility in male dogs. Primary infertility refers to the condition where the dog has never been fertile. The testicles often are small and composed of abnormal tissue. Dogs with primary infertility exhibit normal sex drives but have an abnormally low sperm count. Some potential causes include failure of development of parts of the male reproductive duct system, errors in metabolism involving reproductive hormones, abnormalities in sperm cell formation, failure of the testicles to descend (bilateral cryptorchidism), and absence of germinal epithelial cells in the seminiferous tubules ("Sertoli-cell-only" syndrome).

Acquired infertility occurs when an environmental cause results in a decline in fertility in a previously normal dog. Age is the most common cause of a decline in fertility in male dogs. Atrophy of the testes is a common occurrence in dogs greater than 10 years of age. The presence of a fever is a second common cause. An increase in the temperature of the testes results in decreased sperm motility and, eventually, decreased sperm production. This is reversible after a return to normal temperature and health. Environmental stressors such as excessive breeding, change in living conditions, heavy dog show schedules, and psychological trauma can all be causes of temporary infertility in the male dog.

Infectious diseases: Any part of the male reproductive tract can become infected with pathogenic bacteria or other microbes. Infection of the testes is referred to as orchitis; infection of the penis and prepuce is called balanoposthitis. Canine brucellosis is also a serious disorder in male dogs. As in bitches, many dogs affected with this disease often exhibit no clinical signs. It is a potentially disastrous disease due to the fact that it is transmitted via semen during breeding. Clinical signs that may occur in the male include epididymitis (inflamed epididymis), orchitis, prostatitis (inflamed prostrate gland), pain of the scrotum, infertility, and lymph node enlargement. All male dogs used for breeding should be screened for this disease and eliminated from the breeding program if found to be infected.

Neonatal Health Problems

Orphaned puppies: Although the care of puppies is best left up to the mother, there are situations in which the owner must act as the mother to newborn puppies. This is often temporary—if, for example the dam is ill or has had a cesarean section. In other cases, the death of the mother results in one or more orphaned puppies that require complete care. The needs of these puppies are the same as for any other newborns. One of the most important aspects to consider is that orphans no longer have the warmth of the bitch available. Therefore, the ambient temperature of the whelping area must be kept slightly higher (Table 4.2).

Orphans can be fed using either a commercial puppy formula or a homemade formula (see Chapter 18). For the first few days, puppies should be fed every 2 to 3 hours. This can be decreased gradually to every 4 to 5 hours until the puppies are 3 weeks of age. From 3 to 6 weeks, they should be fed at least 4 times per day. Formula can be administered using a stomach tube or bottle.

TABLE 4.2	Ambient Temperatures for Orphaned Puppies	
	Age of Puppies	Temperature at Floor (degrees F)
	0–7 Days	85–95
	7–14 Days	80–85
	14–21 Days	75–80
	>21 Days	70

Using a stomach tube requires training and special care during insertion but allows accurate monitoring of the amount of formula that is fed and decreases the chance of aspiration. Many owners prefer to use a nursing bottle, but this method is more time-consuming, and, if the nipple delivers milk too quickly, aspiration can occur. If a feeding tube is used, training from either a veterinarian or an experienced breeder should be obtained.

During the first 4 to 5 days, orphaned puppies should be weighed daily as a means of monitoring health. It is the goal when caring for orphans that they achieve near-normal rates of weight gain. For the first 2 weeks of life, the puppies must also be stimulated to urinate and defecate by stroking the belly and the genital and anal areas with a washcloth dampened with warm water. At 3 weeks of age, puppies can be introduced to semisolid food and gradually weaned, just as if the mother were present.

Chilling: Normal, healthy litters will lie together in a heap to conserve warmth. If the puppies are lying widely separated from each other, the litter box temperature may be too hot. If, however, all of the puppies are heaped together and there is a lone puppy lying outside the group, this may be a sign of illness. General signs of sick neonates include limpness when being held, the absence of activated sleep, absent or weak suckling reflex, low weight gain or even weight loss, and excessive crying. During the first 2 weeks of life, puppies do not thermoregulate efficiently. A healthy puppy can maintain its body temperature only 10 to 12 degrees F above its surroundings and requires outside heat to maintain normal body temperature. Hypothermia in newborns is one of the chief causes for neonatal morbidity and death. A chilled puppy will have a decreased internal body temperature, falling as low as 78 to 85 degrees F. As the core temperature drops, the body's metabolism becomes depressed, the digestive system slows down, and heart and respiration rates decrease. A chilled puppy will initially be noisy and overactive. However, as hypothermia progresses, the puppy becomes increasingly quiet and limp. Over time, the puppy loses all normal reflexes. Death will occur if hypothermia is not treated promptly.

A puppy that has been chilled must be warmed very slowly. The best method is to use human body heat. This can be done by holding the puppy close to the body, under an arm or shirt, or in a pocket. Chilled puppies should not be placed on a heating pad or under a heat lamp. This will result in heating the extremities more quickly than the body's core. The increased metabolic rate of the extremities cannot be supported by the heart and lungs, and inadequate blood supply to the extremities results in tissue starvation. Similarly, a chilled puppy should not be immediately fed. As the puppy warms and becomes more active, a glucose solution or honey/water solution may be fed by stomach tube to provide energy and prevent dehydration. Chilling is best prevented by closely monitoring the mothering behaviors of the bitch and providing a whelping box that is free of drafts and allows puppies access to an artificial heat source, if necessary.

Infectious diseases: There are several infectious diseases that can affect newborn puppies. The term "fading puppy syndrome" has been used for many years to describe the sudden death of puppies less than 3 weeks of age. Until recently, a cause was not known for this disorder. It is currently believed that infection with canine herpesvirus (CHV) is responsible. This virus causes infectious tracheobronchitis in adult dogs, which is a relatively mild disorder that is usually self-limiting (see Chapter 11). However, when contracted by neonatal puppies, CHV is invariably fatal. Puppies can contract the disease as they pass through the birth canal, from the nasal secretions of the mother, or from contact with infected siblings. If the puppies are born with an adequate level of maternal immunity, they usually will be protected against the severe effects of the virus. CHV infection usually is only seen in the first litter of puppies of a bitch. After this, older females usually develop an antibody titer capable of protecting subsequent litters. Signs of CHV in puppies that are younger than 3 to 4 weeks include excessive crying, refusal to eat, depression, and the production of soft, yellow-green feces. The virus is usually fatal within 12 to 24 hours of the first onset of these signs. A unique characteristic of CHV is that the virus is extremely temperature sensitive and can only replicate in a temperature range of 95 to 96 degrees F. If body temperature is greater than this range, the virus will not cause serious damage to the body. Although the body temperature of adult dogs is naturally higher than the temperature at which CHV replicates, neonatal puppies are not capable of closely controlling body temperature and frequently show a temperature that supports the growth of this virus. As a result, chilled puppies are at increased risk for contracting CHV. Because this virus is rapidly fatal in young puppies, treatment is usually futile. There is no vaccine that is universally protective against this virus, and the best prevention is to immunize the bitch prior to breeding, provide a clean whelping environment, and prevent chilling of puppies.

Conclusions

Companion animal professionals must possess an understanding of canine reproductive anatomy and physiology, the female estrous cycle, gestation, parturition, and neonatal care of puppies when involved in the care of breeding animals. A second aspect of dog breeding that requires study is genetics and breeding programs. In addition, selective breeding for many generations has resulted in the predisposition of many breeds for certain inherited disorders. The following chapter reviews the basic principles of genetics in the dog and examines the benefits and disadvantages of various breeding programs.

Cited References

1. Holst, P.A. *Canine Reproduction: A Breeder's Guide.* Alpine Publications, Inc., Loveland, Colorado. (1985).

2. Concannon, P.W. **Canine pregnancy and parturition.** Veterinary Clinics of North America: Small Animal Practice, 16:453-475. (1986)

3. Concannon, P.W., Hansel, W., and McEntee, K. **Changes in LH, progesterone and sexual behavior associated with preovulatory lutenization in the bitch.** Biology and Reproduction, 17:604-615. (1977)

4. Sokolowski, J.H. **Prostaglandin-F2-alpha-THAM for medical treatment of endometriosis, metritis, and pyometra in the bitch.** Journal of the American Animal Hospital Association, 16:119-122. (1980)

5. Currier, R.W., Raithel, W.F., Martin, R.J., and Potter, M.E. **Canine brucellosis.** Journal of the American Veterinary Medical Association, 180:187-198. (1982)

5 Genetics and Breeding Programs

UNDERSTANDING THE PHYSIOLOGY AND ENDOCRINOL-OGY of reproduction is essential for successful dog breeding. In addition, knowledge of the general principles of genetics, advantages and disadvantages of different breeding systems, and the risks of producing genetically inherited disorders is important to dog breeders, veterinary technicians, and veterinarians. This information is used to select breeding animals and aid in producing healthy puppies that possess the desired conformation (body type) and temperament for their breed.

Basic Genetic Principles

Chromosomes and genes: The Austrian monk Gregor Mendel (1822-1884) is recognized as the father of genetics and was responsible for determining the physical basis of inheritance. Although little was known about cellular causes of inheritance during Mendel's time, his work with garden peas produced the basic laws of this field. It is now known that the nucleus of every cell, containing the **chromosomes**, is the "genetic storehouse" of the body. Chromosomes come in different shapes and sizes but always occur in matched pairs, called **homologous** chromosomes. Each dog possesses one pair of sex chromosomes and 38 pairs of autosomes. The autosomes carry traits that can be transmitted to either sex. In mammals, the female has two sex chromosomes that are essentially identical, designated as the X chromosomes (XX). Males, in contrast, have one X chromosome and one Y chromosome (XY).

In an individual animal, one member of each chromosome pair was inherited from each parent. Every species has a characteristic number of chromosomes. The dog has 78 (39 pairs), as do the wolf and coyote. Although different breeds of dogs have very different physical appearances, all dogs (*Canis familiaris*) have the same number, size, and shape of chromosomes. The differences that are seen are due to the genes within the chromosomes, which cannot be observed through normal methods of microscopy. The genes, located along the length of the chromosomes, are the basic units of inheritance. Biochemically, they contain a code for the manufacture of the proteins that direct the development of organisms and all the life processes. The genes are composed primarily of DNA and, like the chromosomes, exist as pairs. Genes at the same locus (site) in homologous chromosomes will influence the same trait. Physically, genes are recognized only by their end effect. For example, in dogs, the gene at the B locus codes for either black or brown coat color.

If alternate ways of influencing a given trait exist, these are called the **alleles** of a gene. The two alleles for the B locus are designated as B and b. The B allele codes for black and the b allele codes for brown. A dog will inherit one of the three possible combinations of these two alleles, BB, Bb, or bb. If the two alleles are identical (and therefore influence the trait in the same way), the individual is **homozygous** for that locus (BB or bb). If the two alleles are different, the individual is **heterozygous** for that trait (Bb).

Although in many cases there exist only two gene variations (i.e. two alleles) for a particular trait, some genes have multiple alleles. When this occurs, a dog still can possess only two of the possible alleles since there are only two homologous chromosomes capable of bearing the alleles. For example, the gene that codes for coat spots in dogs is designated as the S series. There are four alleles for this gene that code for either no spotting (S); chest, toes, and tail spotting (s^i); piebald spotting (s^p); or all-white coat (s^w). A dog could have any one of the 10 possible combination pairs of these alleles at that locus.

Inheritance of genetic material: Meiosis occurs within the reproductive organs of males and females and results in the production of the gametes (ova and sperm). Gametes are unique because they contain only one set of homologous chromosomes (39 total chromosomes). When the sperm of the male and the ova of the female join during fertilization, the chromosome number is restored to 78, with each parent contributing one chromosome in homologous pairs. Genetically, this means that one allele for each trait is contributed by the dam and one allele is contributed by the sire. The inheritance of genetic material is therefore equally shared by the two parents.

In mammals, the inheritance of gender is determined by the male parent. As discussed previously, the female sex chromosomes are essentially alike (XX), while the male's sex chromosomes are different (XY). As a result, all of the ova produced by females contain a single X sex chromosome; 50 percent of the sperm produced by males contains an X chromosome and 50 percent contains a Y chromosome. During reproduction, if an ovum is fertilized with a sperm that contains an X chromosome, a female fetus will develop (XX). If the ovum is fertilized with a sperm containing a Y chromosome, a male puppy will develop (XY). Therefore, in dogs (and all mammals), the male parent always determines the sex of the offspring.

Predicting outcomes using the Punnett square: A simple method that can be used to predict the genetic outcome of a particular mating is called the Punnett square (Figure 5.1). The square is composed of all of the possible alleles for a trait or traits that can be contributed by one parent in the top row and all of the possible alleles that can be contributed by the gametes of the second parent in the left column. All possible combinations of alleles that can occur in the offspring are depicted in the intersecting squares. The proportion that each combination contributes to the entire diagram represents the predicted ratio that that combination will occur. It is important to recognize that the predicted ratio only represents the proportions of each **genotype** that are predicted by chance combinations. Within a single litter of puppies, these ratios may or may not be achieved. However, when data from many litters are collected, statistical analysis will reveal these predicted ratios. A simple example is the inheritance of sex. The two alleles that can be contributed by the male are either X or Y and are depicted in the first row. The female contributes only X chromosomes. The resultant inner squares show that the expected gender ratio of male and female combinations is 50:50.

Dominant and recessive genes: The set of genes that an individual inherits from its parents represents the individual's genotype. The dog's **phenotype** is the external visible expression of the genotype. Depending on the type of gene action that is in effect, the genotype may or may not be discernible by the dog's phenotype. Complete dominance is an example of such gene action. Complete dominance occurs when one of the possible alleles for a gene is capable of totally masking expression of the other allele that is carried on its homologous chromosome. The masking allele is called the dominant allele; the one that is masked is called the recessive allele. The dominant allele can be present either singly (heterozygous) or in duplicate (homozygous), and expression of the trait will be the same. The recessive gene must be present in duplicate (homozygous) for phenotypic expression.

Traditional genetic nomenclature denotes the dominant gene with an uppercase letter and the recessive gene with a lowercase letter. The inheritance of black or chocolate (brown) coat color in Labrador Retrievers is an example of this type of gene action. In the case of the B series of coat color, a dog that is BB or Bb will have a black coat. A dog with the genotype of bb, on the other hand, will have a brown coat (Table 5.1). In the case of a black Labrador Retriever, its outward appearance would not provide information about the dog's genotype, since the dog could be either BB or Bb. In contrast, because the gene action of this series is complete dominance, all chocolate Labrador Retrievers are known to have the genotype of bb.

Incomplete dominance: Incomplete dominance occurs when the heterozygous state produces an intermediate phenotype. As a result, when incomplete dominance is in effect, it is possible to determine genotype by observing the dog's phenotype. The inheritance of the merle coat color in dogs is an example of this type of gene action. This coat pattern, designated as the M series, causes a reduced (diluted) coat pigment in irregular areas of the body. Australian shepherds are a breed that exhibit this coat color, and the

FIGURE 5.1   Punnett Square: Inheritance of sex

	X	**Y**
X	XX	XY
X	XX	XY

Predicted Ratios:
50% Male
50% Female

TABLE 5.1 Major Coat Color Genes in the Dog

Gene Series	Allele	Effect	Breed Examples
A	A	uniformly colored hair shaft	Irish Setter, Weimaraner
	a^g	black banded hair shaft	Norwegian Elkhound
	a^s	black saddle	Airedale Terrier, German Shepherd Dog
	a^t	tan points	Rottweiler
	a^y	sable (banded hair shaft with red/yellow/ black)	Collie, English Springer Spaniel
B	B	black	Labrador Retriever, Newfoundland
	b	brown (chocolate, liver)	Labrador Retriever, Chesapeake Bay Retriever
C	C	red	Basenji, Golden Retriever, Cocker Spaniel
	c^{ch}	golden yellow (buff)	Golden Retriever, Cocker Spaniel
D	D	full expression of color	Golden Retriever, Samoyed
	d	dilution of color	Weimaraner, Doberman Pinscher
E	E	extension of color (black)	Basenji, Bedlington Terrier
	E^m	black mask	Norwegian Elkhound, Great Dane
	e	yellow	Golden Retriever, Labrador Retriever
	e^{br}	brindle	Great Dane
G	G	progressive graying	Kerry Blue Terrier, Poodle
	g	nonprogressive graying	Cocker Spaniel, Dalmatian
M	M	merle	Collie, Great Dane
	m	non-merle (full color)	Cocker Spaniel, Samoyed, Poodle
S	S	solid color	Bedlington Terrier, Irish Setter, Poodle
	s^i	Irish white spot pattern	Basenji, Collie, Cocker Spaniel
	s^p	piebald white spot pattern	Basset Hound, Newfoundland, English Springer Spaniel
	s^w	all-white coat	Samoyed, Dalmatian
T	T	ticking (color spots)	Dalmatian, Basset Hound
	t	no ticking	Great Dane, Basenji

desired merle coat is a blotchy pattern of flecks and patches of color (Figure 5.2). Dogs with the genotype mm show full expression of coat color (i.e. no merle pattern). Dogs that are homozygous for M (MM) are almost completely white due to extensive dilution and restriction of pigment in the hairs of the coat. Dogs with this genotype often also have undesirable defects such as deafness and sight impairments. Dogs that are heterozygous for the merle series (Mm) exhibit an intermediate color pattern, the desired merle pattern. Breeding two merle dogs (Mm) usually is not recommended because 25 percent of the puppies produced from such a cross would be the highly diluted MM coloring and may be born with associated physical problems (Figure 5.3).

Epistasis: Complete and incomplete dominance gene actions involve interactions between genes that are located at the same locus (alleles). When genes at different loci interact, the gene action is called epistasis. This means

FIGURE 5.2   Merle coat pattern (Australian Shepherd)

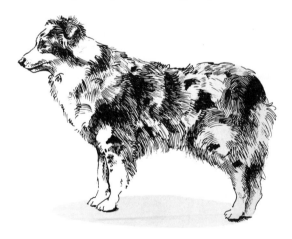

FIGURE 5.3   Punnett Square: Inheritance of merle coat pattern

	M	**m**
M	MM (white, health problems)	Mm (merle coat pattern)
m	Mm (merle coat pattern)	mm (full color)

Predicted Ratios:
50% Merle
25% Full color
25% White

that the visible or phenotypic expression of the genotype at one locus will depend not only on the alleles at that locus but also on the genotype of a second locus. For some traits, the genotype of one locus is capable of completely masking the phenotypic expression of the genotype of another locus. In other cases, the effect of one gene may be to alter the expression of another. An example is the epistatic interaction of the B series (black or brown coat color) with the D series (dilution factor). The gene action of the B series is complete dominance. A black dog has a genotype of either BB or Bb, while a brown dog has a genotype of bb. The gene action of the D series is also complete dominance. The D allele is dominant and does not cause color dilution when present in the homozygous or heterozygous state (DD or Dd). Dogs that are homozygous recessive (dd) have uniformly decreased pigment in the hairs of the coat. This causes a black coat genotype (BB or Bb) to be blue and a brown coat genotype (bb) to be fawn. A breed that exhibits this type of coat color inheritance is the Doberman Pinscher. Figure 5.4 illustrates the expected coat colors that result from breeding two black Dobermans that are heterozygous for coat color and dilution (BbDd). As is illustrated, a variety of coat colors may be seen in the puppies that are produced.

Crossing-over and gene linkage: The process of meiosis involves the transmission of chromosomes to gametes as entire units. However, occasionally, a piece of chromosome material may transpose with a similar piece from its homologous partner during the production of gametes. This process is called crossing-over, and the end result is that a piece of genetic material that originally came from the animal's dam becomes associated with the chromosome that was originally inherited from its sire. This becomes important in breeding programs because it confuses the line of inheritance patterns when an affected trait is being studied.

FIGURE 5.4   Punnett Square: Inheritance of coat color in Doberman Pinschers

	BD	**Bd**	**bD**	**bd**
BD	BBDD (black)	BBDd (black)	BbDD (black)	BbDd (black)
Bd	BBDd (black)	BBdd (blue)	BbDd (black)	Bbdd (blue)
bD	BbDD (black)	BbDd (black)	bbDD (red)	bbDd (red)
bd	BbDd (black)	Bbdd (blue)	bbDd (red)	bbdd (fawn)

Predicted Ratios:
9/16 (56.25%) Black
3/16 (18.75%) Red
3/16 (18.75%) Blue
1/16 (6.25%) Fawn

Gene linkage refers to the tendency for certain traits to be inherited together. Genes that are carried on the same chromosome are said to be linked, and the traits that they affect will tend to be inherited together. In breeding programs, one of the ways undesirable traits often become established in a line is through linkage with another trait that is desirable. The closer that genes are located on a chromosome, the greater the likelihood that they will consistently be inherited together. Crossing-over can break up this linked inheritance of traits and is more likely with genes that are located far apart on the chromosome than with genes that are located close together.

Sex linkage: Genes that are located on the sex chromosomes are called the sex-linked genes. The Y chromosome is basically inert, primarily carrying genes that determine some male characteristics. Almost all sex-linked traits are carried on the X chromosome and follow the inheritance patterns of this chromosome. In males, the genes on the X chromosome will always be expressed because there exists no homologous X chromosome in that gender. Males always inherit their X chromosome from their dam. In the case of a recessive trait, a dam that is heterozygous for the trait (i.e., a "carrier") will not express it but will pass it on to 50 percent of her sons. Similarly, 50 percent of a carrier female's daughters will be carriers. An affected sire will produce carrier daughters, and when a carrier female is bred to an affected male, half of all the puppies will be affected (Figure 5.5a-c). In humans, the genes for color blindness and male-pattern baldness are carried on the X chromosome. In dogs, several blood-clotting disorders are sex-linked. As a result, certain types of hemophilia are expressed primarily in male dogs and infrequently in females.

Polygenic inheritance: Many of the traits that are observed in an animal are influenced by more than a single gene. Rather, multiple genes are involved, each of which has a relatively small effect on the trait. Together they result in the phenotype that is expressed. Polygenically influenced traits will not show clear demarcation between animals. For example, dogs are not either long or short in body but show many degrees of body length. These fine divisions are not easily measured, and it is difficult to explain them in terms of the presence or absence of one or two specific genes. Hair length is another example. The L series codes for either a short coat (LL or Ll) or a long coat (ll). However, continuous variation exists between coat lengths because of a series of modifying polygenes that add or subtract length from the main effects of the major genotype. It is difficult for breeders to manipulate polygenes through selective breeding programs because numerous genes may be involved and many cannot be readily identified. The influence of polygenes on certain traits can be changed slowly over many generations but not through one or two individual matings.

Selection of Breeding Animals

A primary goal of breeders of purebred dogs is to improve the conformation, movement, coat type, and temperament of the dogs that they produce. Most are striving to produce dogs that meet the accepted standard of excellence for their breed. Purebred breed registries prohibit breeding animals outside of

FIGURE 5.5a   Punnett Square: Inheritance of sex-linked traits (carrier dam/unaffected sire)

	X	Y
X*	X*X	X*Y
X	XX	XY

Predicted Ratios:
25% Carrier Females
25% Affected Males
25% Healthy Females
25% Healthy Males
*Denotes affected gene

FIGURE 5.5b   Punnett Square: Inheritance of sex-linked traits (healthy dam/affected sire)

	X*	Y
X	X*X	XY
X	X*X	XY

Predicted Ratios:
50% Carrier Females (All Females)
50% Healthy Males
*Denotes affected gene

FIGURE 5.5c   Punnett Square: Inheritance of sex-linked traits (carrier dam/affected sire)

	X*	Y
X*	X*X*	X*Y
X	XX*	XY

Predicted Ratios:
25% Affected Females
25% Carrier Females
25% Affected Males
25% Healthy Males
*Denotes affected gene

the breed's registry. As a result, most breeders work with dogs of known heritage within a particular lineage. Their objectives are accomplished through the selection of superior breeding animals and the development of a systematic breeding program.

Within a breed, the gene pairs that are responsible for breed type all exist as homozygous pairs. For example, the genes that make a Doberman Pinscher look like a Doberman and not a Miniature Poodle were originally selected over a number of generations until the desired traits occurred consistently in all of the dogs that were produced. The group of dogs initially registered as foundation stock for a particular breed will determine the degree of heterogeneity and homogeneity that are observed within the breed for all generations to follow. The genes that are present in homozygous form (and, therefore, show little variation from generation to generation) are called the nonvariable gene pairs of the breed. This means that within any breed, there are certain traits that will always breed true. The greater the number of homozygous traits within a breed (and, subsequently, the more limited the gene pool), the greater the uniformity of individuals within that breed. In contrast, the variable gene pairs, along with occasional gene mutations, are the genes that produce individual variation within the breed.

The dog's pedigree: A purebred dog's pedigree is considered to be the "blueprint" of his or her genetic background (Figure 5.6). The standard format for pedigrees lists the sire's name above and the dam's name below the dog's name. In the example provided, OTCH Topbrass Cisco Kid is the sire and Topbrass Misdemeanor TD is the dam of Topbrass AutumnGold UDT WC. Reading from left to right provides the parents in each preceding generation. Cisco's father is Poika of Handjem and his dam is Valentine Torch of Topbrass. Misdemeanor's parents are AFCH Holway Barty and Ch. Sunstream Gypsy of Topbrass.

When a dog is bred for the first time, the only genetic information that the breeder has available, other than the animal's phenotype, is its pedigree. The pedigree is useful in several ways. First, it can provide information about the type of breeding system that has been used in past generations. If a genetic breeding system has been employed, the degree of linebreeding and inbreeding can be determined. Both inbreeding and linebreeding increase homozygosity. An inbreeding coefficient can be calculated from the pedigree and represents the number of common ancestors that are present in proportion to the number of possible positions in the pedigree. This number provides breeders with an estimate of a dog's degree of inbreeding and can be used for comparisons between individuals within a breed or line. This value is also a measure of the percentage of all the variable gene pairs in an animal that are homozygous due to inheritance from common ancestors. The presence of common ancestors, even in later generations, increases the inbreeding coefficient. Therefore, it is advantageous to examine a pedigree that has as many generations represented as possible.

Within limitations, a dog's pedigree may also provide an indication of the qualities the dog is expected to have. Although descriptive information is not included on the pedigree, if the breeder or owner knew any of the dog's ancestors or had information available concerning their conformation and/or performance, this information could be used in the selection process. Most experienced breeders are knowledgeable about multiple generations of their breed and line and can discern a great deal of information about a dog just by examining its pedigree.

Although the pedigree is helpful, it has certain limitations as a selection tool. A typical pedigree shows only the names and titles of the dog's ancestors. Detailed information about the ancestor's appearance or working ability are not provided on the pedigree. For example, a dog that has a hunting title has successfully performed all of the requirements for that title. However, his or her individual strengths and weakness are not revealed. Similarly, the presence of a conformation championship (designated by the prefix CH) indicates that the dog's appearance met the breed standard and the dog was successfully exhibited at dog shows. However, the championship title on the pedigree does not indicate structural strengths or weaknesses. Also, if the pedigree is "shallow" (i.e., contains only three to four generations), complete information of the dog's heritage is not known. If inbreeding or linebreeding

FIGURE 5.6   Sample pedigree: Topbrass AutumnGold UDT WC: Topbrass Retrievers, Jackie and Joe Mertens

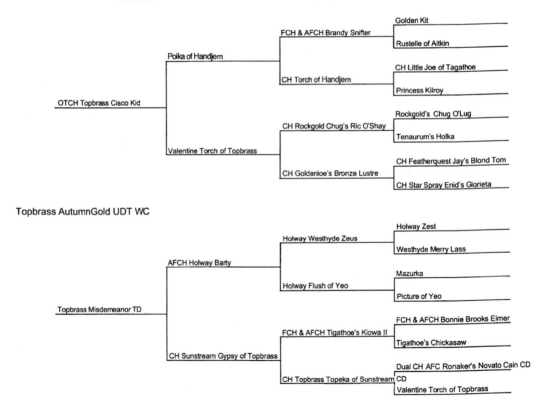

were used in earlier generations, an inbreeding coefficient calculated from the most recent three or four generations would not accurately reflect the dog's true degree of genetic homozygosity.

An "open" pedigree is one in which the name of each ancestor appears only one time. A dog with a three-generation open pedigree has inherited qualities from 14 different ancestors. This indicates that the dog's genotype is relatively heterozygous, compared to a dog of the same breed that has common ancestors present in the pedigree. It is difficult to start a breeding program with a dog that has an open pedigree because there are many possible gene combinations due to the high number of variable gene pairs. The selection for desired traits would proceed very slowly because many possible combinations of genes (traits) exist.

It is advantageous to begin a breeding program with a dog that is linebred because its pedigree will show that the dog possesses the accumulation of the genes of two or more selected ancestors. Naturally, it is hoped that these ancestors possessed desirable rather than undesirable traits. Selecting a dog whose pedigree shows several common ancestors (on paternal and maternal sides of the pedigree) ensures that the gene pool is somewhat limited to the genes contributed by these ancestors. Because they are present on both sides of the pedigree, this ensures that there is homozygosity in the genes the common ancestors have contributed. The goal of the breeder is to select common ancestors that possess desirable traits and that the breeder wishes to "fix" in the line as nonvariable gene pairs.

Performance testing: Studying pedigrees provides a means of genotypic selection. Performance testing, on the other hand, is a phenotypic method of selecting dogs for breeding that relies upon the evaluation of select physical traits or working ability. One of the most common examples of performance testing is exhibiting dogs in the conformation show ring with the intent of earning points and an eventual breed championship title. In this case, the performance that is evaluated is the dog's appearance and movement relative to the ideal standard for its breed. Dogs that obtain the title of champion are often selected for breeding.

Health and freedom from genetic diseases are also important, often used performance criteria. For example, Canine hip dysplasia (CHD) is a common developmental skeletal disorder seen in many large and giant breeds (see Chapter 12). If a breeder is attempting to eliminate CHD from a line of dogs, only dogs that are free of the disorder are selected for breeding. Performance testing may also include selecting dogs based on their success in various working events. For example, a breeder of Labrador Retrievers may be interested in improving the hunting ability of the line and so may select only those dogs for breeding who have achieved a Junior Hunter title. Similarly, a breeder of Whippets may decide that only dogs who have excelled in lure coursing events will be used for breeding.

Like the pedigree, there are certain limitations to the use of performance testing. First, because animals are being selected using phenotypic criteria, the success of this method depends on the extent to which the trait is genetically determined. While some physical traits such as coat type, color, and even body structure have very high heritabilities, other traits such as hunting success or the presence of an outgoing, friendly temperament may have lower heritabilities. For example, a dog that has excelled in hunting trials may have inherited the desirable degree of working ability from its parents, but its success is also a reflection of the training techniques that were used and the selection of hunt tests in areas that are best suited to its particular strengths.

A second factor is the breeder's accuracy in making a decision. For example if a breeder is using head type as the performance criteria and wishes to select dogs for breeding who have a head type that most closely approximates the breed's ideal, it is imperative for success that the breeder is an excellent judge of head type. This factor becomes very important when subjective evaluations of performance criteria are in effect.

Progeny testing: Progeny testing is simply performance testing a dog's progeny. Breeding stock is selected based on the success of the puppies a male or female has produced. Although selections are made using phenotypic criteria, progeny testing is actually a type of genotypic selection because individuals who are homozygous for desired traits are more likely to be selected. A dog that is homozygous for a desired trait (or, more realistically, for a large proportion of the polygenes that influence a desired trait) has a greater potential for passing the trait on to offspring compared to an individual who is heterozygous for the same traits. Used consistently, progeny testing is a powerful tool for increasing homozygosity within a line.

Several factors must be considered when progeny testing is used as a selection tool. First, the pedigree and the phenotypic qualities of the mate or mates to which the dog was bred must be considered when evaluating the progeny. Because 50 percent of the genes are contributed by the mate, the qualities of one parent will affect the evaluation of the other. Second, all of the progeny that have been produced should be evaluated. If success in the conformation ring is the selection criteria, all of the dogs that have been produced by the dog in question must be evaluated in this manner. Within a purebred line of dogs, it is not uncommon to have one or two outstanding animals in a litter. If only the animals that are trained and exhibited at dog shows or trials are evaluated for progeny testing, an assessment of the parents' breeding success will be inaccurate. As with performance testing, progeny testing must also consider environmental influences. These are even more difficult to assess because multiple dogs living in a variety of environments must be evaluated.

Progeny testing provides a useful method for determining a male or female's ability to pass on desired traits to his or her offspring, and it can improve the homozygosity of a purebred line. However, there are several disadvantages to this method of selection. First, it is very time consuming and labor intensive. Second, because some of the traits breeders are interested in improving cannot be evaluated until the dog is an adult, selecting an individual based on the merits of his or her offspring becomes impractical. For example, the Orthopedic Foundation of Animals (OFA) evaluates and certifies the health of dogs' hips when they are 2 years of age or older. If progeny testing for the absence of CHD is used, the parent may be beyond prime breeding age by the time the offspring can be evaluated. Similarly, certain performance tests, such as hunting tests, entail up to several years of training and conditioning before a dog is capable of competing.

There are also ethical questions that must be addressed when using progeny testing. Because the overpopulation of dogs and cats is a significant societal problem, strong arguments can be made against producing a litter of puppies with the intent of using their performance to evaluate the quality of one or both parents. Many breeders resolve these conflicts by using progeny testing as a supplementary selection tool, secondary to the use of pedigrees and performance testing.

Types of Breeding Systems

Several types of breeding systems can be used to aid in the selection of breeding animals and the development of a pedigree line. There are three primary types of genotypic breeding systems: inbreeding, linebreeding, and outcrossing. Nongenetic breeding systems include positive assortative, negative assortative, and crossbreeding.

Inbreeding refers to mating closely related individuals, such as sire and daughter, brother and sister, or cousin and cousin. The intent of this system is to accumulate the genetic contributions of one or several outstanding ancestors on both the paternal and the maternal sides of the pedigree. Genetically, this increases the chance of having the genes that were carried by that ancestor reproduced in the litter that is being bred. Technically, inbreeding is any mating that results in a higher inbreeding coefficient than the value that is average for the breed. A breed's average inbreeding coefficient is influenced by the number of animals that made up the original foundation stock and the number of litters that are bred and registered each year. For example, the Labrador Retriever has a relatively low average inbreeding coefficient (approximately 10 percent) because the breed had a large number of foundation animals and is widely popular. In contrast, an inbreeding coefficient of 10 percent is considered very low for the Irish Water Spaniel. This breed was developed from a relatively small gene pool, and a relatively small number of litters are produced annually.

Linebreeding represents a moderate form of inbreeding. Geneticists make no distinction between inbreeding and linebreeding, and often use the terms interchangeably. Dog breeders, on the other hand, identify linebreeding as breeding related individuals who are removed by greater than one generation (Figure 5.7). Such pairs include grandsire and granddaughter, and second/third cousins. Like inbreeding, the ultimate goal of linebreeding is to accumulate the genetic contribution of one or more select ancestors. For example, the pedigree in Figure 5.7 is linebred on NAFC AFC Topbrass Cotton and on his father, AFC Holway Barty. Because matings are made between distantly related individuals, the accumulation of common ancestors on each side of the dog's pedigree proceeds more slowly than with inbreeding.

Both inbreeding and linebreeding increase the number of homozygous gene pairs in dogs. As the number of times that common ancestors appear in the pedigree increase, the number of different hereditary combinations that can occur are reduced, and there is an increased probability that any gene will be homozygous by descent. As a result, highly linebred or inbred litters contain individuals that are very uniform in appearance and temperament. Because both dominant and recessive genes are affected by inbreeding and linebreeding, the expression of recessive traits also increases with the inbreeding coefficient. Since many deleterious gene effects are recessive, this can result in the expression of undesirable traits that were not seen in previous generations. In some cases, this may be advantageous because inbreeding exposes both the good and bad genes in the line. Breeders may use inbreeding to expose deleterious recessive genes and ultimately remove dogs that carry these genes from their breeding stock.

Moderate linebreeding is the genetic system of choice for many breeders of purebred dogs. The success of a linebreeding program depends on the selection of outstanding ancestors that possess many desirable traits and who are homozygous for a large proportion of the genes that control these traits. If in-

FIGURE 5.7   Linebred pedigree: Topbrass Retrievers, Jackie and Joe Mertens

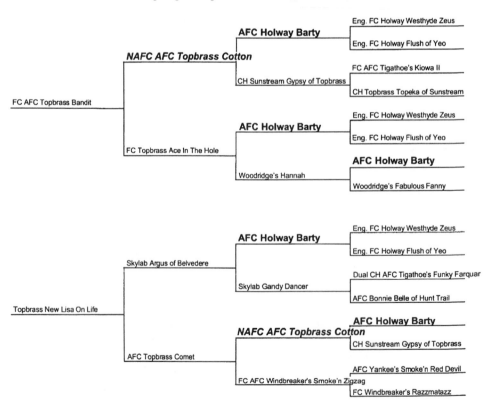

breeding is used, it must be used cautiously because of the potential to rapidly increase the inbreeding coefficient and expose deleterious recessives that may adversely affect health and reproductive success.

Outcrossing entails mating unrelated individuals, one or both of which are inbred or linebred (Figure 5.8). The sire of this dog, Topbrass Hustle Russell, is linebred on NAFC FC Topbrass Cotton. The dam is not linebred and has no ancestors in common with the sire. The purpose of an outcross is to introduce one or more traits into a line that dogs in that line currently lack. Breeders may also conduct an outcross to increase heterozygosity if deleterious recessives have been identified and have been difficult to eliminate from the line. In production animals, heterozygosity often is referred to as **hybrid vigor**. Although the heterozygosity produced by an outcross does not produce a consistent breeding dog, it is a successful method for producing select individuals who possess the desired traits of each parent. Breeders often will use a single outcross with the purpose of correcting a problem they have identified within their line. The dogs that are produced from this mating are selected for the desired traits then slowly bred back into the line with the intent of "fixing" the new traits in the purebred line.

Because they rely heavily on pedigrees and lineage as a selection tool, in-

FIGURE 5.8   Outcross pedigree: Topbrass Retrievers, Jackie and Joe Mertens

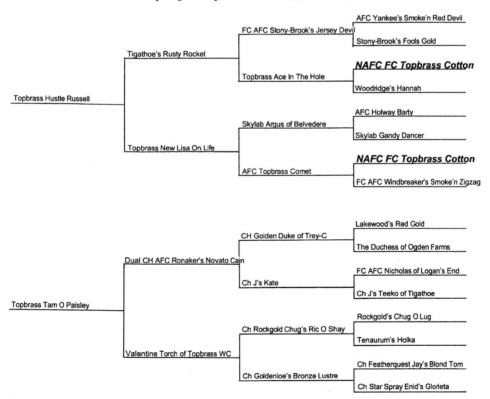

breeding, linebreeding, and outcrossing are all considered to be genotypic systems. In contrast, nongenetic breeding systems use phenotypic selection criteria without consideration of the dog's pedigree or lineage. Positive assortative breeding (also called "like-to-like") involves the selection of breeding pairs based solely on phenotypic qualities, with no consideration of genotype (pedigree). A male and a female who possess the same desirable traits are chosen as a breeding pair. The intent is to increase the chance that the offspring will possess the trait or traits that are found in both parents. However, some individuals may share desirable characteristics that are determined by a different set of genes. This is especially true for traits that have a polygenic inheritance, such as body type, size, and conformation. Because the dog's genotype is not considered, positive assortative breeding systems rely upon the chance occurrence that the desirable traits in each parent are determined by the same set of genes. Success is hit or miss and will be due to the chance occurrence that the two parents have similar genotypes.

Negative assortative breeding (also called divergent breeding) is based on trying to correct the faults or undesirable traits in one dog by pairing it with a mate who displays the contrasting virtue. One example is pairing an oversize male with an undersize female with the intent of producing pups of the proper size to meet the breed standard. Although this system seems quite logical, it does not work well. Like an outcross, negative assortative breeding usually results in increased heterozygosity. In addition, because the parents are phenotypically dissimilar, many of the traits that were desirable in one parent may be, in effect, lost because of the increased heterozygosity in the puppies. Luck may produce a few good animals, but these dogs will not breed true unless they are linebred.

Crossbreeding refers to mating dogs of two different breeds with the intent of creating a new breed or eliminating a problem in one of the breeds. For example, the Bullmastiff was originally created by selecting breeding pairs of Bulldogs and Mastiffs. During the middle 19th century in England, landowners were concerned with keeping their estates free from depredation by poachers. Gamekeepers of these estates wanted to develop a guard dog that was large, strong, and protective. The Mastiff was large and powerful but not aggressive enough, while the Bulldog was strong and aggressive but too small to work an entire estate. After several generations of crossbreeding, the Bullmastiff was created, a perfect dog for their purpose. Many breeds that are popular companion animals today originated through the selective crossbreeding of earlier breeds or breed types (see Chapter 2). Today, the American Kennel Club and other purebred breed registries regulate the practice of crossbreeding by establishing strict guidelines for the introduction of newly recognized breeds of dogs.

Genetically Influenced Disorders in Dogs

Dogs, like other species, are subject to the inheritance of defective and even lethal genes. Many genetic defects appear to be the result of polygenic inheritance rather than a single-gene or chromosome defect. As a result, inheritance patterns often are difficult to discern, and many disorders believed to be genetically influenced in dogs do not have established modes of inheritance. Dominantly inherited defects usually have extreme effects, and affected animals often die in utero or shortly after birth. The majority of genes responsible for inherited disorders are recessive and are passed onto offspring by parents that are heterozygous for the defective gene.

Most breeds of dogs have a set of inherited disorders that occur in greater frequency in that breed than in the general population of dogs. Contrary to popular belief, however, mixed-breed dogs are not immune to genetically determined health problems. Although the more limited gene pool and greater homozygosity of purebreds result in increased incidence of some disorders, mixed-breed dogs are still capable of inheriting the same defects that are seen in purebreds. The following section reviews several genetically determined disorders in dogs and, when known, their mode of inheritance.

Hemophilia A: This blood disorder is caused by a recessive, sex-linked gene and is the most common bleeding disorder observed in dogs.[1] It is caused by a lack of the blood-clotting component, Factor VIII. Clinical signs include episodes of recurrent subcutaneous bleeding, internal hemorrhages, and anemia. Because the defective gene is found on the X chromosome, males are clinically affected and females are carriers. Hemophilia A has been reported in many popular breeds of dogs, including the Beagle, Bulldog, Collie, German Shepherd Dog, Golden Retriever, Greyhound, Labrador Retriever, Poodle, and Shetland Sheepdog.

Von Willebrand's disease (VWD): This disorder is similar to Hemophilia A because the cause of signs is also a lack of clotting Factor VIII. However, the mode of inheritance of VWD is not sex-linked. It appears that an autosomal dominant gene that is lethal when in the homozygous state is responsible.[2] Signs include **hematomas**, lameness due to joint bleeding, and recurrent nosebleeds. Although VWD has been reported in many breeds of dogs, German Shepherd Dogs, Golden Retrievers, Doberman Pinschers, Airedale Terriers, and Miniature Schnauzers are reported to show a higher incidence of this disorder than the total dog population.

Progressive retinal atrophy, peripheral type (PRA): This ocular disorder is caused by an autosomal recessive gene. It was first identified and studied in Gordon and Irish Setters but is now known to occur in many breeds.[3] Early signs are defective night vision followed by the progressive loss of day vision. Changes to the retina characteristic of PRA may be seen when the dog is only a puppy, but clinical signs of vision loss may not be apparent until the dog is 6 to 10 years of age. Because many owners do not recognize the signs, and dogs are not consistently tested for PRA, many affected dogs have been used for breeding. Concerned breeders of susceptible breeds will screen all potential breeding animals for PRA. This practice is contributing to a decrease in the incidence of this disorder in the canine population. Highly susceptible breeds include the Irish Setter, Cardigan and Pembroke Welsh Corgis, English Cocker Spaniel, Gordon Setter, and Norwegian Elkhound.

Copper toxicosis: This disorder was first identified in Bedlington Terriers and is characterized by an inability to normally metabolize copper. Over time, the mineral accumulates in the liver, causing tissue damage and loss of functional liver cells. Cirrhosis develops as scar tissue replaces damaged cells. Studies with Bedlington Terriers have revealed that the disorder is inherited as an autosomal recessive trait in that breed.[4] Copper toxicosis is one of the first genetic disorders to be studied in the Canine Genome project. These studies have enabled researchers to identify a genetic marker linked to the gene that causes copper toxicosis in this breed. A commercial test has recently been developed that can analyze DNA samples taken from cheek swabs and determine the dog's genotype for this disorder (i.e., clear, affected, or carrier). Prior to this time, the only method available to confirm a dog's status was either through multiple test breedings or liver biopsies on individual animals. Other breeds that may be susceptible to copper toxicosis are the Cocker Spaniel, Doberman Pinscher, and West Highland White Terrier.

Chondrodysplastic dwarfism: This syndrome is a type of growth disorder that results in short-legged animals that have normal or near normal body size. Although it has been reported sporadically in several breeds, such as Miniature Poodles and Cocker Spaniels, it has been studied most extensively in Alaskan Malamutes.[5] Affected dogs possess front and hind limbs that have an assembly similar to that of a Basset Hound. The mode of inheritance in this breed is a simple autosomal recessive gene. Affected dogs usually do not have a shortened life span, but there is an associated hemolytic anemia with the disease. This is apparently caused by an impaired ability to absorb intestinal zinc. Oral supplementation with zinc usually resolves the anemia, but it must be provided throughout life to prevent recurrence.

Canine hip dysplasia (CHD): This disorder is characterized by abnormal formation of the hip joint and varying degrees of lameness, pain, and crippling (see Chapter 12). It is observed with greatest incidence in large breeds, but few breeds are completely free of CHD. Canine hip dysplasia shows polygenic inheritance, with multiple genes affecting the shape of the joint, the size of the associated muscle mass, and the congruity of the head of the femur and the pelvis. In addition, rate of growth and other environmental factors can affect the phenotypic expression of this disease.

Cryptorchidism: This condition occurs in male dogs when one (unilateral cryptorchidism) or both (bilateral cryptorchidism) of the dog's testicles fail to descend into the scrotum. Because cryptorchidism has been shown to occur within lines and families of purebred dogs, it is strongly suspected to be hereditary. The problem is believed to be polygenic in nature. Breeds with an increased incidence include the Border Terrier, Cocker Spaniel, English Cocker Spaniel, Miniature Schnauzer, Pomeranian, Silky Terrier, and Whippet.

Conclusions

An understanding of basic genetics, inheritance patterns, and types of breeding systems is essential for professional breeders and professionals who are involved in the promotion of purebred dogs. Selective breeding has resulted in the development of more than 300 different breeds of dogs. A second very important group of dogs in our communities are those designated as "random-bred" or "mix-breed," having no directly known lineage. Dogs come from a variety of sources and in a variety of sizes, shapes, and temperaments. The following chapter examines the relationships we have with this most popular family pet, and it explores the responsibilities, benefits, and problems that accompany breeding, pet selection, and ownership.

Cited References

1. Dodds, W.J. **Inherited bleeding disorders.** Canine Practice, 5:49-58. (1978)

2. Dodds, W.J. **Further studies of canine Von Willebrand's disease.** Journal of Laboratory and Clinical Medicine, 76:713-721. (1970)

3. Hodgeman, S.F.J., Parr, H.B., Rasbridge, W.J., and Steel, J.D. **Progressive retinal atrophy in dogs. 1. The disease in Irish Setters (red).** Veterinary Record, 61:185-190. (1949)

4. Johnson, G.F., Sternlieb, I., Twedt, D.C., Grushoff, P.S., and Scheinberg, I.H. **Inheritance of copper toxicosis in Bedlington Terriers.** American Journal of Veterinary Research, 41:1865-1866. (1980)

5. Fletch, S.M., Pinkerton, P.H., and Brueckner, P.J. **The Alaskan Malamute chondrodysplasia (dwarfism-anemia) syndrome: a review.** Journal of the American Animal Hospital Association, 11:353-361. (1975)

6 Dog Ownership: Benefits and Responsibilities

RECENT ESTIMATES INDICATE that pet owners in the United States share their lives and homes with more than 55 million dogs.[1] Approximately 38 percent of households own at least one dog, the majority of whom are kept as social companions. As society has moved from small rural communities to increasingly large and metropolitan urban and suburban centers, the dog's role as a working partner has diminished. This change has been accompanied by the development of a new and equally important role for *Canis familiaris,* that of the social companion. This chapter will explore this relationship and will examine the responsibilities, benefits, and ambiguities that accompany pet ownership.

The Human-Dog Bond

It is difficult to overstate the significance that animals, and in particular dogs, have in today's society. Images and concepts of our relationships with both nature and animals are an integral part of our language, folklore, and cultural traditions. Children are introduced to the animal world at a young age through the use of animal toys, books, television programs, and the ubiquitous presence of animal characters on items ranging from bedroom furniture to dinnerware. The media frequently capitalize on our animal interests by using elegant purebred dogs or adorable puppies to sell their products or to portray the positive characteristics of politicians and celebrities. Our interest in animals and the natural environment also is well evidenced by the complex, often intense relationships pet owners have with their dogs. It has been postulated that in a society that is increasingly urbanized and removed from the natural environment, keeping dogs as pets represents a continuance of our relationship with nature and our need to retain strong interactions with animals.[2]

In Western society today, the most often cited reason people keep dogs is for companionship. The dog is unique in this respect, because most other domesticated species (with the exception of the cat) are kept primarily for economic or practical reasons. During the past 25 years, the relationships people have with their companion animals have been studied in great detail. Both anecdotal and empirical data show that dogs provide a number of important psychosocial and health benefits to their human companions. Although the mere presence of a pet can have stress-reducing effects, it appears that the greatest benefits are conferred by the existence of a strong, sustainable relationship, or bond, between the dog and the owner.

Attachment: It is generally accepted that the phenomenon of attachment is at least partially responsible for the development of a lasting human-dog bond. Attachment behaviors occur in all social species and are first manifested in young animals during normal bonding to their dam. These behavior patterns are eventually generalized to include relationships with siblings, fathers, extended family, and mates. Attachment behaviors are actions used by an individual that have the effect of keeping another individual in close proximity. For example, the high-pitched crying that a young puppy emits when isolated has the effect of drawing the mother (or new owner) back to the puppy. High-pitched vocalization and hyperactivity are typical responses to isolation in most social species and are designed to reunite separated individuals. Similarly, pleasurable experiences in the form of visual, vocal, and tactile stimulation serve to positively reinforce proximity.

Both dogs and humans are social species that display hierarchical social organizations, engage in attachment behaviors, and have complex nonverbal communication patterns. These similarities facilitate the development of two-way relationships between owners and their dogs. Factors that affect the degree of attachment an individual feels include physical proximity; duration of time spent together; sharing of emotional experiences; and intensity of pleasurable visual, vocal, and tactile signals. A high degree of attachment is signified by an animal that shows stress or anxiety upon separation from its owner and subsequently expresses happiness and relaxation when reunited (see Chapter 8). Likewise, dog owners often feel anxious and distressed when their companion animal is lost or away, and they encourage close proximity by allowing their pet to sleep in the bedroom, share food, and engage in regular and pleasurable play and exercise periods.

Nurturing: In addition to the need for attachment, several other basic needs play a role in the development of the human-dog bond. Nurturing and caretaking behaviors are an important expression of love and affection in humans. The importance of having opportunities to nurture is illustrated by the finding that when people are no longer allowed or able to care for others, the incidence of depression, decreased health, and increased vulnerability to chronic disease increases.[3] Raising and caring for a dog provides an outlet for nurturing. It is a popular perception that pets act as child substitutes for owners and in doing so may replace normal human social interactions or even prevent owners from forming normal attachments to other humans. However, studies of the relationships owners have with their dogs have shown that while the human-dog relationship has some similarities to the human-child bond, the majority of pet owners are normal individuals whose dog actually augments and improves human social relationships.

Touch: The development of the bond between a person and a dog also is affected by the sense of touch. Petting an animal is one of the few acceptable outlets for adults in our society to touch another living being in an affectionate, relaxing way. Touch is an important method of communication between people and dogs. Although verbal interactions are important, dogs lack the capability for complex speech patterns. Nonverbal communication such as body postures, facial expressions, eye contact, and touch are all used when owners interact with their dogs. As a highly social species, the dog uses similar nonverbal cues and is capable of understanding and reacting to human signals. Likewise, the ability of dogs to communicate nonverbally and the capacity of humans to understand and respond to their dog's signals facilitate the development of reciprocal interactions that often are complex. For example, a study of dog owners in a public setting found that the majority of owners interacted with their dogs frequently and openly.[4] More than 90 percent admitted to talking to their pets, and 80 percent stated they talked to their pet as if it were another person. Observations showed that touch, in the form of scratching, patting, and stroking, was the most common mode of communication used, even more frequently than verbal communication. Interestingly, no difference in the frequency, amount, or kind of touch occurred between men and women. Apparently, companion animals are a means through which both genders can express and receive affection openly.

Stress reduction: A dog's ability to reduce human stress is an important contributor to the human-animal bond. Talking to an animal is more relaxing than talking to another person. Blood pressure and heart rate normally increase during conversations with other people. However, both of these measurements fall when people speak to and stroke a friendly dog.[5] This difference may exist because human subjects usually anticipate being judged or evaluated when talking to another human but do not have this perception when talking to a companion animal. The opportunity to provide and receive comforting touch, to engage in nonjudgmental speech, and to fully express oneself without worry of another's reaction may all strongly affect the strength of the relationship that develops between owner and dog.

Other factors: Owners themselves provide numerous reasons for loving their dogs. A survey designed to determine dog owner satisfaction required participants to rate their own dog and a hypothetical "ideal" dog in terms of a series of behavior traits.[6] Owners identified expressiveness, enjoyment of walks and exercise, loyalty/affection, welcoming behavior, and attentiveness as the most desirable traits in both their own and the hypothetical "ideal" dog. Other traits seen as desirable, but not absolutely necessary, were playfulness, friendliness to other people or other dogs, and territorial behavior. This study illustrated that most of the traits that were important in establishing a strong bond involved close proximity and frequent contact between the owner and the dog. A recent study of 37 dog owners who had adopted dogs from an animal shelter found that the degree to which the dog conformed to the owner's perception of an ideal dog was a predictor of the strength of attachment the owner felt.[7] Together, these studies indicate that both the owner's expectations and the dog's behavior are important for the development of a strong and lasting bond (Table 6.1).

TABLE 6.1	Factors Affecting the Development of a Strong Bond between Owners and Their Dogs
	✓ Need for attachment in humans and dogs
	✓ Regular and positive interactions (proximity)
	✓ Need for nurturing and caretaking
	✓ Communication through touch; enjoyment of petting
	✓ Mutual understanding of nonverbal communication
	✓ Reduction of stress in the presence of a dog
	✓ Mutual engagement in play and exercise

Dogs as companions (the canine side of the bond): Because the human-dog bond is a two-way relationship, species-typical behavior must be considered when examining the relationship between owners and their dogs. *Canis familiaris* has several attributes that facilitate bonding with humans. The dog is a diurnal species (active during the day while sleeping at night), so it is active at the same time as most humans. Dogs also possess a social organization and a set of communication patterns similar to those of humans (see chapters 1 and 8). Some of the most important behaviors are those that convey attachment and affection to conspecifics (either humans or other dogs). These include lowered body posture, retracted ears, soliciting and offering touch, licking, and facial greeting. Dogs show a ritualized set of greeting behaviors, will seek out their owners for contact, and are typically responsive to their owner's activity. Most importantly, dogs provide what researchers (and owners) describe as unconditional or nonjudgmental love. In other words, a dog loves its owner regardless of appearance, level of income, or manner of dress. By providing the owners with feelings of unconditional affection, dogs naturally enhance the strength of the attachment that is felt.

Unlike many mammals, the dog possesses an extraordinary level of playfulness. While the young of many species demonstrate play, dogs are unique because they continue to engage in play as adults. This characteristic brings much joy and pleasure to many owners. A study of pet owners in Switzerland found that dog owners reported spending an average of 17.5 hours per week interacting (playing) with their pets. Another survey reported that 95 percent of owners played often with their dogs, and 80 percent agreed with the statement: "My dog gives me an outlet for playfulness." The dog's willingness to play with its owners, capability of learning complex games, and enjoyment of shared exercise all facilitate positive and frequent interactions with owners.

Characteristics of dog owners (the human side of the bond): Not surprisingly, if a person had a pet during childhood, he or she is more likely to be a pet owner as an adult, and the type (species) of pet owned during childhood strongly influences the pet that is chosen.[8] Adults who had pets as children often possess a more positive attitude toward animals and a better understanding of animal behavior and communication than non-owners. In today's society, the typical pet owner owns a home, is employed, and has a slightly higher average income than the non-owner. Pet ownership is highest among families with young children.[9] However, feelings of attachment to the dog are comparatively lower in families that have children. Single, divorced, and widowed individuals report the highest degrees of attachment to their pets. In childless families, owners also interact with their dogs more frequently and in a more complex manner than do individuals in families with children. Epidemiological studies have shown that pet owners are more likely to consume alcoholic beverages, to eat take-out meals frequently, and to consume meat several times more per week than non-owners.[10] Pet owners were also more likely to be physically active. Although pet ownership has been associated with health benefits, these data indicate that pet owners do not necessarily have a consistently more healthy lifestyle than non-owners. This lends support to the theory that dog ownership by itself may offer some important health benefits and is not merely a reflection of certain attributes that people who choose to share their lives with pets are more likely to possess.

Similarities between the relationship that people have with their pets and those they have with other humans have led to an examination of the types of relationships pet owners have with other people in their lives. Although it is true that dog owners may differ somewhat in their relationships to other people compared with non-owners, this difference is not of the type typically predicted. A common perception of pet owners is that they are, for some reason, unable or unwilling to form normal relationships with other people and so transfer their social needs to their companion animals. However, the data do not support this claim. Survey studies show that many owners rate their relationship with their dog as important as those they have with human family members or friends. However, in most cases the relationship with the pet exists in addition to, not in replacement of, other human relationships.[11,12] The socializing effects of pets and their ability to facilitate interactions with other people are well documented.

In addition, recent evidence indicates that happiness within a "pet relationship" is positively correlated with happiness and satisfaction in human relationships. A large study of more than 1,100 married women found that 13 percent of the dog owners who were not attached to their pets reported they were unhappy, while only 6 percent of attached pet owners reported unhappiness.[13] A significantly larger number of owners who were not attached to their pets also reported that their spouse did not serve as a satisfactory confidant, compared with attached female owners. Earlier research showed that having low affection for dogs is associated with low affection for other people, rather than the opposite effect.[14] In particular, men who did not have affection for animals were shown to demonstrate a low desire for affection from other people.

There may be some truth to the belief that some people are "dog people" and others are "cat people." Compared with cat owners, dog owners spend more time with their pets and frequently engage in activities such as grooming, playing, and walking.[15] In addition, dog owners are more willing to seek and spend money on veterinary care than cat owners. Another study of dog and cat owners found that, within the home, interactive behaviors were greater between owners and their dogs than owners and their cats.[16] This was accompanied by higher levels of behavioral and physical intimacy. In the cat's defense, however, more cat owners than dog owners admitted to sleeping with their pets!

Benefits of Companion Animals

There is no doubt that dogs are a significant component in the lives of many people. The dog often is considered to be a part of the family and is treated with the love and respect given to all other family members. The human-dog bond is a unique relationship. During the past 15 years, researchers have taken an active interest in investigating the effects of this relationship and are discovering something dog owners will say they have known all along: Pet ownership is good for human health. Not only do we derive much pleasure and joy from our pets, but they also are good for our physical and psychological well-being. These benefits begin in early childhood and persist long into old age (Table 6.2).

Adults and their dogs: The ability of dogs to reduce stress in their owner's life has been recognized for quite some time. Controlled research studies have shown that blood pressure and heart rate both decrease while people are petting and talking to a friendly dog.[17,18] In humans, gentle touch affects the central nervous system by decreasing sympathetic arousal. Stimulation of the sympathetic nervous system, commonly referred to as the fight/flight response, causes an elevation in heart rate, blood pressure, and vascular resistance. Sympathetic activity decreases when a person is more relaxed as opposed to being aroused. It is possible that touching and petting a friendly dog may cause a physiological response in the sympathetic nervous system that leads to decreased feelings of anxiety and stress. Interestingly, this stress-reducing effect occurs with the simple presence of the dog and can occur even

---

TABLE 6.2   Benefits of Dog Ownership

✓ Reduction of stress (↓blood pressure, ↓heart rate)
✓ Focus for attention and caretaking
✓ Opportunities for exercise and play
✓ Companionship and decreased loneliness
✓ Stimulus for social interactions with other people
✓ Sense of responsibility; enhanced feelings of self-worth and competence

without tactile or verbal interaction between the person and the animal.

The physiological and psychological benefits of companion animal ownership can be explained to some degree by the various functions pets play in our lives. Two researchers, Aaron Katcher and Alan Beck, identified seven important functions of companion animals and examined how these functions might affect physical and emotional health.[19] These functions are: companionship, something to care for and nurture, something to keep one busy, something to touch and fondle, a focus of attention, safety, and exercise. The first three of these roles have the effect of decreasing depression and feelings of isolation; the remaining four are expected to reduce feelings of stress and anxiety. Because they often accompany their owners in public, dogs also act as social catalysts for interactions with other people, a stimulus for exercise, and an outlet for play and humor. Controlled studies have shown that people walking with their dogs take longer walks, interact with more people, and have longer conversations with strangers than those walking alone.[20,21]

Children and their dogs: Interactions with companion animals have been shown to provide distinct benefits to growing children. For young children, a friendly dog offers tactile comfort in the form of petting and stroking, and can provide a learning experience to the child about feelings of softness and gentleness. As the child grows and matures, the family dog can offer a relationship that continues to be a source of nonjudgmental affection and love. The dog may function as an emotional security blanket or a "transitional object," providing comfort and alleviating stress. The opportunity to receive nonjudgmental love allows children to learn how to give and receive affection without the risk of rejection. Play also becomes an important function of dogs for children. The family dog often is included in fantasy games and may act as an important bridge between the child's play world and reality. For older children, dogs can provide an opportunity to learn responsibility. Caring for an animal and being responsible for its exercise, training, and feeding have multiple benefits. Increases in self-esteem, competence, and feelings of autonomy can all be positive results of caring properly for a dog.

On a grander scale, it has been suggested that early and positive associations with animals can provide children with an enhanced understanding and inherent respect for all living beings. Childhood appears to be a crucial period during which positive experiences with animals may have a profound effect on attitudes later in life. A final benefit of interactions with dogs involves social interactions with other children and adults. As with adults, dogs have the ability to act as social catalysts, helping initiate conversations and interactions with others. This function may be especially important for children as they develop and learn how to behave properly in social settings.

Elderly and their dogs: A second subpopulation that receives many benefits from companion animals is the elderly. Dogs can provide elderly owners with all of the same benefits they provide to other adults. However, as an aging person's lifestyle changes, the importance of the role a pet plays may increase significantly. The companionship of a dog can help decrease the loneliness that often is associated with the loss of friends, relatives, and even a spouse. Advancing age may begin to limit an individual's mobility, resulting in prolonged confinement to the home. The presence of a pet in the home can provide a diversion from boredom and a constructive focus of attention. In addition to the need for companionship, it is important to realize that the elderly often have limited opportunities to give and receive affectionate touch. An older person may benefit greatly from a loving dog who can provide warmth, affection, and humor. Having a pet that is dependent for care, food, and attention also provides structure and motivation in an older person's life.

Animal-assisted therapy: Not surprisingly, dogs have a great deal to offer people who are disabled or sick. The involvement of animals with physically and mentally disabled people with the direct intent of improving emotional or physiological health is called animal-assisted therapy (AAT). This concept has been in existence for more than 100 years, but it is only in the last 20 to 30 years that AAT has gained widespread acceptance and has attracted the interest of a large number of researchers and health care professionals. During the 1960s, Dr. Boris Levinson, a psychologist, began to regularly include animals in his therapy sessions with patients and to document and publish his results.[22,23] Levinson believed that pets could act as transitional objects for many patients, especially children. By developing an affectionate, trusting relationship with the pet, the patient eventually learned to extend these feelings to the therapist. Patients who were exceptionally responsive to AAT were those who were nonverbal, inhibited, withdrawn, or culturally disadvantaged. Levinson's work served as the impetus for many health professionals to examine AAT as an appropriate adjunct therapy in a number of different medical fields.

AAT programs are now incorporated into a wide variety of therapeutic settings. Schools for mentally retarded children and adults use animals in their teaching programs. Pets provide positive learning experiences for the mentally retarded and contribute to the attainment of social skills, such as cooperation and communication with others. Programs for the medically ill are found in many hospitals. One of the most rewarding and successful hospital programs targets children's wards. A visiting dog functions to "deinstitutionalize" the hospital setting and helps to relieve the stress and fear many children feel while they are hospitalized.

Another prevalent setting for AAT programs is in nursing homes and long-term care facilities for the elderly. Many residents are required to give up their pets when they enter a nursing facility. In addition, their opportunities to form new attachments to animals and other people often become limited. Feelings of depression, decreased self-esteem, and isolation are not uncommon in elderly patients who are confined to nursing homes. The introduction of dogs into these environments, either in the form of visitation programs or as resident animals, has met with great success. Elderly residents have been found to be more responsive to the staff and to other people, and to show improved emotional states when in the presence of pets. Other benefits of pets in nursing homes include providing an outlet for reminiscing and stimulating humor and play. In the case of resident animals, pets also can offer opportunities for elderly patients to nurture and accept responsibility.

Dogs and the disabled: AAT programs are not the only manner in which dogs are able to aid special populations of people. Dogs can be trained to perform a variety of services that allow the physically disabled to function more independently in society. Dog guides for the sight-impaired are the most well-known type of service dog. A blind person's mobility and independence are greatly enhanced with the aid of a guide dog. Household chores, public transportation, employment, and social activities that once may have required the help of another person are all attainable with the aid of these highly trained dogs. In addition to their aid in dealing with the physical environment, guide dogs provide emotional benefits as well. Guide dogs are reported to contribute to increased self-esteem in their owners and to act as potent social facilitators when traveling in public places.[24]

Dogs also are trained to aid the hearing impaired. Hearing ear dogs are now afforded the same rights to public access as are guide dogs for the blind. These dogs are specially trained to aid their hearing-impaired owners by alerting them to relevant sounds in the environment. For example, many will respond to doorbells, smoke alarms, telephones, alarm clocks, and the cry of a baby. Service dogs for the handicapped work to increase the mobility and independent living skills of people who are physically disabled. Most individuals who have service dogs are in a wheelchair or on crutches. Service dogs are trained to retrieve dropped items, pull wheelchairs up ramps, open doors with a device attached to their harness, and carry a variety of objects. In addition, they are trained to act as a strong brace for support should their owner fall. Service dogs greatly increase the independence of a disabled person. They enable their owners to travel and function in public places that may previously have been inaccessible. As with hearing ear dogs, most states have added service dogs for the disabled to the list of animals allowed full access to public facilities and public transportation.

Dogs and Recreation

In addition to spending vacations, celebrating special events, and sharing daily activities with their dogs, many people become involved in a pet-related hobby such as dog shows, obedience trials, field trials, fly-ball tournaments, and agility trials. A variety of organizations sponsor these events, enabling enthusiasts to work with their dogs toward a number of different goals or titles. The level of involvement on the part of the owner can range from that of a weekend hobbyist to a full-time occupation, as in the case of professional handlers and trainers (Table 6.3).

The American Kennel Club (AKC) is the largest purebred dog registry in existence in the United States (see Chapter 2). This organization maintains the standards and registries of more than 130 recognized breeds of dogs. The AKC also develops and enforces the rules and regulations governing dogs shows, obedience trials, tracking tests, field trials, hunting tests, and several other informal events. The United Kennel Club (UKC) is a second breed registry in the United States. Although it is quite a bit smaller than AKC, UKC recognizes and maintains a registry for purebred breeds and also sanctions dog shows and working dog events.

Dog shows are commonly referred to as "conformation" or "breed" shows. These events were developed with the purpose of exhibiting purebred animals and improving the quality of purebred breeds of dogs. They provide a medium in which purebred dog breeders and enthusiasts can exhibit their dogs and receive critical evaluation of the dog's conformity to the breed standard. The intended goal is that breeders will use this evaluation system to make decisions regarding breeding programs, thus leading to improvements in the breed. Each dog is evaluated according to its ability to meet the established breed standard that has been accepted by the parent breed club and the AKC. Factors such as proper gait, head type, body conformation, coat type and color, eye and nose pigmentation, and temperament are taken into

TABLE 6.3   Dog-Related Sports and Activities

Event	Eligibility
AKC Dog Shows (Conformation)	Purebred Dogs (AKC Recognized); Intact Males and Females Only
UKC Dog Shows (Conformation)	Purebred Dogs (UKC Recognized); Intact Males and Females Only
AKC Obedience Trials	Purebred Dogs (AKC Recognized); Neutered and Intact Animals
UKC Obedience Trials	Purebred and Mixed Breeds; Neutered and Intact Animals
Canine Good Citizen Tests	Purebred and Mixed-Breed Dogs; Neutered and Intact Animals
Field Trials and Hunting Tests	Purebred Dogs of Sporting and Hound Breeds
Lure Coursing	Sight Hound Breeds
Water Rescue Tests	Newfoundland
Terrier Trials (Certificate of Gameness)	Most Terrier Breeds
Herding Instinct Tests	All Herding Breeds; Some Working Breeds
Agility	Purebred and Mixed-Breed Dogs; Neutered and Intact Animals
Fly Ball	Purebred and Mixed-Breed Dogs; Neutered and Intact Animals

consideration. The attainment of the title of Champion denotes a dog who has earned a minimum of 15 points and has placed first over a substantial number of dogs on at least two occasions. In addition to providing a system for evaluating dogs, shows are also a pleasant opportunity for breeders to exchange information with each other, study the changes occurring in their breed, and meet and socialize with friends who have similar interests.

Obedience trials were developed to demonstrate the ability of the dog to be a true companion to humans and to be trained to behave in the home, in public places, and in the presence of other dogs. Unlike conformation shows, dogs who have been spayed or neutered, or who have disqualifying breed faults may still be shown in obedience competitions. Dogs entered in these competitions perform a prescribed set of exercises that are evaluated by a licensed judge. Several titles may be earned by dogs trained in obedience, progressing from a basic level of training to more advanced and difficult exercises. These titles are: Companion Dog (CD), Companion Dog Excellent (CDX), Utility Dog (UD), Utility Dog Excellent (UDX), and Obedience Trial Champion (OTCH). Obedience titles (CD, CDX and UD) are earned through three successful completions of the test, judged by a licensed obedience judge. Recently, the AKC has added an informal degree called the Canine Good Citizen (CGC) award. Both purebred and random-bred dogs are eligible for the CGC test, which is designed to demonstrate good manners and obedience in public settings.

Dogs entered in AKC tracking tests must prove their ability to follow a trail left by a single person (track layer) and to find one or more articles that were dropped by that person. The first title that can be earned is called the Tracking Dog title (TD) and involves a track that is between 440 and 500 yards in length and is 30 minutes to 2 hours old. The highest level of tracking, the Tracking Dog Excellent (TDX) involves a track that is 800 to 1,000 yards in length and 3 to 5 hours old. This track also will include a variety of obstacles and cross-tracks laid by persons other than the track layer. Each dog and handler team is evaluated by two judges, who assess the dog's ability to follow the track without guidance from the handler and to indicate the items that were dropped by the track layer. Tracking titles are earned after one successful completion of a track at a licensed tracking test.

Field trials and hunting tests are held separately for different breeds, depending on the type of hunting task the breed originally was developed to perform. For example, the hound breeds have trials that entail the pursuit of rabbits or hares, with the dogs running in either packs or pairs (braces). Dogs entered in these tests are judged according to their ability and desire to follow the trail of the game. Pointing breed trials evaluate the dog's ability to find and indicate game by stopping and pointing. Retrieving events, on the other hand, test the dog's ability to retrieve shot game from land and water. Spaniel trials test the dog's ability to find birds within shotgun range of the hunter and to flush and retrieve the game when commanded by the handler. In addition to AKC field trials, many parent breed clubs have developed their own tests for evaluating a dog's hunting capabilities. For example, the Golden Retriever Club of America and the Labrador Retriever Club of America each award Working Certificate (WC) and Working Certificate Excellent (WCX) titles to dogs who demonstrate natural instinct to retrieve birds on land and from the water.

Many national breed clubs offer events designed to test the natural ability of a dog to perform the original task for which the breed was developed. For example, the Newfoundland Club of America sponsors water rescue competitions. In these events, the dogs are required to tow their owners back to land from deep water or go to the aid of the handler after the handler falls from a boat. Lure coursing is an event sponsored by the American Sight Hound Field Association. Sight hound breeds such as Greyhounds and Whippets participate in this sport and compete in races in which they chase a simulated rabbit over a predesignated course. The American Working Terrier Association offers a Certificate of Gameness (CG) to dogs of the terrier breeds who demonstrate a willingness to go to ground to hunt out rats or mice. Herding instinct tests are designed to test the natural ability of dogs of the herding breeds to work livestock. These are just a few of the many activities available for dog enthusiasts. As every dog breed was originally developed for a specific purpose, there exist many types of tests to evaluate the ability of individual dogs to demonstrate their instinct to perform the tasks of their heritage.

Two dog activities gaining in popularity that allow participation of both purebred and mixed-breed dogs are agility and fly-ball competitions. Agility dogs are trained to maneuver through a course containing a variety of obstacles. Examples of some of these obstacles include hurdles and jumps, bridges, weave poles, and tunnels. Fly-ball competitions involve relay races in which each dog on a team must jump a series of hurdles then hit a lever that will throw a tennis ball into the air. The dog must then retrieve the ball to the owner, returning over the jumps. Titles can be earned by individual dogs in each of these competitions.

Bonds That Fail: The Pet Overpopulation Problem

In a discussion concerning the theoretical basis of the human-companion animal bond, Bernard Rollin states, "If we are indeed bonded to [companion animals], are we keeping our end of the bargain?"[25] It is widely accepted that dogs and other pets are an important part of our society, but it is also a fact that many bonds between owners and their companion animals do not develop fully or are terminated prematurely. It is estimated that between 8 and 12 percent of the total population of dogs and cats enter shelters each year, and 30 to 60 percent of these animals are ultimately euthanized.[26] Although many owners say they believe a new home will be found when they relinquish their pet, animal shelters are forced to euthanize many dogs and cats just to provide room for the daily influx of unwanted animals. The majority of pets killed at shelters are either surrendered by their owners or are strays who have owners living in the community. Therefore, most of the animals taken to shelters are products of broken bonds with human owners, as opposed to feral animals who have no past relationship with humans.

Results of a survey conducted at animal shelters in eight geographical areas in the United States provide some insight into the histories of the pets that are given up.[27] The majority of owners obtained their pets from relatives, friends, or neighbors, rather than from professional breeders or pet shops. Moreover, a direct relationship was observed between the amount of money spent for the pet and the length of time the pet was kept. These data indicate that pet owners may work harder at relationships they perceive to be of greater initial value than at those that are entered into with little forethought or are obtained free of charge. Almost three-fourths of the pets (72 percent) had been acquired for nonutilitarian purposes. The most often cited reasons for obtaining the pet were companionship or to provide a home for an animal in need. It appears that most of the owners had expectations for the development of a positive bond with their animal, but, for a variety of reasons, this relationship did not occur.

The two leading reasons cited for giving up the pet were lifestyle changes, such as moving or divorce, and behavior problems. A majority of the owners expressed regret at leaving their pet and 59 percent stated they would keep the pet if the problem could be solved or the situation changed. Although it was not explored further in the survey, it is possible the owner's original expectations concerning the amount of time, training, and attention required by the pet were unrealistic. Pet owner education in areas of pet selection, health care, behavior, and training are a necessary part of the solution to this problem. While as a society we greatly value the relationships we have with our companion animals, we also have a long way to go before solving the pet overpopulation problem and improving the chances that dog-owner relationships will stay intact throughout the natural life of the pet.

Selecting the Right Dog

A strong human-dog bond may fail to develop if owners have unrealistic or unreasonable expectations concerning their pet's needs or behavior. Providing information about pet selection before an animal is brought into a new home can create more realistic expectations and facilitate proper training and care once a dog is obtained. An individual's living situation and lifestyles, differences between breeds and breed types, and advantages and disadvantages of puppies and adult dogs are all important factors to consider (Table 6.4).

TABLE 6.4　　Factors to Consider When Selecting a Dog

✓ **Living Situation** (house vs. apartment; stability)
✓ **Time Commitment** (work hours; travel schedule; time spent at home)
✓ **Lifestyle of Owner** (activity level; significant others; other hobbies)
✓ **Cost** (food; training equipment; grooming; toys; veterinary expenses)
✓ **Age of Dog** (puppy; young adult; mature adult)
✓ **Breed** (size; activity level; coat type; temperament; trainability)
✓ **Source** (purebred breeder; animal shelter; newspaper ad)

The process of selective breeding and the need to develop working dogs for different purposes led to the creation of more than 300 different breeds of dogs (see Chapter 2). Obvious breed differences in size, body conformation, color, coat type, and athletic ability are factors most owners naturally consider. However, even more important are the considerable breed differences in behavior and temperament. All of these factors must be considered when selecting a dog that will be well suited for the owner's living environment, lifestyle, and personality. The first question that should be asked is whether or not the owner desires a dog, as opposed to some other type of companion animal, to share his or her life. The cat is currently equal in popularity to the dog as a companion animal and may be a more appropriate pet for some people.

Dog or cat? There are several important differences between dogs and cats. By nature, the dog is a very social species. The dog's wild ancestor is the wolf, *Canis lupus,* who is a pack-living animal (see Chapter 1). In contrast, the domestic cat, *Felis silvestris catus,* is by nature a more solitary creature. Its primary wild ancestor is the African wild cat, *Felis silvestris lybica,* a species that lives a comparatively solitary life. When cats do form pairs or small communal-living groups, the relationships that are established do not have the same interactive, functional pack structure as those of the dog. This difference in lifestyle has resulted in two pets that relate somewhat differently with their human caretakers. While dogs have a strong tendency to integrate themselves intimately into the family structure within the household, cats do not develop pack structure in the same sense and so are typically perceived as being more independent or even aloof. The social requirements of the dog lead to a stronger reliance on proximity and interaction with the owners. In general, dogs tend to bond more strongly to their owners and are less tolerant or accepting of separation or isolation.

There are also some practical differences between dogs and cats that may affect a person's choice of pet. Because of their natural elimination habits, cats are easier to house-train than dogs. Most cats learn to use an indoor litter box within several days. Teaching a young puppy to urinate and defecate outside usually takes several weeks, and most young dogs are not completely reliable until they are 6 months of age or older. Cats require less exercise than dogs. In general, most indoor cats can be exercised through various games they develop with their owner or other cats. In contrast, all dogs require some level of daily outdoor exercise. An owner's living situation may dictate whether a dog or cat can be kept. Apartment dwelling is naturally better suited for cats than dogs. However, many committed city dwellers are able to provide frequent, regular exercise for their dogs through daily walks or excursions to a park. The cost of keeping a pet also may be an important consideration for some owners. While there is not too much difference in upkeep requirements between a cat and a small dog, the cost of keeping a large or giant breed of dog can be substantially higher.

What does a dog need? Once the decision to acquire a dog has been made, several factors should be considered. Accepting the responsibility for a companion animal is a commitment, and current lifestyles tend to be very busy. The time commitment a dog requires must be integrated into a person's normal daily routine. Most new dog owners underestimate the amount of time a dog requires. As a social animal, a dog is happiest when its pack is together, so it requires regular and frequent amounts of time and attention. This includes time devoted to general care and feeding, playtime, exercise time, and, of course, training time. Given the dog's highly social nature and the recent increase in popularity of certain high-energy breeds, it is not surprising that dog trainers and behaviorists report that many behavior problems are caused by boredom, lack of exercise, or separation stress.

A fenced yard can be a benefit for dogs both because of the safety it provides and because it offers an opportunity for exercise. However, a fenced yard is no substitute for daily walks or excursions to a public place for socialization. Most dogs who are kept in yards for excessive periods of time develop habits such as digging, barking, or territorial defense. In addition, because of their desire for social contact, most dogs do not happily tolerate long-term separation from their owners, even in a yard or pen. The stability of the owner's living situation must also be considered. If renting, lease requirements must clearly allow keeping a dog. Moreover, if an individual is considering moving in the near future, the time is probably not right to obtain a dog. The Humane Society of the United States reports that the most common reason for pet relinquishment at shelters is a move or landlord dispute.

The owner's lifestyle also should be considered. Are regular hours kept or does work keep the owner away from home for long, inconsistent time periods? Dogs do not tolerate isolation as easily as cats, and the need for a regular exercise, feeding, and attention schedule is very important. Are there other people to consider? If there is a family, obtaining a dog should be a decision made by the entire family, not just one person. The cost of the dog must be considered, too. This includes not only food expenses but also routine and emergency veterinary care, grooming, equipment, toys, training, and boarding costs.

Adult or puppy? The next question is whether an adult dog or a puppy is the best choice. If a puppy is obtained, the best time to bring a puppy into a new home is when it is between 7 and 12 weeks of age (see Chapter 7). This age coincides with the second half of the primary socialization period, a time during which the puppy is forming primary social attachments. Having the puppy during this time period is a distinct advantage because it allows bonding to human caretakers and gradual acclimatization to the new home environment at a time when the puppy is behaviorally flexible and responsive. A second advantage to obtaining a young dog is that behavior patterns (i.e. bad habits) have not yet been established, giving the owner the opportunity to begin training and prevent problems before they develop. However, for the same reason, the time commitment for puppies is quite high in terms of care, training, and feeding schedule. Puppies need to be taught to urinate and defecate outside the home, to develop house manners, and to inhibit some natural puppy behaviors such as nipping, chasing, and rough play. Because puppies often react to young children in much the same manner they interact with other puppies, obtaining a puppy when there are babies or toddlers in the home usually is not recommended.

There are several advantages to obtaining an adult dog as a companion animal. In many cases, an adult will already be house-trained and may have had obedience training with the previous owner. If this is the case, the initial time commitment on the part of the owners will be somewhat less than with a puppy. Because the period of excess energy, play nipping, and house-breaking is past, an adult is a better choice when there are young children in the home. As a disadvantage, an adult dog may already have some behavior problems that are well established and may be difficult to modify, especially if the dog's background is not known. However, in many cases, consistency and patience in training result in an adult animal that fits in beautifully with the new family.

Purebred or random-bred? While selective breeding and the establishment of purebred dog registries have given us more than 300 different breeds of dogs, there are also a large number of dogs that do not possess a known lineage. These individuals are commonly called random-bred or mix-breed dogs. Some prospective owners have definite preferences concerning size, appearance, and temperament and so will often select one or several breeds they are interested in. Others have more general requirements and may be interested in adopting a random-bred puppy or adult from a local shelter. Almost all of the breeds of dogs that are in existence today were originally developed to fulfill a specific working function (see Chapter 2). The establishment of breed registries and studbooks created breeds that showed consistency in appearance and temperament from generation to generation. This consistency is a distinct advantage for owners who have requirements regarding adult size, coat type, energy level, and temperament. Reputable breeders of purebred dogs will have a thorough knowledge of both their breed and their particular line, and can provide valuable information to prospective owners regarding their dog's success as a potential pet, working companion, or show dog.

Although the predictability and consistency of a purebred dog are distinct advantages, the line breeding and limitation of the gene pool that created the breed may be seen as disadvantages in some cases. Almost every breed of purebred dog has associated with it one or more genetically inherited disorders. For example, many large and giant breeds have a higher incidence of Canine Hip Dysplasia than the general population of dogs. Other examples of breed-related disorders are copper toxicosis in Bedlington Terriers and progressive retinal atrophy in Irish Setters (see Chapter 5). Experienced breeders are aware of potential breed-specific disorders and will screen breeding animals and conduct any testing available to identify carriers. It is also important to realize that purebreds do not have a corner on the genetic anomaly market. Although limited gene pools and inbreeding do produce increased chances of deleterious recessives occurring in the homozygous state, there is no guarantee that a mixed breed of dog will not develop a genetically inherited disorder. Cost is a second disadvantage of purebred dogs and one that may limit availability to certain owners. Depending on the breed's popularity and the reason the owner is purchasing the puppy (i.e. for a pet, working animal, or show animal), the cost of a purebred puppy can vary greatly. Some purebred breed rescue organizations provide dogs to good homes at relatively low costs, depending on the owner's ability to pay.

Obtaining a random-bred puppy or adult from an animal shelter is an excellent, less costly way of obtaining a good family pet. The current overpopulation of dogs results in many dogs needing good, loving homes. Owners often can find a puppy or young adolescent dog at a shelter that will meet all of their requirements for a happy, healthy family pet. Lack of predictability is a potential problem, especially if nothing is known about the dog's heritage or previous care. If a puppy is obtained, ultimate size and appearance may be difficult to ascertain. However, the advantages of many random-bred dogs and the fact that a dog that may otherwise have been euthanized is finding a home can make this slight risk worthwhile.

Where to go? There are several sources of both purebred and random-bred dogs. Almost all communities have a kennel club that provides a breeders referral service. These services often are listed in the phone book or in the pet advertisements of local papers. In most cases, the breeders referral service will answer questions about breeds and direct potential buyers to local breeders and purebred rescue organizations. If a purebred dog is sought, buyers should find a breeder who has an established reputation, is knowledgeable about both the attributes and the faults of their breed, and is genuinely concerned with improving the breed.

Retail pet stores are another source of purebred dogs. However, this is the least desirable place to purchase a dog. Most of the puppies found in these establishments are purchased from large-scale commercial operations and are shipped at very young ages to various retail "outlets" throughout the country. In many cases, the commercial breeding kennels consist of very crowded, poorly constructed, and unsanitary conditions in which females are housed permanently in small kennels and bred repeatedly throughout their lives. Disease losses often are very high, and the care of puppies and the breeding animals is substandard. Screening for genetically transmitted disorders usually is nonexistent. Once puppies from these kennels reach the stores, they are housed in crates and given minimal human contact. Interestingly, puppies at pet stores often are sold at prices equal to or even higher than the prices requested by reputable breeders. Because they are often located in high-traffic areas such as shopping malls, pet stores selling puppies continue to serve the "impulse buyer" who cannot resist the "cute puppy in the window." For the sake of the animals and because of the risks of disease and genetic disorders, a pet store is a good place to buy pet supplies but not a good source for a dog.

The best place to obtain a random-bred puppy is from a local animal shelter. All shelters provide health screening and require that all their animals be spayed or neutered. In some states, it is mandated by law that all animals adopted from private and municipal shelters be neutered. With the advent of early neutering, many shelters are now spaying and neutering all or most of their animals before they are adopted. Owners usually are requested to provide a donation or partially refundable fee to help offset the costs of caring for and feeding the shelter's animals.

Conclusions

The companionship and unconditional love dogs are capable of providing are underlying reasons so many of us choose to share our homes and lives with one or more dogs. From the small Chihuahua, to the regal Great Dane, to the drooling St. Bernard, every dog has a unique set of characteristics that will make it the perfect pet for a specific person and lifestyle. Having an understanding of these differences and of the factors that should be considered when selecting a pet can result in a match that will endure for many years and bring much joy to the lives of both owner and dog.

In the following part, the behavior of man's best friend is examined in detail. As the dog's naturally social temperament is discussed, the reasons humans so easily coexist with *Canis familiaris* become increasingly evident. However, it is also the dog's natural behavior that leads to many incompatibilities between owners and their dogs. Most behaviors that are termed "problems" are actually normal canine behaviors occurring in a situation that is incompatible with the owner's lifestyle. Unfortunately, it is these very behaviors that are often the cause of owners relinquishing their dogs to animal shelters.

The following chapters will provide information regarding the cause of common behavior problems and methods for their management and prevention. Understanding these behaviors and having information available that can be used to prevent and solve common problems can help maintain positive ties between owners and their dogs and keep dogs in their original homes.

Cited References

1. Humane Society of the United States. **HSUS fact sheet: Pet population statistics, 1997**.

2. Katcher, A.H. **Interactions between people and their pets: Form and function.** In: *Interrelationships Between People and Pets* (B. Fogle, editor), Charles C. Thomas, Springfield, Illinois, pp. 41-67. (1981)

3. Lynch, J. *The Broken Heart: The Medical Consequences of Loneliness*. Basic Books, New York, New York. (1977)

4. Katcher, A.H., Friedmann, E., Goodman, M., and Goodman, L. **Men, women and dogs.** California Veterinarian, 2:14-16. (1983)

5. Grossberg, J. and Alf, E. **Interactions with pet dogs: Effects on human**

cardiovascular response. Journal of the Delta Society, 2:20-27. (1986)

6. Serpell, J.A. **The personality of the dog and its influence on the pet-owner bond.** In: *New Perspectives on Our Lives with Companion Animals* (A.H. Katcher and A.M. Beck, editors), University of Philadelphia Press, Philadelphia, Pennsylvania, pp. 57-63. (1983)

7. Serpell, J.A. **Evidence for an association between pet behavior and owner attachment levels.** Applied Animal Behavior Science, 47:49-60. (1996)

8. Kidd, A.H. and Kidd, R.M. **Factors in adults' attitudes toward pets.** Psychological Reports, 65:903-910. (1989)

9. Albert, A. and Bulcroft, K. **Pets, families and the life course.** Journal of Marriage and the Family, 50:543-552. (1988)

10. Anderson, W., Reid, P., and Jennings, G.L. **Pet ownership and risk factors for cardiovascular disease.** Medical Journal of Australia, 157:298-301. (1992)

11. Barker, S.B. and Barker, R.T. **The human-canine bond: Closer than family ties?** Journal of Mental Health Counseling, 10:46-56. (1988)

12. Cain, A.O. **A study of pets in the family system.** In: *New Perspectives on Our Lives with Companion Animals* (A.H. Katcher and A.M. Beck, editors), University of Pennsylvania Press, Philadelphia, Pennsylvania, pp. 72-81. (1983)

13. Ory, M. and Goldberg, E. **Pet possession and life satisfaction.** In: *New Perspectives on Our Lives with Companion Animals* (A. Katcher and A. Beck, editors), University of Pennsylvania Press, Philadelphia, Pennsylvania. (1983)

14. Brown, L.T., Shaw, T.G., and Kirland, K.D. **Affection for people as a function of affection for dogs.** Psychological Reports, 31:957-958. (1972)

15. Albert, A. and Bulcroft, K. **Pets and urban life.** Anthrozoos, 1:9-23. (1987)

16. Miller, M. and Lage, D. **Observed pet-owner in-home interactions: Species differences and association with the pet relationship scale.** Anthrozoos, 4:49-54. (1990)

17. Friedmann, E., Katcher, A.H., Thomas, S.A., Lynch, J.J., and Messent, P.R. **Social interaction and blood pressure: Influence of animal companions.** Journal of Nervous and Mental Disease, 171:461-465. (1983)

18. Katcher, A.H., Friedmann, E., Beck, A.M., and Lynch, J. **Looking, talking, and blood pressure: The physiological consequences of interaction with the living environment.** In: *New Perspectives on Our Lives with Companion Animals* (A.H. Katcher and A.M. Beck, editors), University of Pennsylvania Press, Philadelphia, Pennsylvania, pp. 351-362. (1983)

19. Katcher, A.H. and Beck, A.M. **Health and caring for living things.** In: *Animals and People Sharing the World* (A.R. Rowan, editor), University Press of New England, Hanover, New Hampshire, pp. 53-73. (1988)

20. Messent, P.R. **Facilitation of social interaction by companion animals.** In: *New Perspective on our Lives with Companion Animals* (A.H. Katcher, and A.M. Beck, editors), University of Pennsylvania Press, Philadelphia, Pennsylvania, pp. 37-46. (1983)

21. Serpell, J.A. **Beneficial effects of pet ownership on some aspects of human health and behaviour.** Journal of the Royal Society of Medicine, 84:717-720. (1991)

22. Levinson, B.M. *Pets and Human Development.* Charles C. Thomas Company, Springfield, Illinois. (1972)

23. Levinson, B.M. *Pet-Oriented Child Psychotherapy.* Charles C. Thomas Company, Springfield, Illinois. (1969)

24. Hart, L., Hart, B.L., and Bergin, B. **Socializing effects of service dogs for people with disabilities.** Anthrozoos, 1:41-44. (1987)

25. Kidd, A.H. and Kidd, R.M. **Seeking a theory of the human/companion animal bond.** Anthrozoos, 1:140-157. (1987)

26. Humane Society of the United States, **HSUS fact sheet: Pet population statistics, 1996.**

27. Arkow, P.S. and Dow, S. **The ties that do not bind: A study of the human-animal bonds that fail.** In: *The Pet Connection* (R.K. Anderson, B.L. Hart, and L.A. Hart, editors), Center to Study Human-Animal Relationships and Environments, University of Minnesota, Minneapolis, Minnesota, pp. 348-354. (1984)

Part 2 Behavior: Communicating with Man's Best Friend

7   Developmental Behavior: Puppy to Adult

THE DEVELOPMENTAL BEHAVIOR of the domestic dog has been extensively studied for about 50 years. During the 1940s, a series of studies was conducted at the Roscoe B. Jackson Memorial Laboratory in Bar Harbor, Maine, that examined the relationship between genetics and social behavior in dogs. An important outcome of these studies was the identification of particular developmental periods during which puppies are exceptionally sensitive to environmental influences on behavior. This work resulted in the concept that early experiences are important in terms of their effects on later behavior. Further research defined these "critical periods" in greater detail and provided a time frame for the development of species-specific behavior in the dog. Early behavioral development of the dog can be divided into four stages: the neonatal period, transitional period, socialization period, and juvenile period.

Neonatal Period (Birth to 14 Days)

The neonatal period is characterized by a set of behaviors that are adapted for the puppy's acquisition of food, warmth, and maternal care. The dog is an **altricial** species, meaning that puppies are born in a relatively helpless state. Newborn puppies are unable to see or hear because their eyes are not open and their ears are not functioning. Their motor abilities are limited to crawling short distances. They are unable to regulate internal body temperature and so must depend on an outside source of warmth. Tactile stimulation by the mother is necessary for the stimulation of urination and defecation. Touch and olfaction appear to be the newborn's most well-developed special senses. Neonates are capable of reacting to hot and cold surfaces, and also learn to react to the scent of their mother shortly after birth (Figure 7.1).

Puppies are born with a set of primitive behavior patterns, most of which fade with maturation of the nervous system. The rooting reflex is triggered by maternal licking and is characterized by a "swimming" motion with the front legs as the back legs push forward toward the warm stimulus. This reaction allows the puppy to locate the female's underside and teats shortly after birth. Suckling occurs as soon as the puppy finds the teat for its first meal. This reflex also can be elicited by placing a finger in a pup's mouth. Suckling is accompanied by a treading motion of front limbs, which move against the mammary gland and aid in stimulating milk secretion. During the neonatal period, vocalization patterns are limited to distress calling. These high-frequency, high-pitched cries are accompanied by increased activity and will be

FIGURE 7.1   Newborn puppies

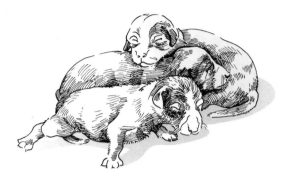

elicited when puppies are either separated from the warmth of the litter or are hungry.

Although the puppies grow very rapidly during the first two weeks of life, their behavior patterns do not change much. Because they are completely dependent on the mother for care, it is probably most advantageous to think of the bitch and her puppies as a functioning unit that must be monitored and maintained together for the first two weeks. The dam has a set of reciprocal behaviors that match the development of her puppies. These include vigorously licking the puppies, lying down on her side to expose her mammary glands, and responding to the cries of her puppies. The dam's maternal capabilities can have a profound effect on the health and well-being of the puppies, especially during the early days following birth.

The learning abilities of puppies appear to be limited during the neonatal period. However, because they are sensitive to olfactory cues and to tactile stimulation, early handling by human caretakers is advantageous. In other mammalian species, early daily handling of neonates has been shown to have positive long-term effects on behavior.[1,2] These include accelerated maturation of the nervous system, increased growth rate, and enhanced development of motor skills, special senses, and problem-solving abilities. A study with newborn puppies found that puppies that were gently handled on a daily basis for the first 5 weeks of life were more confident, exploratory, and socially dominant as adolescents than their non-handled counterparts.[3] These results also indicated that early handling resulted in improvements in stress-resistance, emotional stability, and learning capacity.

Transitional Period (14 to 21 Days)

The transitional period represents a period of rapid physiological change during which the puppy's ability to perceive the outside world and to process information increases dramatically. This is primarily due to the maturation of the sensory organs and neurological system. This period is typically designated as beginning with the opening of the eyes at about 12 to 14 days, and ending about 1 week later when the ear canals open and puppies show their first auditory "startle" response. The deciduous teeth erupt around 20 days, and puppies begin to show an interest in solid food. During this important week, many neonatal behavior patterns slowly disappear and are replaced by behavior patterns of later puppyhood. Puppies begin to stand and walk, and tail wagging is first observed. Anogenital stimulation by the dam is no longer necessary for urination and defecation, and puppies begin to move away from their sleeping area for elimination. Social behaviors start to emerge, including rudimentary play fighting, body postures, and vocalizations.

During the transitional period, puppies are capable of learning, but the rate of learning and the stability of conditioned responses do not reach adult levels until puppies are about 4 to 5 weeks of age. Because puppies are now capable of reacting to olfactory, auditory, and visual stimuli, the introduction of toys and other novel objects into the whelping area is beneficial, even though the puppies are not yet capable of manipulating the objects. Exposing puppies to normal household sounds, smells, and sights; daily handling; petting; and gentle brushing are all advantageous during this stage.

Primary Socialization (3 to 12 Weeks)

The primary socialization period is the most important period of social development for the young dog. It represents a time of very rapid behavioral change and specifically includes the development of species-specific social behaviors. At less than 3 weeks, the puppy's neurological system and special senses are too immature to allow socialization. The onset of primary socialization correlates with the maturation of the puppy's central nervous system and with final myelination of the spinal cord. These changes signify that the puppy is now capable of perceiving and reacting to its environment in the same manner as an adult dog. The upper limit of this period occurs at about 12 weeks and is characterized by a gradually increasing tendency to exhibit reservation when exposed to new stimuli.

Sensitive periods: Like the other periods of development, the primary socialization period was first called a "critical period." However, because the boundaries of these periods in the dog tend to be gradual rather than sudden and because the behaviors or preferences acquired during primary socialization can usually be modified to some degree when the animal is older, the term "sensitive period" has recently replaced "critical period" in the dog.[4] The term "sensitive period" refers to an age range during which certain events are likely to have long-term effects on an individual's development and behavior. After the sensitive period, the individual gradually develops decreased sensitivity to those events. In the case of the primary socialization period, puppies are highly responsive to stimuli that are presented within their environment, to opportunities to learn, and to opportunities to form attachments to other puppies, humans, and other companion animals.

Importance of socialization: Socialization is the process by which an animal develops species-specific social behavior. The dog differs from most other social species in that it can be simultaneously socialized to its own species (conspecifics) and to humans. Adequate socialization to both species and to other forms of environmental stimuli during this sensitive period has value in preventing the development of inappropriate behaviors or deficits in behavior that can seriously hinder the dog's ability to bond with its human caretakers or to interact with other dogs. The puppy learns its species identification during the early portion of primary socialization. The latter part of this sensitive period can be targeted to facilitate the development of social attachments to humans. Dogs that are properly socialized to other dogs and to humans will incorporate both species into their social structure and will tend to direct species-typical behavior patterns, particularly communication patterns, toward both species.

Changes during primary socialization period: A rapid increase in activity and the appearance of increasingly complex behaviors are seen in the early part of primary socialization. When puppies are between 3 and 4 weeks of age, exploratory behaviors increase dramatically. Puppies investigate the whelping area and begin to play with each other and with their mother. Puppies will also readily approach and investigate all novel stimuli without showing any fear. After about 5 weeks, this response diminishes gradually as the puppies begin to show wariness of novel stimuli.

This change makes adaptive sense when considered in terms of the dog's ancestry. Five weeks corresponds to the time at which wolf puppies are making their first excursions away from the security of the den. The development of **xenophobia** or "fear of the new" at this age has significant survival value as it serves to provide protection from potential predators. Site attachment also develops early in the socialization period. Puppies become attached to their sleeping and eating areas and, as they are given access to other areas, appear to form attachment for particular places within the home.

Play between litter mates becomes increasingly complex and is probably very important in the development of social relationships, communication patterns, and other species-specific behaviors. Play fighting rapidly teaches puppies to inhibit their bite and to react appropriately to the distress vocalizations of their litter mates. Facial expressiveness and aggressive vocalizations appear at about 5 weeks of age. These are accompanied by rapid maturation of motor skills as puppies begin to run, climb, and chew. This is also the period during which the first dominance hierarchies develop. Puppies acquire communicative body postures, which signal dominance, submission, play solicitation, and care-seeking. Fragments of sexual behavior such as mounting and pelvic thrusting are also seen during puppy play.

Learning to be a dog: It is very important for puppies to be with litter mates and their dam during the first portion of primary socialization. In addition to learning species-typical behaviors through play, the puppies also experience important interactions with the mother. The dam's interactions with her puppies provide important information about social behavior.

When the puppies play too roughly or become too demanding, the mother will discipline them through the use of growls, body postures, and physical reprimands such as muzzle bites. This discipline teaches the puppies to correctly interpret dominant signals, to inhibit their bites, and to display submissive postures to a dominant dog (Figure 7.2). In general, puppies should remain with their litter until they are 6 to 8 weeks of age. Human handling and interaction should also occur during this time period, but it is imperative that puppies remain with their own species during the early portion of primary socialization for species-specific communication and social behaviors to develop.

Female dogs will naturally start the weaning process when their puppies are 3 to 4 weeks of age. This process will be complete by 7 to 9 weeks, if unimpeded by human intervention. As the bitch starts to wean her puppies, she will begin to walk away while they are nursing, allow nursing for shorter periods of time, and spend more time away from the litter. This gradual onset of increased isolation teaches the puppies self-confidence and allows the development of independence from their mother's care. It is important that this is recognized as a period of gradual lessening of the puppies' attachment to the dam, as opposed to an artificially introduced or abrupt separation.

Placement in new homes: Because puppies need to be with their litter mates during the first part of primary socialization and because socialization to humans and to new places and situations is important during the latter half, placement in new homes is best accomplished when puppies are between 7 and 9 weeks of age. Puppies who are removed from the litter too early often lack the ability to interact and communicate normally with other dogs. In addition, early weaning can cause puppies to become too oriented to humans and may predispose them to over-attachment problems later in life[5] (see Chapter 10).

FIGURE 7.2   Using a muzzle bite to reprimand a puppy

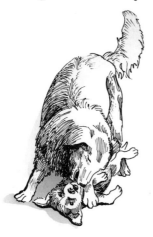

Socialization with humans: Detailed studies of growing puppies have shown that socialization with humans takes place most readily when the puppies are between 5 and 12 weeks of age, with an optimum period between 6 and 8 weeks.[6] Puppies that were allowed to remain with their mother for 14 weeks with no socialization with people showed extreme fear and were largely untrainable as adults. If a dog has had no experience or minimal experience with people by the age of 14 weeks, it will be very difficult to socialize this puppy and difficult for her to develop normal social attachments to people. Therefore, it is important that puppies receive human contact while they are still with their litter, and this contact should continue when they enter their new home.

An important aspect of being a social species is the capacity to form attachments to others of the species social group. In the dog's case, this includes others of their own species, their human caretakers, and any other companion animals that may be present in the household. When puppies are removed from their litter and placed into new homes during the second half of primary socialization, they shift their social attachments from their mother and litter mates to their new human caretakers. Puppies are highly adaptable during this time period and will attach to a wide range of mammals. Therefore, if the dog will be coexisting with a cat, rabbit, gerbil, or other type of family pet, the best time to introduce the new house mates is during primary socialization. In households in which the puppy is going to be an only dog, it is equally important to continue to socialize the puppy to other dogs, preferably puppies that are about the same age.

Fear imprint period: Puppies show the highest level of curiosity and lowest level of hesitancy or fear of new stimuli when they are between 3 and 5 weeks of age. After 5 weeks, they gradually begin to show some uncertainty of new people, objects, or situations. This change reaches a culmination at about 8 to 10 weeks of age, a period that is referred to as "fear imprint." Although the age range of this period is very consistent, puppies vary greatly in the degree to which they demonstrate uncertainty or decreased confidence. While some become quite sensitive and even fearful toward new stimuli, others show little of these signs. It is probable that both genetics and early socialization influence the expression of fear imprint in young puppies. Regardless, because puppies are usually in their new homes during fear imprint, care should be taken not to expose puppies to any traumatic events during this time period.

Socialization procedures: Proper socialization results in a dog who is capable of forming social attachments to other dogs and to humans, adapts well to new situations, and is responsive to training. Conversely, inadequate socialization of a puppy results in a dog that does not form strong attachments, is susceptible to stress, and is threatened by new situations, people, or dogs. In these cases, new experiences may be stressful for the dog throughout his life, regardless of how often he is exposed to them as an adult.

Socialization includes providing a wide variety of positive experiences early in life, preferably during the period of primary socialization (3 to 12 weeks). While still with their litter, puppies can gradually be exposed to a varied environment. After the transition period, as the puppies become more mobile, they can be housed in a wire-fronted enclosure. From the security of this enclosure, the puppies can be exposed to many stimuli. Normal household sights and sounds can be introduced, along with new people, children, and other family pets. Puppies should also be handled and played with frequently. Although the litter is still under the care of the mother during this time, puppies should be separated from the dam and from the other litter mates for short periods of time. The frequency and duration of these separations can be gradually increased as the puppies mature. This functions to introduce a mild separation stress, facilitates bonding to humans, and will aid the puppy in learning to cope with spending time alone later in life.

Socialization procedures can become more varied and extensive once the puppy is in her new home at 7 to 9 weeks of age. Although 12 weeks is identified as the "end" of primary socialization, the time period of up to 4 months is generally accepted as a good period during which to socialize a new puppy. There is evidence that suggests that dogs benefit the most if socialization continues throughout the juvenile period. Providing a wide variety of experiences at a young age has the effect of developing a dog that is accepting of new situations later in life and does not react fearfully to new experiences. An increase in the dog's general ability to adapt to novel situations and stimuli occurs.

One of the best methods of socializing a new puppy is through participation in a puppy kindergarten class. Most communities have this type of class available, either through private dog training schools or training clubs. These classes are beneficial and are able to provide positive exposure to new dogs, people, and places. In addition, because puppies are capable of learning at a rapid rate during this time period, primary socialization represents a time during which obedience training can begin. Most puppy kindergarten classes include an introduction to basic obedience commands (see Chapter 9). Teaching the puppy household manners, introducing car rides, taking walks in the neighborhood, and providing opportunities with friendly adults and children all contribute to the development of a happy, well-adjusted adult dog. These procedures can continue well into the juvenile period as the dog begins to acquire adult behaviors.

Juvenile Period (Secondary Socialization)

The juvenile period extends from the end of primary socialization to sexual maturity. This is a period of refining existing capabilities and increasing coordination as the dog matures physically. Motor skills become more coordinated and adultlike, and attention span gradually increases. The dog's permanent teeth begin to replace the deciduous teeth at about 4 to 5 months of age and are usually fully erupted by 6 months of age. Around 3 to 4 months of age puppies will increase exploratory behaviors and will become more confident and independent. Gradual changes in behavior also are seen in response to learning and as a result of previous experiences (see Chapter 9).

Sexually related behaviors develop with the onset of puberty. Female dogs become sexually mature between 6 and 16 months, depending on size and breed. Male dogs generally reach sexual maturity when they are 10 to 12 months of age. Although dogs are reproductively mature by the time they are 1 year of age, social behaviors continue to develop and change until dogs are 18 months or older. With the onset of puberty, androgen-facilitated behaviors such as urine marking, aggression, inclination to roam, and mounting begin to occur in males. Other adult behaviors such as territorial, protective, and dominance aggression develop after sexual maturity in both male and female dogs (see Chapter 8).

Conclusions

The young dog progresses through four periods of behavioral development. These periods facilitate the development of normal social behaviors and provide opportunities for owners to teach their new puppy to form positive attachments to their human caretakers and to react positively to new experiences later in life. The social behavior of the dog and its significance to the dog's integration into human society are examined in detail in the following chapter.

Cited References

1. Levine, S. **Maternal and environmental influences on the adrenalcortical response to stress in weanling rats.** Science, 135:795-796. (1962)

2. Denenberg, V.H. **A consideration of the usefulness of the critical period hypothesis as applied to the stimulation of rodents in infancy.** In: *Early Experience and Behaviour* (G. Newton and S. Levine, editors), Charles Thomas, Springfield, Illinois, pp. 142-167. (1968)

3. Fox, M.W. *The Dog: Its Domestication and Behavior.* Garland STPM Press, New York, New York. (1978)

4. Bateson, P. **How do sensitive periods arise and what are they for?** Animal Behaviour, 27:470-486. (1979)

5. Borchelt, P.L. **Separation-elicited behavior problems in dogs.** In: *New Perspectives on Our Lives with Companion Animals* (A.H. Katcher and A.M. Beck, editors), University of Pennsylvania Press, Philadelphia, Pennsylvania, pp. 187-196. (1983)

6. Freedman, D.G., King, J.A., and Elliot, O. **Critical periods in the social development of dogs.** Science, 133:1016-1017. (1961)

8 Understanding Normal Canine Behavior

THE DOMESTIC DOG, *Canis familiaris*, belongs to the taxonomic family Canidae. Also included in this family are wolves, coyotes, jackals, and foxes. It is generally accepted that the dog has descended from one or more subspecies of the wolf (see Chapter 1). It is to this ancestry that the dog's inherently social nature can be attributed. The dog has been domesticated for more than 12,000 years, however, and selective breeding has modified the dog's behavior, temperament, and appearance. Studying wolf behavior provides a basis for studying the domestic dog's behavior, but, in the long run, the best information about the behavior of dogs comes from the expert itself, *Canis familiaris*.

The Dog's Social Heritage

The dog's wild ancestor, the wolf, is known to be a highly social, predatory species. However, wide variations in the types of prey that are hunted and social systems that are established are seen in different subspecies of wolf. In general, wild canids are highly flexible and can organize into several types of social groups, depending on the ecology in which they live and the size and availability of their prey species.[1] The most common social system of *Canis lupus* is the pack. Packs consist of small groups of related individuals who remain together throughout the year. Complex hierarchal relationships exist between individuals, and only one pair of animals usually breed (the alpha male and female). All members of the pack work together to raise young, scavenge and hunt for food, protect the den, and demarcate territory.

Maintaining a cohesive group that works well together with minimal strife or fighting is essential for survival in a harsh environment. The major concerns of wolves include obtaining food, raising young and protecting themselves from other predators. These objectives are best achieved if the pack works well together as a unit and minimizes the amount of energy and time spent on fighting or aggressive behaviors between members. Social ranking is a social system that has evolved to achieve this goal. In addition to facilitating cooperative behaviors, this type of system minimizes strife and provides security for the entire pack. In this manner, a hierarchal system increases the chances of survival of each individual.

In wolf packs, social ranking is achieved through single-sex hierarchies. Cross-sex dominance relationships are weak or even nonexistent. The structure of these hierarchies is pyramidal, with the greatest degree of dominance conflict occurring between high-ranking individuals. The alpha male and female are at the top of each hierarchy. Dominant (high-ranking) animals are generally mature wolves who maintain pack order and security. These individuals demonstrate dominant body postures toward lower ranking animals, drive lower ranking individuals away from preferred sleeping areas, initiate pack activities such as hunting and travel, and usually eat first after a hunt or at a scavenge site. It is important to realize that interactions between high- and low-ranking members of a pack are not antagonistic or adversarial in nature. Rather, these relationships have the function of establishing cohesiveness and security in the pack and reducing intragroup aggression. A series of ritualized and stereotypic behaviors aid in maintaining the social order and facilitating cooperation between members of the pack.

The domestic dog has inherited the social nature of its wolf ancestor. Like wolves, dogs possess the need to live within a secure, orderly social group. However, the dog's social group consists of his or her human caretakers and other pets in the household. In multiple-dog households, dogs usually develop social relationships with the other dogs present. Hierarchies typically develop within groups of dogs that are housed together, depending somewhat on breed and individual temperament. Like the wolf, these hierarchies are single-sex. Dominance disputes rarely occur between two animals of the opposite sex. Dogs with high status display dominant body postures toward subordinates and tend to steal toys or food from dogs of lesser rank. They choose the best sleeping and resting areas, initiate many socially facilitated activities in the home and yard, and actively seek and compete for their owner's attention. Generally, there is a close relationship between age and status, with older dogs having and retaining the higher status in a group.

Until recently, pack behavior was widely accepted as a sufficient model for explaining the domestic dog's behavior and its relationship with its human caretakers. However, studies of dogs in recent years have shown that the dog is not simply a neotenized wolf. Rather, the social behavior of *Canis familiaris* is unique. Over the course of 12,000 years, humans have dramatically modified and controlled the dog's ecology and breeding. During this time, the forces of natural selection that normally guide the evolution of a species have not been in effect. Humans have provided food, shelter, and protection for the dog. These changes have effectively eliminated the selective forces of prey availability and competition with other predators. Breeding also has been under the control of humans. The restricted mating of only alpha pairs has been replaced by selective breeding for particular physical and behavioral characteristics. The dog has essentially co-evolved with its human caretakers, and this evolution has included almost complete dependence upon humans for care and survival. These changes, along with the genetic influences of selective breeding, have resulted in social behaviors that are unique to the domestic dog. Important components of the behavior of *Canis familiaris* include elements of dominance and submission, patterns of communication, various types of aggression, and breed-specific behavior patterns.

The Concepts of Dominance and Submission

The model of social hierarchies is effective in explaining much of the behavior observed in many social species. Dominant and subordinate relationships constitute the designated roles of individuals within a pack. The concept of dominance was first used to describe the linear pecking order of domestic fowl. It was later expanded to apply to many social-living species, including the wolf. Dominance is identified as occurring when an animal actively seeks out competition for social rank, either through the use of ritualized communication patterns or overt aggression. Within a social group, a dominant animal is the target of the least amount of aggressive threats, initiates aggression and displays of dominance with impunity, offers few submissive postures to other animals, and evokes deference and submissive displays from other animals.[2] Although the concept of dominance is often over-used (and even abused) in discussions of canine behavior, this model provides a useful method for explaining many (but not all) of the dog's social interactions.

During domestication, artificial selection produced animals that were more trainable and dependent than their wild ancestors. This enhanced trainability is associated with neoteny and the perpetuation of a subordinate nature into adulthood (see Chapter 1). Practically speaking, this means that most dogs are innately subordinate and do not develop into dominant animals as they mature. As individuals, dogs vary greatly in the degree of dominant behavior that they demonstrate. Similarly, while dominance hierarchies appear to be very important in maintaining pack structure within wolf packs, it is less clear that the domestic dog's social structure is strictly hierarchal in nature. Although dogs with dominant temperaments do exist and must be raised and handled appropriately, not all dogs demonstrate dominance or have the potential to show dominance aggression. Moreover, the dominance model of social interactions has often been inappropriately applied to aspects of a dog's behavior that are unrelated to dominant or submissive relationships.[2]

Characteristics of a dominant temperament in dogs include both innate temperament traits and behavior patterns that are displayed toward other dogs and humans. Puppies that have a dominant temperament tend to be highly exploratory, bold, and inquisitive. Within the litter, they often gain possession of food and toys, and initiate and control play sessions with other puppies. As the dog matures, characteristics of dominance become more pronounced. Signs include showing dominant body postures during play, resisting attempts at restraint or control, demonstrating possessiveness over desired resources such as food, toys, or sleeping areas, and initiating all interactions with the owner. Depending on the dog's breed and individual temperament, these signs may be accompanied by increased displays of aggression. Typically, dominance characteristics become fully manifested when the dog reaches social maturity, between 12 and 24 months of age. It is important that obedience training is introduced at a young age in dogs with a dominant temperament. This can ensure that the owner's leadership status is well-established and can prevent the development of a relationship in which the dog feels compelled to directly challenge the owner for dominant status (see chapters 9 and 10).

By comparison, puppies that are naturally subordinate will avoid competing for resources with their more dominant litter mates, readily relinquish toys, food, and sleeping areas to more dominant puppies, and are often described as "followers" rather than "leaders" in the litter. Dominance challenges are often nonexistent in such dogs, even as they mature. Training usually involves teaching good habits and preventing unwanted behaviors rather than actively establishing leadership.

The process of domestication has resulted in a tempering of the need for dominance ranking in dogs. The selection for neotenized features and temperament characteristics has resulted in a species in which many individuals are simply "born subordinate." As a result, many dogs will never display signs of dominance toward their owners, even upon reaching social maturity. For many dogs, dominance challenges are not an issue because they never develop a strong need to compete for social status. For example, some breeds, such as beagles and fox hounds, were developed to work in very large packs and, as a result, show little need for social hierarchies. In contrast, some of the working breeds have been developed to guard and protect, and so are more dominant animals by nature. Individuals of these breeds have a greater predisposition to develop dominant behaviors and a need for social ranking as they reach maturity.

Communication Patterns

Intraspecies communication signals are essential for the formation of social bonds and the maintenance of a cohesive pack structure. The dog, like its wolf ancestor, has a set of highly developed communication patterns. These include visual, olfactory, and auditory cues that are universal among members of *Canis familiaris*. Dogs recognize and understand each other regardless of breed, size, differences in coat length, or cosmetic surgical changes such as ear cropping or tail docking. Moreover, dogs display the same signals to their human caretakers that they use to interact with other dogs. Many of these cues are very subtle, but they have some similarities with human communication patterns and often are relatively easy for owners to interpret. Conversely, canine behavior also can be misunderstood if interpreted solely from the perspective of human motivations. Although some popular training manuals encourage dog owners to attempt to imitate many of the dog's visual and auditory signals when communicating with their dogs, recent work shows that this is not an effective means of communication. Humans are incapable of reproducing the subtle nuances of these cues and, basically, make poor dog substitutes. Understanding the dog's communication patterns and reacting appropriately as a human allow the development of effective communication between owner and dog, without the need to attempt to imitate the dog's own species-specific behaviors.

Scent cues (olfaction): Scent has several advantages as a communication tool for a social species. Smells remain in the environment for a long period of time and can convey information about territory, gender, and reproductive stage, even after the animal has left the immediate area. The fact that all dogs, regardless of appearance, recognize each other as conspecifics indicates that more reliance is placed upon olfaction for species recognition than upon visual cues. Sniffing is a major component of greeting behavior between dogs and provides information about the dog's sex, age, emotional state, and, possibly, social status. Dogs use several types of odors for communication. These include urine, fecal, and anal gland secretions and individual body odor.

Urine is used both to identify an individual and to mark territory. In wolves, raised-leg urination (RLU) is used to scent-mark with urine. Within a pack, dominant animals demonstrate RLUs more frequently than subordinate individuals, and the frequency of this type of urination increases when changes in the dominance order occur. There is also evidence that urine marks within a pack's territory deter other wolves from traveling in the area.[3] Like wolves, dogs use RLUs to scent-mark with urine. However, unlike wolves, in which only dominant animals use RLUs, all intact adult male dogs demonstrate RLUs. The RLU is associated with sexual maturity. Males that are neutered before puberty usually do not demonstrate RLUs even after becoming mature. Females also urine-mark, with an increase during the period of estrus, and some demonstrate a form of RLU. The urine of the estrus bitch contains pheromones that probably are metabolites of estrogen and are capable of attracting male dogs from great distances.

Urination patterns used to mark territory involve frequent squatting or RLUs at numerous sites and the excretion of small volumes of urine. Male dogs often target vertical surfaces and may even display RLUs without the production of urine. Over-marking with urine is frequently seen, especially within gender groups of dogs that live together. Females often stand next to other females as they urinate and immediately urinate over the spot when the first dog walks away. Males over-mark when they detect urine left previously by another dog. Backward scratching of the ground with the hind legs often is observed after urine-marking in males and, less frequently, in females. It is theorized that the disruption of the dirt around the marked area serves as a visual cue and spreads scent around the area. Scratching also may leave additional scent in the area from glands located between the toes and on the foot pads.

All dogs show an interest in the fecal droppings of other dogs and will often over-mark feces with urine. However, it is not known how important feces are for marking territory or identifying individuals. In wolves, defecation does appear to have a function in communication. Wild wolves deposit feces along trails within their pack's territory and on the territory's periphery. Lone wolves appear to use these droppings as signals to avoid entering the territory.[4] However, there is no evidence that dogs use feces in a similar manner. This may be more a function of the environment in which dogs are kept (i.e., walked on lead or confined to homes or fenced yards) than to changes in this behavior pattern. Studies of free-roaming dog populations are needed to further elucidate the role of feces as a communication signal in domestic dogs.

Anal sac secretions are discharged during defecation in all species of canid, including the dog. The anal sacs are a set of two glands located on each side of the anus. They empty into ducts that have openings close to the anal orifice and contain secretions from apocrine and sebaceous glands located within the walls of the ducts. The contents of the anal glands are discharged during defecation and contribute pheromones to the feces and anal region. Recent studies have shown that the anal gland secretions of dogs are highly individual in nature and may provide information about age, sex, and identity.[5,6] It is postulated that these secretions may be important for recognition of the individual and for territory marking. Studies with captive wolf packs indicate that deposition of anal gland secretions in feces is voluntary. Alpha males have the highest rate of secretion, and the rate increases when new wolves are introduced into the pack. This information supports the role of anal glands in territorial marking. Both wolves and dogs also occasionally express their anal glands independently of defecation when they are stressed or frightened.

Visual cues: The dog uses a series of complex, varied visual signals to communicate with other dogs and humans. These include eye contact, facial expressions, and body postures. Many of these cues are similar to those displayed by humans and so are often interpreted by owners to have similar meanings. Although in some cases this is appropriate and helpful, in others there is little or no correlation and the dog's signals may be seriously misinterpreted. For this reason, it is important to understand the species-specific communication signals of the dog and the context in which they are displayed.

Eye contact is an important form of communication in dogs. Dominant animals will initiate direct and prolonged eye contact with other dogs. This is commonly referred to as the "dominant stare." A subordinate animal will avert his gaze from this stare and will avoid direct eye contact with animals of higher rank. For example, when two dogs meet for the first time, they establish eye contact, and the dog that is more dominant will usually maintain contact longer than the more submissive of the two. Similarly, an adult dog will often stare at a puppy who, in turn, averts his gaze and shows submissive body postures. When carried to completion, these patterns of communication facilitate further social interactions and minimize chances of aggression. Conversely, if two dogs meet and one does not lower his gaze, the other may increase the show of dominance by baring his teeth or growling. Continued escalation without an aversion of gaze by one of the dogs can lead to overt aggression and a fight.

Although the dominant stare is important for establishing social ranking, dogs are quite capable of friendly eye contact that does not appear to be related to social ranking. This form of communication often is observed between familiar dogs and between dogs and their owners. Pairs or groups of dogs that live together and have a stable, established social group use dominant/submissive eye contact infrequently. This type of interaction usually is only seen during disputes over a desired resource such as a treasured toy, food, or possibly the owner's attention. More often, friendly and nonthreatening eye contact occurs during greeting, play, and social grooming. In these situations, the general rules applying to eye contact seem to be temporarily suspended. The dog's body postures display no threat, so staring can be used without the risk of confusion and without being interpreted as a dominance threat. Similarly, eye contact is an important component of interactions between dogs and humans. A prolonged and direct stare from a human is interpreted by dogs as a dominant stare, and most dogs react in the same manner they would with another dog. However, dogs who have established a secure, loving relationship with humans often use and accept friendly eye contact to communicate with owners and others. Examples include dogs that are soliciting attention, playing, or begging for food.

The positions of a dog's ears and mouth are important visual signals. When a dog is alert, the ears are shifted up and forward toward the stimulus (Figure 8.1). Similarly, the ears will be up and forward in a dog displaying dominance and will be back and down in a subordinate animal. During greeting and submissive displays, the ears usually are laid back against the head (Figure 8.2). The position of the mouth provides information about a dog's level of confidence and social status. The corners of the mouth are pulled forward into a snarl during displays of dominance aggression. In contrast, the lips are pulled back in the submissive "grin" in dogs displaying passive or active submission (Figure 8.2). During active submission, the dog may attempt to lick the mouth of the more dominant animal.

An animal that is showing dominance or is competing for a higher social status will demonstrate body postures that make it appear larger in size than it is. A dominant dog stands tall on his toes, carries his head high, has an ele-

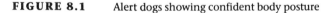

FIGURE 8.1   Alert dogs showing confident body posture

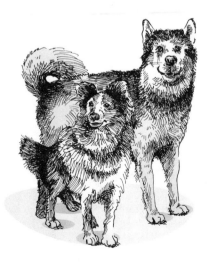

vated tail carriage (depending on the type and length of tail), and shows **pi-loerection** over the shoulders and back (Figures 8.2 and 8.3). As the dog becomes highly stimulated or aggressive, the tail begins to wag at a high frequency. If the display is directed toward another dog, the dominant dog may attempt to place his forepaws over the shoulders of the subordinate dog. Conversely, the body posture of a submissive dog serves to make the body appear smaller than it is. During active submission, a dog crouches low, tucks his tail, avoids eye contact, and may attempt to lick the face of the dominant dog or

FIGURE 8.2   Submissive postures: Active (top) and passive

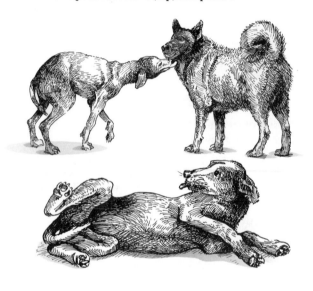

FIGURE 8.3   A dog showing dominance

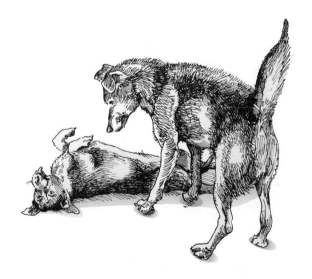

person. Some dogs raise a paw in a signal of appeasement. Many dogs demonstrate active submission during greeting. Extreme submission results in passive postural displays. The dog will lie down and roll partially onto his back, tuck his tail, turn his head away to prevent meeting eye contact, and may dribble urine (Figure 8.2).

Dogs that are extremely fearful and feel threatened show body postures that are a combination of dominance and submission. This often is referred to as "defensive aggression," or the posture of the "fear-biting" dog. Some describe this as depicting ambivalence, because the dog is both insecure and defensive. However, there is some disagreement among behaviorists concerning the frequency and the underlying cause of this posture.[7,8] Most describe the defensive threat posture as occurring in a dog that is fearful and who will attempt to flee before showing aggression. This dog shows the lower body

FIGURE 8.4   Defensive aggressive posture

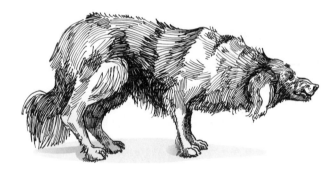

FIGURE 8.5   The play bow—an invitation to play

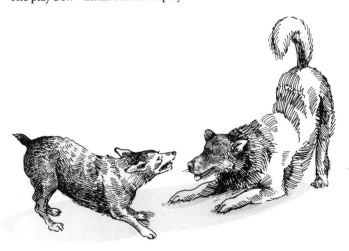

posture of submission but also has raised hackles and will growl or snarl at the threatening person or dog (Figure 8.4).

Another commonly observed body posture in dogs is the play bow (Figure 8.5). This body posture is displayed when a dog meets a person or dog with whom he is familiar or when he is inviting another to play. The dog lowers the forequarters while leaving the back legs extended and the rump raised. Dogs (and humans) interpret this as an invitation to play and often will respond with a similar bow or will immediately begin a chase and "catch-me" game. Other universal play signals include pawing with the front feet, the play "grin," and open-mouth panting. Both puppies and adult dogs use these postures to signal friendly intentions.

An important visual tool of the dog, but one that is poorly understood, is the tail wag. Some believe that tail wagging conveys a state of uncertainly or ambivalence. However, the fact that dogs wag their tails when confidently greeting humans or canine house mates does not support this theory.[9] Another theory maintains that tail wagging originated as a method of distributing the dog's scent more efficiently. Tail wagging may also serve as a visual cue to other dogs, signaling friendly intentions. Again, there are exceptions to this, as in the case of the dominant-aggressive dog whose tail wags rapidly immediately prior to fighting. The best explanation seems to be that tail wagging is a context-specific behavior used in a number of different situations and signals excitability or stimulation. Most owners readily recognize that a relaxed, wagging tail positioned level to or slightly above the dog's back indicates friendliness and confidence. The wagging tail of an anxious or nervous dog is held at a lower level or may even be tucked between the legs. A tail held very high and showing rapid, high-frequency wagging conveys a dominant threat and possibly impending aggression.

Auditory (vocal) cues: Vocal signaling has the advantage of being effective for long distances and when vision is impaired. Dogs are capable of a large range of sounds and use vocal communication frequently. Moreover, particular vocal signals are highly contextual and often convey very different messages depending on the situation in which they are used. Common dog vocalizations include grunts, growls, whines, barks, and howls. Grunts often are heard during greeting or as a sign of contentment or relaxation. Puppies typically grunt while they are feeding or sleeping, but many adult dogs retain this vocalization throughout their lives. Growls are used to signal defensive or offensive aggression or, in a modified form, playfulness. Whines and whimpers are produced by puppies and adolescent dogs to signal hunger, discomfort, or loneliness. Many adult dogs continue to show this type of vocalization in certain situations. Whining often is displayed during attention-seeking, greeting, or displays of submission. Whines and whimpers also may be elicited when a dog is fearful or in pain.

The domestic dog is unique among canids in its use of the bark. Although wolves do bark, they usually exhibit only one or two short barks followed by silence. Repetitive barking is unique to *Canis familiaris*. It has been suggested that during domestication, repetitive barking was desirable because it provided a method of signaling alarm or the approach of intruders. Barking may be a type of neotenized behavior, representing vestiges of puppy and adolescent vocalizations.[10] Dogs most often bark in defense of territory, when playing, when isolated, or as an attention-seeking behavior.

Wolves frequently howl as a form of auditory communication. Although all dogs are capable of howling, not all use this form of vocal communication. Wolves use the howl to seek contact with other pack members when separated or to assemble pack members prior to hunting or travel. Dogs usually howl when they are isolated. Howling in dogs appears to be a remnant of wolf behavior and may convey loneliness and an attempt to bring the dog's social group back together. Some dogs also howl in response to environmental sounds such as sirens, airplanes flying overhead, or certain types of music. The significance of this behavior is unknown. Some think that it may be related to the dog's ability to perceive frequencies of sound that are higher than those perceptible to humans.

Aggression

Aggression is one of the most frequently reported behavior problems in dogs. Often a dog that demonstrates aggression toward other dogs, people, or another species is considered to be abnormal in some way. However, aggression is a functional behavior for the dog and can be motivated by a variety of situations or conflicts. Aggressive behavior in dogs is context dependent. This means that the situation that the dog is in and the stimuli that are presented to the dog strongly influence aggressive responses. For example, a dog that is aggressive at the gate of her yard may not show this behavior in any other situation. Because aggression is a complex behavior with multiple causes, it has been helpful to categorize it into functional types. The most common forms of aggression are dominance, territorial, and possessive. Other forms include pain-elicited, maternal, intermale, and redirected aggression. Predatory behavior often is incorrectly described as a type of aggressive behavior but should be classified as a separate behavior pattern. Methods for solving aggression problems are discussed in Chapter 10.

Dominance aggression: Artificial selection for companion dogs resulted in the neotenization of many physical and behavioral traits (see Chapters 1 and 2). As a result, most dogs are naturally subordinate and demonstrate low levels of aggression. However, one objective in the breeding of some types of dogs was to create an animal that would protect territory or livestock. This selection resulted in dogs that possess an inherently more dominant nature and have increased levels of aggression. Although not all dominant dogs demonstrate dominance aggression, the potential for this type of aggressive response increases in dominant dogs as they reach social maturity.

Dominance aggression is expressed when a dominant dog reacts to an apparent challenge to his social status. In most cases, the circumstances that evoke aggression involve competition for valued resources. In dog-to-dog interactions, these may include food, a toy, a bone, or a favorite sleeping area. Dominance aggression between dogs also may be triggered when two dogs are competing for the attention of their owner. The dominance model predicts that the more dominant dog in a relationship will be more self-confident and will readily obtain desired resources. However, when a lower-ranking animal seeks to increase his or her status or competes for a specific resource, a dominance dispute may rapidly escalate into fighting. Dominance aggression directed toward humans involves circumstances in which the dog perceives the human as a threat to his or her social status. Most typically, this is in response to gestures or body postures that are perceived to be dominant by the dog. These may include standing over, physically reprimanding, or restraining the dog. Attempts to take a possession away may also trigger aggression in a dominant dog.

Territorial aggression: Like dominance and submission, territorial behavior is a normal canine behavior. Dogs that have a more dominant nature or are of a breed that has been selected to guard will display enhanced territorial behaviors. Some may react aggressively to intruders entering their home or yard. This can be explained by the theory that territory is a valuable resource that must be protected and competitively maintained. Although a dog's territory typically encompasses the owner's home and possibly the yard, some dogs demonstrate territorial aggression in areas where they are frequently walked or exercised. Dogs that guard their owner's car when they are inside are also displaying territorial aggression. As in the case of dominance, there are marked breed differences and individual variations in territorial behavior. Mild displays often can be controlled through training. However, if the dog is highly aggressive or if the behavior is encouraged by the owner, this type of aggression can be very difficult to modify once it is established.

In some cases, territorial aggression is motivated by fear or nervousness rather than dominance and self-confidence. A dog that feels vulnerable or unable to escape may learn to use aggression to drive off intruders. This type of territorial defense often is seen in poorly socialized dogs that have been confined to a small area or tied to a doghouse. In these cases, treatment focuses on decreasing the dog's fear and desensitizing the dog to visitors (see Chapter 10).

Possessive aggression: Possessive aggression often is classified as a subcategory of dominance aggression because it involves aggressive displays during competition for valued resources. For the pet dog, such resources typically include toys, food, or the owner's attention. However, some dogs fixate on unusual items such as pieces of tissue, articles of clothing, or even the television remote control. These situations often reflect learned behavior and are associated with a history of object-stealing by the dog. When an owner reacts by chasing or harshly reprimanding the dog, the dog learns to respond by guarding the stolen item.

Possessive aggression also can occur in dogs that have been compelled to guard their food from other animals or have learned to distrust humans who approach their food bowl. These dogs usually guard their food bowl defensively but show no other signs of possessive aggression. In these cases, this may be a learned behavior in response to limited access to food or competition with other animals. Some owners repeatedly remove their dog's food bowl while the dog is eating in the mistaken belief that this is an effective means of asserting dominance. However, this practice only serves to build distrust in the relationship with the dog and may cause the dog to begin to guard the bowl whenever a person approaches. Although all dogs should readily accept owners approaching their food bowls, repeated and arbitrary removal of the bowl sends a message to the dog that her access to food is unpredictable and, therefore, should be guarded.

Other types of aggression: The dog demonstrates two types of aggressive behavior that are gender-specific. Maternal aggression occurs in females with young litters who perceive a person or animal as a threat to their puppies. This type of aggression is not seen in all females and generally decreases after the puppies are several weeks old. Some male dogs demonstrate intermale aggression. This is probably a form of dominance aggression and is typically seen in intact males who greet other males with dominant body postures and stares. While neutering normally decreases the intensity of intermale aggression, it usually does not completely eliminate it.

Pain-elicited aggression occurs when a dog is injured or extremely frightened and reacts aggressively to being handled. This is similar to defensive or nervous aggression in which the dog reacts aggressively only when all attempts to escape have been impeded. Redirected aggression occurs when a dog that is aggressively motivated is prevented from directing aggression toward the targeted dog or human. The dog then "redirects" his aggression toward a person, dog, or even an inanimate object that is in close proximity. A common example of redirected aggression is the case in which a dog guards an entryway and bites the owner while being pulled away from the area.

Predation

Predatory behavior often is mislabeled as a type of aggression. For the wolf and other canids, predation is simply food acquisition, not a form of aggression. In canid species, the predatory sequence includes detection of prey (orientation), eyeing prey, stalking, chasing, grabbing bite, killing bite, dissecting bite, and consuming bite (feeding behavior). In contrast to aggressive behaviors, predatory behavior is typically quite silent and is not accompanied by growling or snarling. Although some dogs yip or bark when in pursuit of game, the killing bite is quiet. Like other behavior patterns, predation has been modified in the domestic dog through the processes of domestication and selective breeding.

In most breeds, the level of predatory response has been significantly reduced. However, in some breeds, certain aspects of predation have been selected and enhanced. For example, many hunting breeds excel at the detection of prey, but the stalk, chase, and bite portions of predation have been truncated from the sequence. In contrast, the stalking and chasing of herding breeds represent another segment of predatory behavior that has been modified through selective breeding. Terrier breeds have a high predatory response that includes the killing bite but not the dissecting or consuming bite. These breeds were developed to go to ground and kill rabbits, rodents, and other game. In all dogs, predatory behavior is not directly associated with hunger, but rather with the presence and movement of prey. Dogs that chase small animals, cars, children, or bikers are all demonstrating portions of the predatory sequence (i.e. stalk and chase).

Breed Differences in Behavior

The behavior of all animals is influenced by both environment and genetics. In the previous chapter the importance of environment during a dog's development was examined. Equally important in determining the behavior of an individual dog is the genetic makeup the dog is born with. Centuries of selective breeding have created numerous breeds of dog, many of which bear little physical resemblance to their wild wolf ancestor (see Chapter 2). In the same manner that selective breeding has affected physical appearance, it has altered behavior. Breed-specific behaviors reflect the varying purposes for which different types of dogs were developed. Some examples of these were described in the preceding paragraphs. Of greatest concern to most pet owners are breed characteristics of level of trainability, reactivity, and aggression.

Contrary to popular belief, genes do not directly code for certain behaviors. In reality, genes simply code for all of the amino acid sequences in an organism's protein molecules. The structural and biochemical effects of these molecules ultimately influence the development, organization, physiology, and behavior of an individual. No specific gene, or even set of genes, has been found that causes aggressive behavior, predatory instinct, or any other type of species-specific behavior pattern.[11] Genes influence behavior by setting limits on the components of a behavior, the time period during development at which it occurs, and the relative thresholds for stimulus and intensity.[12] In their raw forms, these patterns are inherited and instinctual (i.e. not learned), but are subsequently influenced by learning. General consistency exists between all dogs in visual, auditory, and olfactory communication patterns. With few exceptions, individuals of different breeds have no difficulty recognizing one another as members of the same species and instinctively present species-specific communication cues to one another. However, depending on the original function for which a breed or breed type was developed, different dogs display certain behavior patterns or even portions of patterns in variable manners or to varying degrees of intensity.

Physical effects upon behavior: An important way in which genetics influence behavior is through the determination of physical structure. All behavior depends on the physical capabilities of an animal. For example, a dog could not show a dominant stare if it did not have an eye type that allowed this. Similarly, the submissive grin would not be possible without the necessary facial muscles. Since genes are responsible for these structures, it follows that all behavior is physically influenced by genetics. As a species, the domestic dog is highly unusual in the range of structural differences that occur between individuals. A St. Bernard stands 40 inches at the shoulder and can weigh much more than 150 pounds. By comparison, a tiny Chihuahua stands less than 6 inches and weighs less than 5 pounds. The long, slender legs and deep chest of the Greyhound contribute to its ability to hunt using its eyesight. In contrast, the short thick legs of the Basset Hound contribute to this breed's talent as a scent trailer (see Chapter 2). The physical attributes of a particular breed are closely tied to the breed's original function and so influence the behaviors that are necessary to carry out that function.

Recently, it has been suggested that the physical traits of dogs may affect behavior in a second way.[13] Physical alterations in appearance may significantly affect the ability to send and perceive species-specific communication signals. Visually, the dog uses body postures, facial expressions, and eye contact to communicate to others. Some breeds possess physical traits that may interfere with or even prohibit their ability to send or receive these signals. The presence of a thick, abundant coat may impede a dog's ability to show dominant and submissive body postures, hackle raising, or eye contact. Ears that are positioned lower on the head, have a pendulous pinnae (flap), or are artificially cropped may all alter facial expressions. Curled tails and naturally or artificially docked tails inhibit normal tail wagging and distort the visual signal of a raised or lowered tail. Excessive skin folds or hair around the face and eyes may alter ability to show normal facial expressions and eye contact.

The importance of these differences in the ability to communicate with other dogs is not known. However, these changes do interfere with the ability of humans to interpret dogs' signals. It has been suggested that these distortions may not be as important in dog-to-dog interactions because the domestic dog also relies on olfactory signals from other dogs.[14,15]

Inheritance of temperament: In addition to effects upon physical traits, genetics also influence an animal's reactivity, trainability, and ability to learn from the environment. The heritability of temperament in animals was first demonstrated in a classic study of maze learning in rats.[16] Researchers found that certain rats were consistently successful in finding their way through a maze for a food reward, while others were unsuccessful in learning the maze, even after repeated training sessions. The "maze-smart" rats were selected as breeding pairs and mated for several generations. The same process was repeated with "maze-dull" rats. After several generations, two distinct lines of rats developed: those that rapidly learned to run a maze and those that repeatedly failed at maze learning. Statistically significant differences in ability to learn maze running were found in the two lines. Further studies showed that the maze-smart rats were strongly food-motivated and were not intimidated by mechanical devices, while maze-dull rats were less motivated by food and were timid of new environments. This research provided an impetus for the study of the inheritance of learning in other species. Subsequent studies have shown that genetics plays a role in various types of aggression, courtship, and mating behavior, and displays of emotion.

In the mid-1960s, Scott and Fuller studied the genetic basis for temperament differences in five breeds of dogs: Basenjis, Beagles, Cocker Spaniels, Shetland Sheepdogs, and Wire-haired Fox Terriers.[17] Differences between breeds were seen in a number of characteristics, including emotional reactivity, trainability, and problem-solving abilities. Terriers, Basenjis, and Beagles showed greater reactivity to restraint than Shetland Sheepdogs and Cocker Spaniels. Training tests included teaching the dogs to remain quiet while sitting on a scale, walk on a lead, and stay on a table until verbally released. Results of this series of tests suggested that Cocker Spaniels were easiest to train, while Basenjis and Beagles were most difficult to teach these commands. Problem-solving tests showed varying results relative to the type of task that was given to the dog. Scott and Fuller's work provided the basis for the theory that heredity significantly affects the expression of emotional behavior in dogs and that breed differences exist in emotional behavior and trainability.

The inheritance of specific behavior patterns has also been studied in dogs. In one study, the artificial selection for nervous temperament in a group of Pointers produced a line of dogs that were hesitant to explore new areas, tended to freeze in response to novel sounds, and avoided contact with humans.[18] A "non-fearful" line of dogs was bred simultaneously, and individuals of that line did not show these traits. Cross-fostering fearful puppies with normal mothers and normal puppies with fearful mothers showed that maternal behavior minimally affected the level of fearfulness in the puppies. Attempts to decrease nervousness through socialization and training also met with limited success. Recent evidence has shown that inherited differences in temperament may be related to differences in the distributions and quantities of certain types of neurochemicals.[19] Comparisons between herding dogs, livestock-guarding dogs, and sled dogs found that the more lethargic livestock-guarding dogs had lower levels of the neurotransmitter dopamine than levels produced by more reactive Border Collies and sled dogs.

The inheritance of aggressive behavior in dogs is of great interest to companion animal professionals. Breed differences are well documented in the literature, but controlled studies of the inheritance of aggression are lacking. For example, a line of Bernese Mountain Dogs in Holland has been reported to exhibit extreme dominance aggression, while other lines of the same breed do not appear to have this behavior problem. High levels of territorial aggression and nervous aggression have been reported in German Shepherd Dogs. The Cocker Spaniel, English Cocker Spaniel and English Springer Spaniel exhibit a phenomenon that has been commonly referred to as "rage syndrome" or "low threshold aggression." This problem has been shown to be more common in blonde Cockers than in other colors, and particular lines tend to have a higher incidence.[20] A recent study of more than 1,000 English Cocker Spaniels found that this breed does have a relatively high incidence of aggression and that "rage syndrome" appears to be an expression of social dominance.[21] Because of a lack of controlled breeding studies in other breeds, the degree to which aggression is inherited in the domestic dog is unclear.

Controlled breeding programs at institutions that train guide dogs and other types of service dogs have been useful in providing information about the heritability of certain temperament traits in dogs. When Guide Dogs for the Blind, located in San Rafael, California, began its training program, dogs that began the training had a very low success rate.[22] In an attempt to improve their training success, the organization instituted a breeding program that selected successful dogs for breeding. Within a five-year period, the success rate increased from 30 percent to 60 percent. Heritability scores can be calculated from controlled breeding studies such as these. These scores provide an estimate of the proportion of phenotypic variability that is attributable to genetic influences. A study of guide dogs in Australia estimated the heritability of nervousness to be between 0.47 and 0.58. These values are interpreted to mean that between 47 and 58 percent of the variability between dogs in the trait of nervousness can be attributed to genetic factors. Another study of guide dog breeding programs reported that sound sensitivity and body sensitivity were the most highly heritable traits observed in dogs selected for these tasks.[23]

General temperament characteristics of breeds: When selecting a dog for a pet, most prospective owners are interested in breed differences in temperament. A well-publicized study was conducted in the late 1980s that attempted to identify behavior characteristics that would provide maximum discrimination among different breeds of dogs.[24] The study surveyed 96 veterinarians and dog obedience judges regarding the behavior characteristics of 56 popular AKC recognized breeds. Thirteen different behavior characteristics were identified and ranked. Traits that were believed to be specifically important to pet owners were selected. These included dominance, territorial behavior, affection, destructiveness, demand for affection, sociability toward children, and emotional excitability. Tabulated results showed that four major traits exhibited pronounced breed differences. These were excitability, general activity level, tendency to snap at children, and excessive barking. In contrast, ease of housebreaking, destructiveness, and demand for affection showed less pronounced differences between breeds. These results indicate that some behavior traits in dogs may have a stronger genetic influence than others.

The researchers grouped behavior traits into three major components that accounted for most of the variation between breeds: reactivity, aggression, and trainability. Behaviors that were included with reactivity included excitability, demand for affection, tendency to snap at children, and general activity level. Components of the aggression category included territorial defense, watchdog barking, aggression toward dogs, and tendency for dominance over the owner. Obedience training success and housebreaking ease were included within the trainability category. To facilitate practical use of their results, the researchers grouped breeds into a series of 10 categories based on their ratings in excitability and watchdog barking. They subsequently published a book that is intended to help owners in breed selection and that categorizes breeds according to the results of this study.[25]

In Chapter 2, breeds of dogs were categorized according to their original uses to humans. These included spitz, mastiff, sight hound, scent hound, terrier, gundog, livestock-herding, livestock-guarding, and toy breeds. Although breeds and, certainly, individuals vary greatly in specific temperament characteristics and trainability, it is true that a dog's breed has a profound influence on an individual's temperament. Some generalities about temperament and trainability also can be inferred by examining these various groups of dogs.

The spitz breeds include sled dogs and other arctic breeds. Because they were required to work in groups with a team effort, sled dogs were selected to show minimal hierarchal behaviors toward one another. This trait allows them to run as a team and facilitates switching to different positions on the team. However, the fact that usually one lead dog is selected indicates that dominance hierarchies are still present in these dogs to some degree. In addition, most sled dogs were kept primarily as outdoor dogs with a strict "working" relationship with the owner. As a result, these breeds often are referred to as being fairly independent or aloof in their relationships with people. They show low to moderate reactivity, aggression, and trainability.

The mastiff breeds are considered to be the ancestors of many of the working breeds of today that have been developed to protect and guard people and homesteads. Protectiveness is actually a form of territorial behavior (or possessive behavior). Because dogs with a dominant nature are more naturally territorial, individuals of these breeds tend to be relatively dominant. Because they often have been required to actively protect by warning attacking intruders, the working breeds are high in reactivity and moderate to high in aggression. These dogs tend to bond strongly to one owner or family and, when raised in a structured environment, are highly trainable.

Herding breeds were developed to move livestock. Herding instinct is actually a form of predatory behavior. The instinctual predatory sequence is complete and exaggerated up to the chase response. However, the grabbing and killing bite are inhibited and have been strongly selected against in herding dogs. In general, it is difficult to alter biting behavior in individuals that do show a bite response, and so dogs that nip or bite at livestock have not been selected for breeding. Herding breeds are considered to be highly trainable and will bond very strongly to their human caretakers. Because of their need to respond quickly to movements and changes in the behavior of the herd, these breeds also are highly reactive.

Livestock-guarding dogs were developed in central Europe to protect sheep flocks from predators. Most of these dogs are very large in size and white or light tan in color. Examples include the Great Pyrenees, Anatolian, Akbash, and Maremma. Unlike the herding dogs, livestock-guarding dogs have been selected to show little or no predatory behavior. They do not demonstrate prey orientation or stalk in response to movement. In fact, as puppies, most will not even chase a ball or toy. In general, livestock-guarding dogs have low to moderate reactivity, low trainability, and moderate aggression. Although they do have the ability to guard aggressively, much of their effectiveness as a deterrent to wild predators is due simply to their imposing size and presence within the herd.

Certain components of predatory behavior also are seen in retrievers, pointers, setters, and spaniels. Hunting dogs that are bred for indicating and retrieving game are highly trainable, reactive, and possess low levels of aggression. Early studies of the heritability of hunting traits such as pointing ability and performance in field trials indicated that these are very complex characteristics with low heritabilities.[26] However, more recent studies of several hunting breeds showed that hunting eagerness and other traits are heritable and that several important traits tend to be inherited together.[27] Trainability is important in these breeds because their success relies upon responding correctly to signals from the hunter. Predatory sequence in pointers and retrievers includes the grabbing bite (this is part of the retrieve) but not the killing bite or dissecting bite.

Terriers were developed to find and kill small rodents and other animals farmers and ranchers considered to be pest species. These breeds work with little or no direction from their handler and are required to immediately kill the game upon catching it. These two requirements have resulted in breeds that have low to medium trainability, high reactivity, and high levels of aggression. In general, terriers show increased interdog aggression as well as an exaggerated predatory response.

Both the sight hound and scent hound breeds were developed as hunting dogs, but they worked in very different terrains and were used to hunt different game animals. The sight hounds were developed to follow their quarry using eyesight and to chase down and eventually capture their prey. Not only are these dogs built physically for speed, but they also possess a strong predatory chase instinct. In many individuals, the grabbing and killing bite are still part of the predatory sequences. The sight hounds worked independently of the hunter, and, as a result, these breeds are usually considered to be fairly independent or even aloof in nature. However, several sight hounds, such as the Greyhound and Whippet, are also known for their extremely gentle, quiet disposition. Most are relatively silent dogs, since barking while chasing game was not a desirable trait for these breeds.

The scent hounds were developed to trail their quarry using their sense of smell. These dogs are physically built for endurance, not speed, and their body structure is also conducive to traveling long distances with their noses to the ground. These breeds have a low level of reactivity and, generally, are rather lethargic and stoic as pets. They show low levels of aggression and are considered to be low to moderately trainable. Because the trailing breeds were required to signal to the hunter when they were on a scent, most have developed a distinctive howl or bay that is used when hunting.

Many of the toy breeds represent miniaturizations of other breeds. In some cases, they may retain the behavior characteristics of their larger forefathers. In others, a more subordinate nature was selected along with the neotenized features. The toys were probably the first true companion dogs, and many of these breeds reflect this in their strong predisposition to bonding to humans, puppylike behaviors, and high trainability.

Conclusions

Although the dog was originally domesticated from the wolf and has inherited its social nature from this wild ancestor, the domestic dog, *Canis familiaris,* has its own unique set of behavior patterns. Understanding canine communication and how dogs interact with both other dogs and their human caretakers is important for dog owners and professionals who handle and work with dogs on a daily basis. This information also provides the base for understanding canine learning and solving common behavior problems in dogs, topics that are examined in the following two chapters.

Cited References

1. Fox, M.W. *The Dog: Its Domestication and Behavior.* Garland STPM Press, New York, New York. (1978)

2. Borchelt, P.L. and Voith, V.L. **Dominance aggression in dogs.** In: *Readings in Companion Animal Behavior,* (V.L. Voith and P.L. Borchelt, editors), Veterinary Learning Systems, Trenton, New Jersey, pp. 230-239. (1996)

3. Peters, R.P. and Mech, L.D. **Scent-marking in wolves.** American Scientist, 63:628-637. (1975)

4. Mech, L.D. *The Wolf: The Ecology and Behavior of an Endangered Species,* Natural History Press, New York, New York. (1970)

5. Bradshaw, J.W.S., Natynczuk, S.E., and Macdonald, D.W. **Potential applications of anal sac volatiles from domestic dogs.** In: *Chemical Signals in Vertebrates,* Fifth Edition (D.W. MacDonald, D.Muller-Schwarze, and S.E. Natynczuk, editors), Oxford University Press, Oxford, United Kingdom, pp. 640-644. (1990)

6. Natynczuk, S.E. Bradshaw, J.W.S., and Macdonald, D.W. **Chemical constituents of the anal sacs of domestic dogs.** Biochemical Systematics and Ecology, 17:83-87. (1989)

7. Abrantes, R. **The expression of emotions in man and canid.** In: *Canine Development Throughout Life,* Waltham Symposium, No. 8 (A.T.B. Edney, editor), Journal of Small Animal Practice, 28:1030-1036. (1987)

8. Nott, H.M.R. **Social behaviour of the dog.** In: *The Waltham Book of Dog and Cat Behaviour* (C. Thorne, editor), Pergamon Press, Oxford, United Kingdom, pp. 97-114. (1992)

9. Morris, Desmond. *Dog Watching,* Crown Publishers, New York, New York, (1987)

10. Coppinger, R.P. and Feinstein, M. **Why dogs bark.** Smithsonian Magazine, January: 119-129. (1991)

11. Coppinger, R. and Coppinger, L. **Biological basis of behavior of domestic dog breeds.** From: *Readings in Companion Animal Behavior* (V.L. Voith and P.L. Borchelt, editors), Veterinary Learning Systems, Trenton, New Jersey, pp. 9-18. (1996)

12. Estep, D.Q. **The ontogeny of behavior.** In: *Readings in Companion Animal Behavior* (V.L. Voith and P.L. Borchelt, editors), Veterinary Learning Systems, Trenton, New Jersey, pp. 19-31. (1996)

13. Bradshaw, J.W.S., Wickens, S.M., and Goodwin, D. **Dogs and wolves: Do they really speak the same language?** Association of Pet Behaviour Counselors' Newsletter. (1994)

14. Beaver, B.V. **Friendly communications by the dog.** Veterinary Medicine: Small Animal Clinician, 76:647-649. (1981)

15. Blackshaw, J.K. **Human and animal inter-relationships. Review Series 3: Normal behaviour patterns of dogs. Part 1.** Australian Veterinary Practitioner, 15:110-112. (1985)

16. Tryon, R.C. **Genetic differences in maze-learning ability in rats.** In: *39th Yearbook of the National Society for the Study of Education,* Public School Publishing Company, Bloomington, Indiana, pp. 111-119. (1940)

17. Scott, J.P. and Fuller, J.L. *Genetics and the Social Behavior of the Dog.* University of Chicago Press, Chicago, Illinois. (1965)

18. Dykman, R.A., Murphree, O.D., and Reese, W.G. **Familial anthropophobia in pointer dogs?** Archives of Genetics and Psychiatry, 36:988-993. (1979)

19. Arons, C.D. and Shoemaker, W.J. **The distribution of catecholamines and beta-endorphin in the brain of three behaviorally distinct breeds of dogs and their F1 hybrids.** Brain Research, 594:31-39. (1992)

20. Mugford, R.A. **Aggressive behaviour in the English Cocker Spaniel.** The Veterinary Annual, 24:310-314. (1984)

21. Podberscek, A.L. and Serpell, J.A. **The English Cocker Spaniel: Preliminary findings on aggressive behaviour.** Applied Animal Behaviour Science, 47:750-89. (1996)

22. Falt, L. **Inheritance of behaviour in the dog.** In: *Nutrition and Behaviour in Dogs and Cats* (R.S. Anderson, editor), Pergamon Press, Oxford, United Kingdom, pp. 183-187. (1984)

23. Bartlett, C.R. **Heritabilities and genetic correlations between hip dysplasia and temperament traits of seeing-eye dogs.** Master's Thesis, Rutgers University, New Brunswick, New Jersey. (1976)

24. Hart, B.L. and Hart, L.A. **Selecting pet dogs on the basis of cluster analysis of breed behavior profiles and gender.** Journal of the American Veterinary Medical Association, 186: 1181-1185. (1985)

25. Hart, B.L. and Hart, L.A. *The Perfect Puppy: How to Choose Your Dog by Its Behavior.* W.H. Freeman and Company, New York, New York. (1988)

26. Burns, M. and Fraser, M.N. *Genetics of the Dog: The Basis of Successful Breeding.* Oliver and Boyd, Edinburgh, Scotland. (1966)

27. Vangen, O. and Klemetsdal, G. **Genetic studies of Finnish and Norwegian test results in two breeds of hunting dog.** VI World Conference on Animal Production, Helsinki, Sweden, Paper 4.25. (1988)

9 Learning Processes and Training Principles

DOGS BEGIN TO LEARN as soon as they are capable of receiving and processing information. Maturation of the puppy's special senses and neurological system begins during the transitional period of development. By the time of weaning, the puppy's brain is capable of receiving and processing information from all of the special senses. Learning involves an enduring change in behavior in response to stimuli in the environment. It occurs through several processes. The major types of learning observed in dogs include habituation and sensitization, classical conditioning, operant conditioning, and social learning. A dog's ability to learn also is influenced by numerous intrinsic and extrinsic factors. These must be considered when attempting to teach new behaviors or to stop unwanted behaviors in puppies and adult dogs.

Habituation and Sensitization

Habituation: All animals are born with a set of species-specific behavior patterns that serve to protect them from harm. In *Canis familiaris*, this includes visual orientation to new stimuli, followed by either investigation, flight, freeze, or fight responses. These responses had adaptive value for the dog's wolf ancestors because they increased chances of survival in an unpredictable and often hazardous environment. Although domestication has removed most natural hazards, the domestic dog retains these innate responses. Habituation occurs when an animal learns to distinguish between relevant and irrelevant stimuli in the environment. In general, relevant stimuli are those that have the potential to either harm or benefit the animal in some way. Irrelevant stimuli are those that are of no consequence to the animal and so can be screened out from its perceptual world. Habituation occurs when a decrease in responsiveness is produced by the repeated presence of a stimulus that is innocuous or irrelevant to the animal. This allows the dog to sort out which things to ignore in its environment and which to attend to. For example, a new puppy may be initially startled by the sound of the vacuum cleaner running in the house but slowly becomes habituated to the sound after repeated exposures.

Habituation develops in two stages. Short-term habituation occurs when a dog is exposed to the stimuli repeatedly but for a relatively short period of time. For example, exposure to a moving vacuum cleaner in several rooms of the house for a 30-minute period may result in short-term habituation. At the end of this time, the puppy may completely ignore the noise and presence of the vacuum cleaner. However, if the vacuum is reintroduced the following day, the puppy may once again show a startle or fear response. This is called spontaneous recovery. Long-term habituation occurs when many repetitions of the stimulus no longer evoke a response in the dog.

Dog trainers who instruct their clients to socialize their puppies to new places, people, and experiences are actually describing habituation. Taking puppies for numerous car rides, introducing them to different people, and walking with them in new areas are all training methods that result in habituation. Habituation is an important form of learning in young dogs and occurs more readily in puppies than in adults. A lack of habituation, especially in mature dogs, can be a serious problem. Examples of unhabituated fears or anxiety reactions include a dog who is fearful of children, car rides, or other dogs simply as a result of never having been exposed to these stimuli.

Sensitization: This type of learning represents the polar opposite of habituation. Sensitization occurs when repeated exposure to a stimulus results in an increase in responsiveness. In dogs, sensitization usually involves either fearful (freeze or flight) or aggressive (fight) responses. For example, a new puppy who sees a cat for the first time may approach the cat with curiosity. If the cat is not habituated to dogs, she may swat at the puppy. Repeated exposures to this kind of swatting may sensitize the puppy to the cat. Future meetings may elicit a fearful reaction in the puppy, characterized by the puppy attempting to run away (flight) or cower (freeze). Generalization to similar stimuli is common. In this case, the puppy may become fearful of all cats. The effects of sensitization are less stimulus-specific than habituation. This means that any small change in a stimulus can lead to sensitization, even if the dog was previously habituated to the stimulus. For example, the puppy who was habituated to the vacuum cleaner may suddenly become sensitized to the machine if it malfunctions and makes a much louder noise or moves erratically. Similarly, a dog who had been completely habituated to car rides may become sensitized if involved in a traffic accident while riding with her owner. As a general rule of thumb, intense stimuli usually lead to sensitization and weaker stimuli lead to habituation.

Classical Conditioning

Classical conditioning involves learning about relationships between two or more stimuli. The basic elements of this type of learning are a meaningless stimulus that initially elicits no response and a meaningful stimulus that does elicit a response. Consistent pairing of the two stimuli, with the meaningless signal preceding the meaningful signal, leads to classical conditioning. The animal learns that the first stimulus predicts the second and begins to show the same or similar response to the first that it initially showed only to the second. This is called a stimulus-stimulus association and forms the basic axiom of classical conditioning.

In its simplest form, classical conditioning involves innate responses such as fear, anxiety, or pleasure. For example, most dogs show excitement at mealtime. Their anticipation usually is accompanied by increased activity, salivation, and vocalizations. The unconditioned (meaningful) stimulus is simply the presence of the dog's food. A neutral (meaningless) stimulus may be the owner asking "Do you want to eat?" immediately before presenting the dog's food. Initially, this question alone will not evoke a response (i.e. it is a neutral stimulus). However, over time, the dog begins to associate this spoken cue with the bowl of food that immediately follows and responds in the same manner that it does to the actual presence of food. The question "Do you want to eat?" is now a conditioned stimulus because it evokes the same response as the actual presence of food, even if the food bowl is not present (Figure 9.1).

Early research studies of classical conditioning examined only the conditioning of involuntary responses and simple reflexes. However, practical applications of classical conditioning in dog training include more complex responses that have both involuntary and voluntary components. Specifically, techniques that facilitate this type of learning can be used to teach dogs to respond positively to stressful situations. For example, many puppies and adolescent dogs resist grooming because they become overstimulated by handling or by the feel of the brush. The pleasurable emotions that are associated with eating (unconditioned stimulus) can be paired with the presence of the brush (neutral stimulus). If introduced gradually, the dog eventually begins to associate being brushed and handled with food and positive experiences.

The timing with which stimuli are presented to the dog is an important factor in classical conditioning. The neutral (conditioned) stimulus should be presented immediately before and, if possible, overlapping with the unconditioned stimulus. This facilitates the development of a connection between the two stimuli. If the conditioned stimulus is presented after the unconditioned stimulus, learning proceeds slowly, if at all. For example, a dog can learn to eliminate on command through classical conditioning. Unconditioned stimuli include internal signs and external events that trigger eliminative behavior, such as eating, waking up after a nap, or sniffing an area that was previously used for elimination. The conditioned stimuli include taking the dog outside and the owner's command, "hurry up." To facilitate classical conditioning (i.e. create a relationship between the command and other stimuli that signal elimination), the dog should be presented with the com-

---

FIGURE 9.1   Classical conditioning

Unconditioned Stimulus → → → → → →   **Unconditioned Response**
    Food   Activity, Salivation, Vocalization

Conditioned Stimulus → → → → → → →   **Conditioned Response**
   "Do you want to eat?"   Activity, Salivation, Vocalization

mand immediately before urinating or defecating. The command can be repeated several times while the dog is circling or sniffing an area of the yard used for elimination. If, however, the command is not given until the dog is already in the process of elimination, classical conditioning usually will not occur. For greatest success, the pairing of the two stimuli must also be predictable and consistent. The dog always hears the command immediately before eliminating, and the command is always given using the same words and in the same tone of voice.

Operant Conditioning (Instrumental Learning)

Learning that occurs as a result of the effects (or consequences) that the dog's behavior has is called operant conditioning or instrumental learning. This terminology originates from the concept that behaving animals are constantly "operating on" their environment and subsequently alter their behavior in response to the consequences. The basic premise is that positive and negative consequences affect the frequency with which the animal will engage in a behavior in the future. If an action results in a pleasurable consequence (positive reinforcement) or in the cessation of an aversive consequence (negative reinforcement), the probability of the animal repeating the action is increased. If an action is paired with punishment, the probability of the action being repeated is decreased. The process involves learning stimulus-response and response-consequence relations (Figure 9.2). The dog learns an association between (1) a stimuli and (2) a relationship between a response and a consequence.[1]

Reinforcement and punishment: Four types of response-consequence relationships (or contingencies) are possible in operant conditioning. A consequence that causes an increase in behavior is called reinforcement; a consequence that causes a decrease in behavior is called punishment.[2] Positive reinforcement occurs when a behavior produces a pleasant stimulus. For dogs, typical positive reinforcers include food, praise, petting, social interactions, affectionate eye contact, and play. In contrast, a behavior that results in the prevention or termination of an unpleasant stimulus is said to be negatively reinforced. Commonly used negative reinforcers in dog training include collar corrections, verbal reprimands, and harsh eye contact. There are

FIGURE 9.2   Operant conditioning

Unconditioned Stimulus → →	**Unconditioned Response** → →	**Consequence**
Food treat held in front of nose	Sit	Eating food treat
Conditioned Stimulus → → → →	**Conditioned Response** → → → →	**Consequence**
Verbal command "sit"	Sit	Eating food treat

two types of punishment. Positive punishment occurs when a behavior produces an aversive consequence. Typical punishments used with dogs include a sharp word, a swat, a jerk on the lead, or any other stimulus that a particular dog finds unpleasant or aversive. A behavior that results in the prevention or termination of a pleasant stimulus that was already present or was imminent is being negatively punished (Table 9.1).

Practical dog training usually includes some combination of these four response-consequence contingencies. For example, most basic dog obedience classes include instructions for teaching a dog to stay in position while sitting (a sit-stay exercise). Positive reinforcement of this behavior may include providing quiet praise, petting, or food treats while the dog remains in the desired position. Movements from this position are ignored or prevented. In contrast, negative reinforcement of sit-stay involves giving a collar jerk or a harsh reprimand whenever the dog moves away from the correct position. Because negative reinforcement consists of the cessation of the negative stimulus when the desired behavior is offered, the collar corrections or reprimands are continuous when the dog is not in the correct position and immediately stop when the dog sits and stays.

Punishment functions primarily to stop behavior, not to increase the frequency of behavior. Punishment often is used when owners attempt to teach a young puppy not to nip or bite while playing. Using a physical or verbal reprimand (negative stimulus) whenever the dog begins to nip is an example of positive punishment. In contrast, withholding interactions and play with the owner whenever nipping begins constitutes negative punishment. The difference between reinforcement and punishment in these two examples is that reinforcement targets a specific behavior that is desirable (i.e. sit-stay). Punishment is not concerned with increasing behavior but rather with stopping a behavior (Table 9.1).

TABLE 9.1   Reinforcement vs. Punishment

Reinforcing Staying and Punishing Nipping

	Positive (addition of stimulus)	**Negative** (removal of stimulus)
Reinforcement (increases behavior)	Quiet praise, petting, and food treats provided while maintaining sit-stay; movements out of position are ignored	Collar jerks, verbal reprimands given whenever dog moves from sit-stay and terminated when dog maintains stay
Punishment (decreases behavior)	Physical corrections(muzzle shake, swat) or verbal reprimands when puppy begins to nip	Removal of interaction with owner and cessation of play when puppy begins to nip

Escape/avoidance approach: Practical dog training methods developed shortly after World War II were based primarily on the use of negative reinforcement and punishment.[3,4] These programs were the foundation for what became known as "escape-avoidance" training. An aversive stimulus was applied whenever the dog offered unwanted behavior (for example, collar jerks as a consequence for pulling on the lead). During the learning phase the dog could escape this aversive consequence by changing her behavior (not pulling on the lead or staying in position). As the dog learned the contingencies associated with the negative reinforcement, she would begin to avoid the negative stimulus by continually offering the desired behavior and by not engaging in undesirable behaviors. Similarly, the correction-based training methods of this period included various forms of punishment for stopping unwanted behaviors.

Escape-avoidance conditioning relies upon the dog's natural avoidance behaviors. The exact nature of an avoidance response, however, is highly variable.[5] Although most dogs will move away from an aversive stimulus if there is an escape route available, others may show submission, freeze in place, or become aggressive. As a result, the risk is that the response of the dog is not always predictable or desirable. Negative reinforcement only provides the animal with information about what *not* to do but does not provide information about what *to do*. Essentially, the dog learns through the process of elimination. She attempts a variety of different behaviors to escape the aversive stimulus until it is successful in turning off the unpleasant stimulus. In the case of teaching sit-stay, the dog may try to run, lie down submissively, or become fearful or aggressive, rather than freezing (i.e. staying) in response to the collar corrections. In short, negative reinforcement relies on the dog's ability to select an appropriate behavior to escape the negative stimulus. Because stress or fear often are introduced with the use of negative reinforcement and punishment, the elicited behavior may not be the behavior the trainer is attempting to increase. Furthermore, just as in humans, stress and fear often interfere with the dog's ability to learn.

Positive reinforcement approach: New knowledge about canine behavior and learning has led to an increase in the use of positive reinforcement in training and behavior modification programs. Many dog training and behavior books that have been written within the past 10 years focus on positive reinforcement, extinction, and shaping.[6,7,8,9,10,11,12] Positive reinforcement and extinction have been found to be more effective in modifying behavior than negative reinforcement and punishment. Positive reinforcement provides specific information to the dog about the exact behavior that is desired. For example, when teaching a sit-stay, food and praise are provided *only* while the dog is sitting and are simply withheld if the dog moves or changes position. For an exuberant puppy or adolescent, a food treat (an unconditioned stimulus) can initially be used as a prompt to elicit the sit-stay, further increasing the chance of the dog's success (Table 9.1).

Unlike negative reinforcement and punishment, positive reinforcement is not associated with stress, fear, or avoidance behaviors. These emotions can interfere with and even prevent effective learning, ultimately slowing down the training process and damaging the relationship between the dog and her owner. The use of positive reinforcement has the added advantage of enhancing the bond and mutual attachment that exist between owners and their dogs. Positive reinforcement also lends itself well to successive approximation, while negative reinforcement does not. This facilitates teaching complex behaviors and exercises that require a great deal of control. It is beyond the scope of this book to provide instructions for practical dog training. However, the reference list of Part II provides a list of training books that use operant conditioning techniques and emphasize the use of positive reinforcement.

Timing: Just as with classical conditioning, the timing with which stimuli and reinforcers are presented to the dog is an important consideration with operant conditioning. Laboratory studies have shown that the timing of positive and negative reinforcement must occur within 1 second or less after the occurrence of the behavior to be effective as a teaching tool.[13] Learning occurs most rapidly if there is some overlap between the behavior and its consequence. If reinforcement follows the behavior by more than 1 second, the animal often is already engaging in another behavior, and it is this behavior that is reinforced. For example, if positive reinforcement (petting, praise, food treats) is provided while the dog is sitting, this is the behavior that will be reinforced. However, if the owner waits too long and praises the dog as he stands up or lies down, then this movement is reinforced.

Schedules of reinforcement must also be considered. When a dog is initially learning a desired response, learning occurs most rapidly if every correct response that is offered is positively reinforced. This is called a continuous reinforcement schedule. Once the behavior has been established, it is best maintained with an intermittent reinforcement schedule. Intermittent schedules involve reinforcing only some correct responses. An analogy of this concept is gambling behavior in humans. A person who is addicted to the slot machines of Las Vegas is responding to an intermittent schedule of reinforcement. Slot-machine-playing behavior is strongly maintained because it is occasionally and unpredictably reinforced by the arrival of money. Similarly, a dog who has been trained to come when called will continue to offer this behavior in anticipation of possibly receiving reinforcement.

Several types of schedules of intermittent reinforcement can be used. These include fixed ratio, fixed interval, variable ratio and variable interval (Table 9.2). In general all types of intermittent reinforcement schedules produce stronger responses of learned behavior than continuous reinforcement schedules. Interestingly, many problem behaviors in dogs are unknowingly maintained by owners who are using an intermittent schedule of reinforcement. For example, the dog who barks for attention during dinnertime often has been fed tidbits at variable times, reinforcing (and often strengthening) this behavior.

TABLE 9.2	Reinforcement Schedules
Continuous	Reinforcement is provided for every correct response
Variable Interval	Reinforcement is provided at irregular time intervals (For example: A food treat is given to a dog during a sit-stay exercise at 30, 40, 90, 200, and 240 seconds)
Fixed Interval	Reinforcement is provided at regular time intervals (For example: A food treat is given to a dog during a sit-stay exercise at 30, 60, 90, 120, 150, 180, 210, and 240 seconds)
Variable Ratio	Reinforcement is provided after an irregular number of correct responses (For example: A food treat is given to a dog for coming when called after the first, second, fifth, seventh, and twelfth correct response)
Fixed Ratio	Reinforcement is provided after a regular number of correct responses (For example: A food treat is given to a dog for coming when called after the first, fourth, seventh, tenth and thirteenth correct response)

Conditioned reinforcers: Conditioned reinforcers (or secondary reinforcers) are stimuli that have been associated with a primary or biologic reinforcer. Over time, these stimuli take on reinforcing properties of their own and have essentially the same reinforcing capabilities as the primary (or unconditioned) reinforcer. The word "good" is a common example. If the owner tells the dog "good dog" for sitting, then immediately offers a primary reinforcer such as a food treat, the phrase "good dog" becomes associated or "bridged" with the primary reinforcer. The phrase "good dog" very rapidly becomes a secondary reinforcer and will serve as a positive reinforcer, even when not paired with food. It is important, however, to periodically pair the conditioned reinforcer "good dog" with the primary reinforcer to maintain the reinforcement properties of the secondary reinforcer. Several contemporary dog training books provide in-depth information about the use of conditioned reinforcers in practical dog training.[11,12,14]

Social Learning

Social learning is most commonly observed in group-living species in which communication between individuals is an important contributor to survival. The wolf is a social animal whose survival depends on a pack that functions efficiently and protects individual members from danger. Social learning is an important way in which wolves and dogs learn and involves a type of mimicry. Dogs that live together often "teach" one another particular behaviors. Common examples include dogs who learn to roll in noxious-smelling substances or to **coprophagize** (eat feces) by watching a house mate do the same. Social facilitation occurs when one animal displays the same behavior as another because seeing the other animal affects the dog's motivational state. The most common example of this in dogs is feeding behavior. Dogs are strongly affected by the presence of other dogs during mealtimes and many will overconsume when in the presence of other dogs who are eating. It is not unusual for dogs to increase their food intake and even become obese when a new dog is introduced into the home.

Training and Behavior Modification Techniques

A number of training methods and techniques can be used to teach new behaviors and modify problem behavior in dogs. This section reviews methods that use operant conditioning and positive reinforcement. The Part 2 reference list provides several books that examine these techniques in detail and present specific instructions for their use in dog training.

Successive approximation (shaping): Operant conditioning relies upon the consequences of behavior for learning. Therefore, by definition, the dog must first offer the desired behavior so it can be reinforced. However, some of the behaviors owners and trainers wish to teach to their dogs occur at very low frequencies or are not normally part of the dog's behavioral repertoire. An example is waiting for a dog to spontaneously sit in place for 4 minutes so this behavior can be reinforced. This is quite unproductive since most dogs will not spontaneously offer this behavior. For this reason, operant conditioning techniques almost always include the procedure of successive approximation, also called shaping. Shaping entails inducing a dog to offer a part or an approximation of a desired response and successively reinforcing closer approximations as the dog learns. As the dog is successful at each level of response, the criteria for reinforcement are shifted slightly toward the final behavior, and previous forms of the behavior are no longer reinforced.

In the case of teaching a sit-stay, a first-level response would be simply to sit, without requiring stay. When the dog reliably sits on command, the criteria shift and the owner now reinforces sit followed by a 2-second stay in place. This criterion (time) is gradually shifted as the dog is successful, until he is capable of staying for several minutes. A second criterion for the stay would be distance away from the owner. This can be shaped using the same procedure but must be done separately from shaping time intervals. In other words, the trainer concentrates on increasing time while staying close to the dog. Once the dog is reliably staying and an intermittent reinforcement schedule is in place, distance can then be shaped. When the trainer begins to shape distance, he or she will move farther and farther away from the dog but only for very short periods of time. Once both time and distance have been shaped, the two criteria can be combined, and increasing intervals of time with longer distances can be simultaneously shaped.

If failure occurs at any level, the trainer simply drops back down to a lower response level until the dog is again proficient at that level. Successive approximation is a powerful tool because very complex behavior patterns can be achieved and many problem behaviors can be solved without the need of negative reinforcement or punishment (see Chapter 10).

Extinction: Extinction provides an effective method for eliminating unwanted learned associations. For classical conditioning, extinction involves repeatedly presenting the conditioned stimulus by itself without the unconditioned stimulus. This results in a gradual decline (or extinction) of the conditioned response. For example, a dog who jumps up to go for a walk whenever the owner picks up the lead is demonstrating an association between the lead (conditioned stimulus) and going outside for a walk (unconditioned stimulus). Extinction of this behavior is accomplished by the owner picking up the lead at frequent intervals but not following this action by taking the dog for a walk.

Extinction of operantly conditioned behaviors is accomplished by withdrawing reinforcement from the targeted response. In the absence of reinforcement, the frequency with which the dog offers the behavior will decrease, eventually leading to extinction. Typically, when reinforcement is first withdrawn, the dog will show a sudden increase in the behavior. This is called an **extinction burst**. If the behavior is subsequently never reinforced, extinction occurs. Barking for attention is a common problem in dogs that often has been operantly conditioned. The reinforcement for this behavior is the owner's attention. Withdrawing all interactions whenever the dog barks for attention eventually will lead to extinction.

The effectiveness of extinction as a training tool often has been overlooked because owners have typically been instructed to use punishment to stop unwanted behaviors. However, punishment often causes stress, fear, or aggression and is not always successful in eliminating the behavior. In cases in which the dog's behavior is motivated by stress or anxiety, the use of punishment or negative reinforcement is actually counterproductive. Extinction can be used as an effective, humane alternative to punishment for stopping many undesirable behaviors in dogs.

Systematic desensitization: This is a technique often used to habituate established fearful or aggressive reactions in dogs. The fear-inducing (or aggression-inducing) stimulus is presented at a very low level of intensity until habituation is achieved. The level of intensity is then increased slightly, and the dog is exposed to the stimulus until it is desensitized at that intensity. This is repeated in increments until the dog is habituated to the full intensity of the stimulus. For example, the puppy who was sensitized to the vacuum cleaner could undergo a program of systematic desensitization for his fear response. He would gradually be exposed to the cleaner at low levels of intensity, perhaps beginning with an inactive machine at a far distance and gradually activating the vacuum cleaner and coming closer as the puppy habituates at each level.

It is essential to this program that the stimulus is presented at a level that is always lower than the level that elicits a fearful response. A delicate balance of slowly increasing the intensity of the stimulus and avoiding a fearful response must be maintained for success. Systematic desensitization is the technique routinely used to treat dogs who are thunder sensitive or who are shy or fearful with strangers. It is also helpful in the treatment of certain types of aggression (see Chapter 10). Pairing systematic desensitization with counter-conditioning and counter-commanding increases the chances of success of a desensitization program.

Counter-conditioning and counter-commanding: Counter-conditioning refers to teaching a dog to respond to a stimulus in a manner that is incompatible with the response previously evoked by the same stimulus. A new response that is behaviorally, emotionally, or physiologically incompatible with the previously undesired response is chosen. For example, eating is a pleasurable activity for dogs and is incompatible with running away (flight). Counter-conditioning during a systematic desensitization program for fear-flight responses includes feeding the dog food treats at each level of desensitization. As the dog becomes habituated, she begins to associate the presence of the stimulus with the pleasure of eating rather than with fear.

Counter-commanding involves teaching the dog to offer an alternate voluntary response that is incompatible with the previously undesired behaviors. For example, if the sound of the vacuum cleaner caused the sensitized puppy to attempt to flee, a sit-stay could be counter-commanded during the desensitization program. Counter-commanding works best with a dog that has had some obedience training and when the unwanted behavior has a relatively low level of motivation. Positive reinforcement should always be used to counter-condition a response because the goal is to change a situation that was previously unpleasant into a pleasant experience for the dog. As with systematic desensitization, it is essential that the counter-conditioning and counter-commanding take place at levels of intensity at which the sensitized response is not elicited.

Flooding: Flooding is also called "response prevention" and can be used to extinguish certain types of avoidance responses. The traditional extinction procedure of simply removing the association between the response and its consequence may be ineffective in solving avoidance behaviors. This occurs because, once conditioned, the dog never allows himself to again encounter the aversive stimulus. As a result, it is not possible for the dog to learn that the aversive event is no longer present. For example, a dog that hides behind his owner upon seeing a large truck coming down the street may become conditioned to hiding whenever the owner and dog approach the curb. By avoiding the curb, the dog never again is exposed to the truck but also cannot learn that the truck is usually not present (i.e. the curb is actually not predictive of the truck's approach). It is also theorized that avoidance behavior may be reinforced by the fear reduction that occurs when the dog is able to avoid the fear-producing situation.

Flooding involves exposing the animal to the avoidance situation while preventing the avoidance behavior. The dog is "flooded" with the warning cues, but the aversive stimulus does not appear. In the case of the truck-fearful dog, this would involve repeated exposure to the curb in the absence of loud trucks. Flooding can be a precarious technique because it often produces an initial increase in fear. Therefore, it is extremely important to ensure that the aversive stimulus is not present when flooding is taking place. In general, flooding can be successful in situations in which the dog's fear response is not severe and in which the owner is capable of having complete control over the fear-eliciting stimulus.

Influences on Learning

Various external and internal influences affect a dog's motivation to engage in a given behavior and, subsequently, her ability to learn. If a dog's tendency to engage in a desirable behavior is high, that behavior is relatively easy to positively reinforce and attain stimulus control of it (i.e. put the behavior "on command"). However, if the dog's motivation is low, the strength of the reinforcer must be high enough to overcome a naturally weak motivation. Similarly, if the underlying motivation for an unwanted behavior is very high, then a very strong reinforcer is going to be needed to counter-condition an alternate behavior. Before attempting to alter behavior, the dog's motivation for engaging in the behavior should be assessed. Internal factors that affect motivation include the dog's breed, individual temperament, sensitivity, and past experiences. External factors include the types of reinforcers that are available, the learning environment, and attributes of the trainer.

Internal influences on learning: All purebred breeds of dogs were originally developed to serve a specific working function (see Chapter 2). The ease or difficulty of teaching a new behavior to a dog depends somewhat on the extent to which the new behavior is in harmony with the breed's natural instincts. For example, retrievers originally were developed as hunting aids to indicate and retrieve game for the hunter. Retrieving instinct represents a portion of the dog's natural predatory sequence that has been somewhat modified to exaggerate the grab-bite and carry components. As a result, most retrievers can be easily taught to play fetch with a tennis ball, Frisbee, or toy.

In contrast, the retrievers also were selected to be highly sociable and to show low levels of dominance and territorial aggression. Because their motivation to protect is naturally quite low, it is rare to find an individual retriever who can easily be trained to protect a home or business.

Similarly, certain breeds have selective tendencies to engage in behaviors their owners may find undesirable. Border collies originally were bred to work outside with herds of sheep. Their job was to control the herd and move it from place to place. Herding instinct represents the orientation, stalk, and chase portions of the dog's predatory sequence. As a pet in a suburban home, this instinct may manifest itself through chasing children, runners, bikers, or small animals. Because the internal motivation to chase is very high in herding breeds, modifying this behavior may be quite difficult, especially if the dog has no other outlet for chasing.

Regardless of breed, every dog is an individual. A dog's temperament characteristics and past experiences strongly influence his ability to learn new behaviors. Factors that should be considered include the dog's need for dominant-subordinate relationships with his owner and with other dogs, the type and intensity of reactivity that he displays when aroused, his degree of self-confidence or timidity when confronted with novel experiences, and his degree of dependence upon the owner. Past experiences that are important to consider include the amount of socialization (i.e. habituation) the dog experienced during primary socialization and adolescence, the amount and type of prior training experienced, and her prior and current living situation. Dogs also differ significantly in their degree of touch, sight, and sound sensitivity. Sensitivity is affected by breed, individual temperament, and by past experiences.

External influences: When choosing appropriate reinforcers to use in dog training, the dog's level of desire for the reinforcer must be considered. Simply put, it is the dog who always determines what is positively (or negatively) reinforcing, not the trainer. For example, some dogs may happily work for a small piece of cheese, while others will be more strongly motivated by a squeaky toy or tennis ball. A positive reinforcer is also useful only for the duration that the dog will offer the desired behavior in anticipation of receiving it. For example, if food treats are being used, the power of this positive reinforcer will be enhanced if the dog is moderately hungry. Similarly, if social interaction (petting, praise, play) is used as a reinforcer, a dog who has been isolated from the owner for a short period of time is expected to respond to this reinforcer more strongly than one who has had access to her owner's attention for several hours before the training session. Since most dogs will work for several different types of positive reinforcement, changing the reinforcer or alternating between several primary reinforcers is an effective training tool.

The environment in which the dog is trained and the trainer's expertise are also important considerations. All subjects (including humans) learn new tasks most efficiently when they are taught in an area that is quiet and free of distractions. A regular, consistent routine also contributes to rapid learning. The trainer's attitude and level of experience are similarly important. Consistency in providing stimuli (cues) and the ability to provide reinforcers at the appropriate time both contribute to rapid learning.

Conclusions

Dogs learn primarily through habituation, sensitization, classical conditioning, and operant conditioning. In addition, influences such as a dog's breed, sex, age, individual temperament, and former experiences significantly influence learning. An understanding of these learning processes has led to the development of several effective tools for training companion dogs, and for modifying problem behaviors. The following chapter examines several common behavior problems in dogs and presents approaches for solving these problems.

Cited References

1. Reid, P.J. and Borchelt, P.L. **Learning.** In: *Readings in Companion Animal Behavior* (V.L. Voith and P.L. Borchelt, editors), Veterinary Learning Systems, Trenton, New Jersey, pp. 62-71. (1996)

2. Borchelt, P.L. **Punishment.** In: *Readings in Companion Animal Behavior* (V.L. Voith and P.L. Borchelt, editors), Veterinary Learning Systems, Trenton, New Jersey, pp. 72-80. (1996)

3. Koehler, W. *The Koehler Method of Dog Training.* Howell Book House, New York, New York. (1962)

4. Saunders, B. *The Complete Book of Dog Obedience: A Guide for Trainers.* Howell Book House, New York, New York. (1976)

5. Bolles, R.C. **Species-specific defense reactions and avoidance learning.** Psychology Review, 77:32-48. (1970)

6. Fisher, J. *Dogwise: The Natural Way to Train Your Dog.* Souvenir Press, London, United Kingdom. (1992)

7. Rogerson, J. *Your Dog: Its Development, Behaviour, and Training.* Popular Dogs Publishing Company, London, United Kingdom. (1990)

8. Neville, P. *Do Dogs Need Shrinks?* Carol Publishing Group, New York, New York. (1992)

9. Wilkes, G. *A Behavior Sampler.* Sunshine Books, North Bend, Washington. (1994)

10. O'Farrell, V. *Dog's Best Friend: How Not to Be a Problem Owner.* Methuen Press, London, United Kingdom. (1994)

11. Donaldson, J. *Culture Clash: A Revolutionary New Way of Understanding the Relationship between Humans and Domestic Dogs.* James and Kenneth Publishers, Oakland, California. (1996)

12. Reid, P.J. *Excel-erated Learning: Explaining How Dogs Learn and How Best to Teach Them.* James and Kenneth Publishers, Oakland, California. (1996)

13. Skinner, B.F. *The Behavior of Organisms: An Experimental Approach.* Appleton-Century, New York, New York. (1938)

14. Pryor, K. *Karen Pryor on Behavior.* Sunshine Books, North Bend, Washington. (1995)

10 Common Behavior Problems and Solutions

DURING ITS EARLY ASSOCIATIONS with man, the dog served as a talented, indispensable aid for survival. In different areas of the world, dogs were selectively bred to protect homesteads, aid hunters, and move livestock. However, as our culture evolved and modern technology replaced many of the dog's duties, the dog's working role diminished. Today, many dogs live as cherished companions and playmates for young and old alike, and often are considered to be indispensable members of the family. It is, therefore, a paradox that during a time when our bond with *Canis familiaris* is in many ways strong and enduring, owners are still abandoning, giving away, and euthanizing many healthy pets. Each year, animal shelters throughout the United States are forced to euthanize millions of dogs.[1] Moreover, behavior problems are identified by owners as a primary reason for relinquishment of pets to shelters.[2]

Within the last 20 years, knowledge of canine behavior and training has expanded enormously. There has been an increase in the number of practitioners in this field and in the number and sophistication of treatment programs that are used. This chapter provides an overview of the diagnosis and treatment of several types of behavior problems in dogs. These are divided into three major areas: aggression, fears and phobias, and separation anxiety. Since it is beyond the scope of this book to provide a complete review of this topic, several excellent books entirely devoted to canine behavior, training, and the treatment of problems are referred to in the text and are cited in the reference list for Part II.

Identification and Diagnosis: Obtaining a Behavioral History

The normal behavioral repertoire of the dog includes social behaviors that facilitate group cohesiveness, signals of dominance and subordinance, components of predatory behavior, and aggressive behaviors (chapters 7 and 8). These behaviors are normal for all dogs and do not necessarily constitute a problem. All dogs are capable of demonstrating aggression, dominant and subordinate body postures, separation stress, and predatory behavior. However, when these patterns are displayed with an intensity or frequency that is highly incompatible with the owner's lifestyle; when the owner has no control over the dog's actions; or when the dog poses a danger to the owner, his environment, other animals, or himself, these behaviors are then considered to be problematic.

It is also imperative to consider that problem behaviors have different causes, and successful treatment entails careful diagnosis of the underlying motivation. For example, house soiling may be a result of inadequate house-training, the presence of a medical problem, a manifestation of separation anxiety, or marking behavior.[3] Completion of behavior history forms, complete veterinary examinations, and interviews with the owner should always be the first steps taken when diagnosing behavior problems in dogs.[4] Forms should include demographic information about the owner and descriptive data about the dog; the source and length of time the owner has had the dog; and information about the dog's daily care, training, and exercise (Figure 10.1). The form should indicate the onset and duration of the unwanted behavior, the context in which it occurs, which family members (or other people) are involved, and the intensity and frequency with which the behavior is displayed. A thorough medical examination by a veterinarian is warranted if there is any possibility the problem has a medical origin. If possible, the owner's level of motivation and capabilities for dealing with the problem and for implementing the treatment program should be assessed. This knowledge allows the development of an effective treatment plan and provides insight regarding the overall **prognosis**.

Treatment programs for modifying a dog's behavior can have several approaches. In many cases, management of the dog's environment and living situation is combined with a behavior modification program aimed at lessening the motivation for the unwanted behavior, strengthening the motivation to engage in an alternate behavior, or removing the reinforcement for the unwanted behavior. Factors that affect the overall prognosis include the type and number of problems diagnosed, the age of onset and duration, the ability of the owners and family to accept and implement a treatment program, and the degree of risk the animal poses to other dogs, animals, or people. In the case of aggression, it is not unusual for a dog to show different types of aggression in different contexts. For example, a dominant aggressive dog often will also be possessive and territorial. Generally speaking, the more types of aggression or other behavior problems a dog demonstrates, the poorer the overall prognosis for treatment.

Problem Aggression in Dogs

Aggression is the most commonly reported behavior problem in dogs.[5] Between 1 and 3 million people in the United States are bitten by dogs each year and more than half a million of these bites result in serious injury.[6] Children are bitten more often than adults and are particularly susceptible to serious injury or fatality from dog bites.[7] Aggression between dogs is also a serious problem. This may occur between dogs who are strangers or between two or more dogs that live together in the same household. Although intermale aggression is more common, aggression between females or between sexes also occurs. Dogs that chase or attack small animals such as cats, squirrels, or rabbits also are often said to be showing aggression. However, in most cases, this is a manifestation of predatory behavior and is not a true form of aggression (see Chapter 8).

Aggressive behaviors provide important advantages for many species of animal. Competition between group members and between species is part of the process of survival and natural selection. Successful defensive behaviors

---

FIGURE 10.1   Sample behavior history form

BEHAVIOR HISTORY FORM

DATE _____   STUDENT'S NAME/ADDRESS/PHONE _____

DOG'S NAME _____   BREED _____

AGE _____   SEX _____   SPAYED/NEUTERED? _____   AGE NEUTERED: _____

AGE OBTAINED: _____   SOURCE: _____   OTHER ANIMALS IN HOUSEHOLD: _____

PRINCIPLE CARETAKER: _____   SECONDARY CARETAKER(S): _____

TYPE(S) OF EXERCISE PROVIDED: _____   FREQUENCY· _____

ACCESS TO OUTDOORS: _____   BEHAVIOR WHEN OUTDOORS: _____

DOG'S PRINCIPLE LIVING AREA: _____   DOG'S FAVORITE SLEEPING AREA: _____

WHERE IS DOG WHEN NO ONE IS AT HOME? _____   DURATION/FREQUENCY OF TIME ALONE: _____

TYPE OF FOOD: _____   AMOUNT FED: _____   FEEDING SCHEDULE: _____

FOOD BOWL OR TOY POSSESSIVE? _____   REACTIONS: _____   OWNER'S RESPONSE: _____

GAMES PLAYED WITH DOG: _____   TYPE OF TOYS: _____   DOG'S REACTIONS: _____

TYPE OF GROOMING CARE: _____   FREQUENCY: _____   REACTION OF THE DOG: _____

TYPES OF INTERACTIONS THAT THE DOG ENJOYS: _____

TYPES OF INTERACTIONS THAT THE OWNER ENJOYS: _____

REACTION TO OTHER DOGS: _____   REACTION TO NEW PEOPLE: _____

REACTION TO CHILDREN: _____   REACTION TO CATS/SMALL ANIMALS: _____

REACTION TO VISITORS IN HOME: _____   REACTION TO MAILMAN/DELIVERY MEN: _____

REACTION TO VISITORS APPROACHING YARD: _____   APPROACHING CAR: _____

CAR RIDING MANNERS: _____   BEHAVIOR AT VETERINARIAN'S OFFICE: _____

PREVIOUS OBEDIENCE TRAINING: _____   COMMANDS THE DOG RESPONDS TO: _____

===

DESCRIPTION OF BEHAVIOR PROBLEM: _____

AGE OF ONSET: _____   FREQUENCY: _____   DIRECTED TOWARD: _____

SOLUTIONS ATTEMPTED: _____   REACTION OF DOG: _____

DIAGNOSIS: _____   TYPE OF BEHAVIOR MODIFICATION PROGRAM : _____

MATERIALS AND TREATMENT PLAN PROVIDED: _____

FOLLOW-UP SCHEDULE: _____

prevent an animal from becoming a meal for a predator or from losing its territory to competing animals of the same species. For the wolf, competition between pack members is highly ritualized and includes complex patterns of communication. Moreover, most aggressive displays are inhibited and do not usually result in serious fights or injuries. These highly ritualized, precise communication methods have been inherited by our domestic dog (see Chapter 8). However, it is also important to realize that the dog, like her ancestor, is still a lethally equipped predatory species. Therefore, although these ritualized pack behaviors usually serve to minimize injury and reduce conflict between conspecifics, dogs living in the same social group are capable of fighting and injuring each other, and of biting their owners or other people. Moreover, it is theorized that selective breeding for enhanced dominance, territorial behavior, and lowered stimulus thresholds for aggression in some breeds have resulted in animals who are more highly aggressive than their wolf ancestors.[8]

Because aggressive behaviors are a part of every dog's behavioral makeup, individual dogs cannot be classified as being either "aggressive" or "nonaggressive." Every dog, from the smallest toy to the largest working breed, is capable of showing aggressive behavior. In addition, simply labeling a dog as "aggressive" provides no information about the context in which the aggression occurs or the factors that precipitate it and is not helpful in developing an effective treatment program. In the past, aggressive behavior in dogs has been classified according to several schemes. These have included dividing types of aggression according to its focus (i.e. the owner, strangers, visitors to the home, or other dogs)or the type of defense behaviors the dog shows, or determining if the behavior was learned or inherited.[9,10] However, none of these classification methods was useful in treating aggression because none addressed the underlying cause of the behavior.

Today, the most widely used method of diagnosing and classifying problem aggression relies upon determining the function the aggression has for the dog. A functional classification approach takes into account the context in which the aggression occurs as well as the types of behavior patterns and body postures the dog exhibits. This allows deduction of the underlying motivation for the behavior and facilitates the development of an effective treatment program. The most common forms of aggression include dominance, possessive, and territorial. Other forms include pain-elicited, maternal, intermale, and redirected aggression (Table 10.1). Diagnosis and treatment programs for dominance, territorial, and possessive aggression are reviewed in the following section. For a more thorough review of this topic, refer to the list of readings provided for Part 2.

Dominance aggression: Dominance aggression has been reported to comprise between 20 and 30 percent of the caseload of professional behaviorists, veterinarians, and trainers.[11] This type of aggression may be directed toward humans or toward other dogs (intraspecies) and ranges from mild posturing and growling to direct attacks and uninhibited biting. Obtaining a complete behavioral history of the dog's behavior and relationship with the owners is

TABLE 10.1   Types of Aggression in Dogs

Classification	Description	Type of Treatment Program
Dominance	Directed toward owners or other dogs in household in response to challenges to social status (several manifestations are possible)	Counter-conditioning subordinate behaviors; systematic desensitization to reintroduce eliciting factors; control access to all desired resources
Possessive	Directed toward owners or other dogs in household in response to competition for a valued resource	Treat underlying cause (dominance; learned food-guarding); operant conditioning (give; leave it; come)
Territorial	Directed toward visiting humans or animals; aggression intensifies at areas of entry or exit	Decrease motivation; counter-condition controlled behaviors away from entrance or exit areas; systematic desensitization
Pain-elicited	Directed toward owners or other humans; occurs in response to injury or physical reprimands	Remove cause; eliminate use of escape-avoidance training methods
Maternal	Directed toward humans or other animals in response to approach or handling of young (females only)	Usually self-limiting; counter-conditioning and systematic desensitization
Intermale	Sexually motivated aggression between male dogs (usually intact)	Neutering; counter-conditioning; operant conditioning (sit, down, leave it)
Redirected	Directed toward humans or other dogs when prevented access to the primary stimulus that elicited the aggression	Treat underlying cause of aggression; operant conditioning for control (sit, down, come)

necessary to distinguish between dominance-related aggression and other forms of aggression. Dominance aggression is typically elicited only in specific circumstances, and these circumstances differ among dogs.[12,13] Owners often become proficient at predicting the circumstances that will evoke an aggressive response in the dog and so can provide valuable diagnostic information to the behaviorist or trainer.

Typically, dominance aggression is expressed when a dominant dog reacts to an apparent challenge to his social status or to the loss of control of a valued resource. In dog-to-dog interactions valued items may include food, a toy, a bone, or a favorite sleeping area. Dominance aggression between dogs may also be triggered when two dogs are competing for the attention of their owner. Dominance aggression directed toward humans involves circumstances in which the dog perceives the human to be a threat to his social status. Most typically, this is in response to gestures or body postures that are perceived to be dominant by the dog. These may include standing over, physically reprimanding, or restraining the dog. Attempts to take a possession away also may trigger an aggressive response.

When there is no confrontation, a dominant aggressive dog is usually friendly and self-confident. In fact, owners often describe the dog as being a wonderful, enjoyable pet, except in certain circumstances. In some cases, dominant aggressive dogs only show aggression toward certain family members and appear to have a subordinate relationship with others. It appears that dominant dogs show little or no aggression to a person over whom they are clearly dominant or to whom they are clearly submissive. Individuals who never assert themselves or do not interact with the dog are rarely threatened. Similarly, dogs exhibiting dominance aggression usually are not aggressive toward strangers or visitors to the home. This occurs because the visitor is not part of the dog's normal social group and is often perceived by dominant-aggressive dogs as a stimulus for play and attention, but not as a member of his social group. Although dominant aggressive dogs can be very assertive and pushy with visitors, they usually only direct aggression toward them if they remain in the home for an extended period or attempt to directly challenge the dog's status.

The majority of dogs that are presented for dominance aggression are intact males, and purebred dogs more often are represented than mixed-breed dogs.[14] In contrast, most female dogs that exhibit dominance aggression are spayed. There is some evidence that spaying may result in an increase in dominance aggression in females that were already showing signs of aggression.[15] However, these data do not indicate that spaying causes dominance aggression and do not suggest that keeping a female pet intact will prevent aggression. Dominance aggression typically first manifests itself in males and females when the dog reaches sexual maturity (about 9 months to 1 year) or social maturity (1 to 2 years). A recent study has shown that dominance aggression is more prevalent in dogs that were seriously ill as puppies than in those that were healthy throughout growth.[16] These dogs also were more likely to show fear-related behaviors. It was postulated that inadequate or restricted socialization (i.e., a lack of habituation) due to illness may have contributed to the development of these problems.

The goals of treatment for dominance aggression are to modify the dog's behavior and manage the environment to ensure the safety of the owner, other people, and other dogs. Ideally, the dog can eventually be exposed to the context that previously elicited aggression without showing an aggressive response. If the dominance is directed toward the owner, this involves establishing a more subordinate relationship of the dog to the owner. When dominance aggression is directed toward other dogs, treatment involves supporting the normal pack structure (if possible) and, more importantly, managing the multidog household in a manner that prevents or redirects aggressive displays between dogs. If the dog is an intact male, castration is recommended. This results in a decrease in the level of aggression in many males, but not all dominant aggressive dogs respond noticeably.[17]

Physical punishment has been shown to be ineffective in the treatment of aggression and in many circumstances serves to exacerbate the problem.[18] Pain has long been recognized as an elicitor of aggression, and reprimands often are perceived as a challenge by a dominant dog. Similarly, using physical punishment when a dominant dog shows aggression toward another dog can result in redirected aggression toward the owner and further escalates the conflict between the two dogs. Case studies of dominant aggressive dogs have shown that owner attempts to discipline a dominant dog are a common cause of aggression and bites to owners.[12] Therefore, if the owner has been using physical reprimands, dominance rolls, or direct challenges to the dog, these procedures should be discontinued.

The most effective way to treat dominance aggression involves the gradual introduction of interactions between the owner and dog in which the owner is dominant and the dog is submissive. This is accomplished through a program that uses systematic desensitization and counter-conditioning (see Chapter 9). Each program must be tailored specifically to address the context and intensity of the dog's aggression, and the lifestyle and capabilities of the owner. Every dog is unique, and owners differ in their motivation and ability to modify the dog's environment and implement a consistent training program.

Counter-conditioning and counter-commanding are used to teach the dog to show elements of subordinate behavior (see Chapter 9). Most typically, a down-stay or sit-stay exercise is taught using operant conditioning and positive reinforcement. These exercises then precede the dog's access to all valued resources such as meals, toys, walks outside, and interactions with the owner. A basic rule of all treatment programs for dominance aggression is that the dog is placed in nonconfrontational situations in which all food, playtime, attention, and other valued resources are available only as reinforcements for subordinate behavior. Obedience training is helpful if used to teach the dog to respond to commands, to allow handling, and to relinquish possessions. However, most basic obedience classes available to pet owners do not adequately address dominance aggression problems, and individualized treatment is necessary in the majority of cases.

Not all cases of dominance aggression can be treated successfully. The degree of danger to the owner and the family, and the limitations of the owner must be considered. Some dominant aggressive dogs are unresponsive to treatment, even when a detailed training program is used and when the owners are dedicated and consistent. In other cases, the owners may be unwilling or unable to commit to a complete behavior modification program or live in a situation in which the dog may continue to be a danger to the owners, to their children, or to others. In such cases, options such as carefully placing the dog in another home or euthanasia must be considered. Some owners may wish to consider using pharmacologic therapy in conjunction with the behavior modification program. A veterinary behaviorist should always be consulted if considering adjunctive drug therapy.

Possessive aggression: Possessive aggression often is associated with dominance aggression and is manifested as aggressive displays during competition for valued resources. For the pet dog, such resources typically include toys, food, or the owner's attention. However, some dogs fixate on unusual items such as pieces of tissue, articles of clothing, or even the television remote control. These situations often reflect learned behavior and are associated with a history of object-stealing by the dog. When an owner reacts by chasing or harshly reprimanding the dog, the dog learns to respond by guarding the stolen item. Possessive aggression also can occur in dogs that have been compelled to guard their food from other animals or have learned to distrust humans who approach their food bowl. These dogs usually guard their food bowl defensively but show no other signs of possessive aggression (see Chapter 8).

If dominance aggression also is present, the treatment program for possessive aggression first involves identifying and treating dominance. Part of the program also should address possessive aggression. Specifically, all objects that the dog guards or steals must be removed, and access to these objects is supervised by the owner. The dog is taught to relinquish possessions using a "give" command and to refrain from picking up objects using a "leave it" command. As discussed previously, operant conditioning using positive reinforcement and successive approximation can be used to safely and successfully teach these commands.[19] When dogs are possessive over food bowls or toys with other dogs in the family, but not with humans, this often can be solved through simple management procedures. It is normal canine behavior for dogs to guard food from pack members, and dominant animals often will steal objects from subordinate members even if they have little interest in the item themselves. It appears that this is another form of stereotypic "posturing" within a pack structure. Simply feeding the dogs in separate areas, disallowing the sharing of food bowls, and careful selection of the types of toys the dogs have unsupervised access to usually solve these problems. In most cases, owners should be advised to remove any toys that are used for retrieving or "find it" games and only have these toys available for the duration of the game. Removing chew bones that are highly desirable or providing them when the dogs can either be separated or supervised also helps prevent possessive fighting between dogs.

Territorial aggression: When intruders approach or enter their territory, many dogs show orienting behaviors and bark but do not become aggressive. This is a natural behavior and only becomes a problem when the dog becomes uncontrollable or aggressive. Areas that pet dogs are most likely to consider home territory include the owner's house, yard, car, and possibly other areas where the dog is frequently walked or confined. For confident dogs, territory is a valuable resource that must be protected and competitively maintained. For fearful or nervous dogs, territorial aggression is a learned behavior that has proved to be effective in driving off intruders. This type of territorial defense often is seen in poorly socialized dogs that have been confined to a small area or tied to a doghouse. Like possessive aggression, territorial aggression often is seen in dogs that are also dominant aggressive. These three behaviors—dominance, territorial and possessive aggression—are referred to as the "dominance triad."

When territorial behaviors are associated with dominance, the behavior modification program to treat dominance aggression also should address the dog's territorial behaviors. Territorial aggression is most prevalent in dogs who are kept tied outside for long periods of time, are confined to a small yard, or who have been encouraged by their owners to guard entryways or yards. In these cases, exposure to eliciting stimuli can be prevented or moderated simply by bringing the dog into the house or changing the way in which the dog is managed within the home. During the treatment program, dogs that tend to guard certain doors or windows in the house should not be allowed free access to those areas. This is an important component of treatment because there is the potential for an aggressive response on each occasion the dog has unsupervised access to guarded areas. A unique characteristic of territorial behavior is that it is always immediately reinforced when the intended target moves away. An example is the dog who barks and growls each day at the mail carrier as he or she approaches the house to deliver mail. As the intended target (the mail carrier) deposits the mail and departs, the dog's agitation decreases, thus reinforcing the barking and growling behaviors.

Counter-conditioning/commanding and systematic desensitization are effective techniques for use with territorial behaviors. The dog is first taught a behavior that is incompatible with charging the door and barking. A typical response is to come to the owner and sit. A reliable response to the command for this behavior must be instilled before attempting to desensitize the dog to the approach of visitors to the house. When the dog's response is reliable, a systematic desensitization program is introduced, starting with the approach of family members or friends to the guarded area. As the dog begins to associate the presence of visitors with responding to the counter command and receiving positive reinforcement for that response, the stimuli can gradually be intensified.

A program of counter-conditioning and desensitization can be coupled with efforts to decrease the dog's motivation to guard and increase her motivation to greet visitors in a friendly manner. This is accomplished through classical conditioning (see Chapter 8). The arrival of the owners or visitors at the doorway can be paired with food treats or even the dog's dinner. Classical conditioning eventually results in the dog associating visitors with positive response rather than negative. At first, the owner provides all of the reinforcement for quiet and controlled behavior at the door, but eventually visitors can be asked to reinforce the dog's appropriate behaviors as they enter. Over time, the dog associates visitors with the arrival of her dinner, food treats, and positive attention.

In cases in which the dog exhibits territorial aggression because of nervousness or fear, it is important to institute a very gradual desensitization program to visitors. In such a program, the intensity of the stimulus (i.e., visitors entering the home) should never be introduced at a level that elicits the fearful response. Complete success may be achieved in some cases, and the dog becomes calm and friendly toward visitors. In many cases, however, especially if the dog has a very strong reinforcement history for fear-induced territorial aggression, the goal may be simply to decrease the dog's aggression or to teach the dog to move to another room whenever visitors arrive.

Fears and Phobias

Fear is a natural, normal part of the dog's behavioral repertoire and has adaptive function for all animals. In all species, certain fear responses are innate and are important for survival. In wolves, **xenophobia,** or fear of unfamiliar animals and objects, has its onset shortly after the wolf pups are capable of traveling away from the den and exploring nearby territory. The tendency to run back to the security of the den and to adult pack members in response to unfamiliar animals or situations has distinctive survival value in a wild environment. The domestic dog has inherited this tendency, but generations of selective breeding have significantly decreased its intensity. Socialization techniques that allow dogs to habituate to new people, places, and other dogs during primary and secondary socialization are effective in preventing fear-related problems in most domestic dogs (see Chapter 7). However, fearful behaviors can become problematic when triggered by harmless stimuli or when the behavior occurs at an intensity or a frequency that impacts the dog's safety, quality of life, or relationship with his or her owners.

Companion animal behaviorists and trainers report that fears and phobias are common behavior problems in dogs and make up a substantial proportion of the cases they see. A survey of more than 2,000 dog owners showed that almost 38 percent of dogs were fearful of loud noises, 22 percent were fearful of unfamiliar adults, 33 percent were fearful of children, and 14 percent were fearful of other dogs.[20] Approximately one-third of the pets presented to a college of veterinary medicine behavior clinic were found to have fear-related problems. In addition, studies with guide dogs have shown that fear is one of the most common reasons for rejecting potential dogs from training.[21,22]

Signs and causes of fear-related behaviors: Fear-related problems vary significantly in the type of stimulus that elicits the fear and the intensity of the reaction. Some dogs exhibit general fears of a relatively low magnitude, but they are triggered by a wide range of stimuli. These dogs often are referred to as being shy or timid. Others exhibit specific fears, for example, toward a certain type of person or a particular location. Phobias are fear responses that occur at a much greater intensity than the situation or potential danger warrants. An example is the dog who becomes so agitated and frantic upon hearing fireworks that he is in danger of injuring himself in his attempts to escape. Although behavior modification often is helpful in treating fear-related behaviors, the long-term prognosis is variable and depends on the age of onset, the duration and the intensity of the fearful response, the ability to control the eliciting stimuli, and the dog's temperament and prior experiences.

When confronted with fearful stimuli, dogs exhibit one or a combination of three possible reactions. These are freezing, fleeing, or fighting. Freezing responses include panting, trembling, attempting to stay close to the owner, crouching, or lying immobile. Fleeing behaviors include all attempts to run away or avoid the stimulus. Dogs that react aggressively usually will demonstrate growling, snapping at air, or biting. This behavior may be followed by an attempt to flee. Some fearful dogs only become aggressive if all attempts to flee have been impeded.

Fears and phobias can develop at any age. In some cases their origins can be traced to a specific traumatic event; in others the owner is unable to identify any specific incident that triggered the change in behavior. In some cases, there is a significant genetic influence. Early studies of the genetic inheritance of behavior in dogs found that 52 percent of nervous dogs in a laboratory colony were directly descended from a single female who had shown fear-induced aggression.[23] It is known that nervous behavior in dogs can be increased through selective breeding (see Chapter 5). Certain breeds appear to show a higher incidence of timidity or fear-related behaviors. These include herding breeds such as Shetland Sheepdogs, German Shepherd Dogs, Belgian Sheepdogs, and several toy breeds. There is also anecdotal evidence from breeders that certain lines within breeds produce dogs who have a tendency toward fearful behavior.[20]

Early experience has a profound effect on the development of fearful behaviors in dogs, especially during primary and secondary socialization. An experiment with Scottish Terriers found that puppies who were raised for 7 months with little to no human contact showed extreme fear reactions when confronted with an unfamiliar person.[24] Repeated handling in an attempt to habituate the young dogs met with little success. Further studies showed that handling during primary socialization (3 to 12 weeks) is essential for the development of normal nonfearful behaviors in growing puppies (see Chapter 7). Moreover, exposing puppies to frequent handling and even to mild stressors during the first few weeks of life has been shown to produce individuals that are less easily frightened and that habituate more readily to novel stimuli than puppies that were not handled.[25] The same study showed that nervous behavior of the mother significantly influenced the development of fearful behaviors in her puppies. Socialization (habituation) during the primary socialization period is very important for the development of puppies who are comfortable and friendly toward new people and in new environments. Many fear-related problems can be prevented simply through proper socialization of a young dog to people, places, and experiences during the primary and secondary socialization periods (7 weeks to 6 months of age).

Reinforcement of fear: One of the primary difficulties in solving fears and phobias in dogs is that these behaviors often are strongly reinforced each time the dog engages in them. Whenever a fearful experience leads the dog to attempt to escape (flee), and the dog is successful in doing so, this behavior is automatically reinforced. For example, a dog who was once frightened by a young neighbor boy banging two metal garbage cans together learned to run into the garage whenever the boy approached. The association between the boy and the loud noise (classical conditioning) caused the dog to continue to show this behavior even when the boy did not make any loud noises. Running into the garage essentially prevented exposure to the noise (regardless of whether or not the boy had any intention of being noisy). The behavior was reinforced each time it occurred because the dog was avoiding exposure to the unpleasant stimulus (i.e., running away was negatively reinforced) (see Chapter 9).

A second way in which fearful responses can be reinforced involves the owner's reaction to the dog's behavior. When a fearful experience prompts the owner to make a misguided effort to comfort the dog with attention or food treats, the behavior (fear) usually is reinforced. This is a common reaction of owners and is certainly a normal, understandable response. Similarly, punishment is not effective since this serves only to intensify fear and escape behaviors.

Common fears in dogs: Fearful behaviors or phobias in dogs can be divided into four general categories: fear of new places or situations, fear of unfamiliar people, fear of unfamiliar dogs, and noise phobias. Some dogs exhibit only one specific type of fear, while others may show several apparently unrelated fear responses or phobias.

Agoraphobia, or fear of new places and experiences, is seen most commonly in dogs who live in kennels or in house pets that have been inadequately socialized. It is not uncommon for owners to report that the dog's only trips away from the home involve infrequent visits to either the veterinarian's office, the grooming shop, or a boarding kennel. Similarly, dogs from large breeding kennels may have had little or no experiences away from their kennel setting. In these cases, age has a significant effect on the prognosis, with older adult dogs being less responsive to treatment than young adolescents. In some situations, dogs become agoraphobic as a result of an unpleasant or traumatic experience. In one case study, a dog became unwilling to leave the house to go for her regular (and previously enjoyable) walks around the neighborhood after having been attacked and badly bitten by a neighbor's loose dog. The ability of dogs to eventually overcome situational fears varies greatly, and many will retain a certain level of timidity for the remainder of their lives.

Dogs that are timid or fearful when meeting new people usually have not been adequately socialized to different types and ages of people. A typical example is a dog who is owned by a quiet, elderly couple and shows nervous or fearful behavior when approached by young children. Similarly, the fear of other dogs occurs primarily as a result of a lack of socialization. Such dogs have not learned normal intraspecies communication patterns and may be unable to either send or perceive normal canine communication signals. Certainly, a traumatic event such as being attacked by another dog as a puppy can cause the development of a fearful response, but this is much less common than many owners perceive it to be. When inadequate socialization as a young dog is the cause of fear of people and/or other dogs, the prognosis for complete recovery is moderate to poor.[26] Some dogs will attempt to flee, while others learn to react defensively by fighting or biting when approached by unfamiliar dogs or people. Fear is a common cause of interdog and human-directed aggression, which often is misdiagnosed as dominance aggression. For this reason, a thorough behavioral history and interview with the owners are necessary for accurate diagnosis and treatment.

Noise phobias make up the largest proportion of fear-related problems in dogs.[22] The most common stimuli are thunder, gunshots, and fireworks. Although many noise phobias can be managed successfully with a behavior modification program, the prognosis varies greatly depending on the individual, the duration of the phobia, the ability to control exposure to the stimulus, and success in finding an effective artificial stimulus to use during the exposure exercises. Fear of thunderstorms typically develops in mature adults and gradually increases in intensity as the dog ages. Dogs with thunderstorm phobias usually display a gradient of fearful behavior that is directly proportional to the intensity of the storm. Owners report that the dog begins to pace nervously and stays close as the weather becomes dark and there are signs of an approaching storm. One of the problems in treating thunderstorm phobia is the number of stimuli the dog may be reacting to. These often include wind, rain, changes in atmospheric pressure and ionization, lightning, and odors. Because the easiest stimulus to replicate is auditory (i.e., thunder), this is what owners usually focus on and is the cue used in desensitization programs.

Treatment of fears and phobias: The first step in the treatment of a fear-related behavior problem is to completely identify the attributes of all stimuli that elicit a fear response in the dog. It is usually beneficial to encourage the owner to list all possible situations in which the dog has the potential for showing fear or timidity. The techniques that are most helpful in treating fear in dogs include habituation, systematic desensitization, counter-conditioning, shaping, and flooding (see Chapter 9).

Once the stimuli that elicit fear in the dog have been identified, the owner and trainer can develop a gradient of these stimuli that progresses from the least fearful to the most fearful in the dog's perception. This is the systematic desensitization portion of the program. An example is a dog who is afraid of unfamiliar children, particularly children younger than the age of 5 years (Table 10.2). Systematic desensitization is most successful when paired with counter-conditioning. For dogs that experience fear and flight responses to people, the use of food treats or a desired toy and counter-commanding sit/stay are most successful.

The owner begins the program with the stimulus of lowest intensity. If the dog shows no fear when exposed, this "non-fear" or relaxed response is reinforced with food treats, petting, or playtime with a toy. If fear is induced, the stimulus is immediately removed. After waiting a period of time, the program can begin once again but with a stimulus of lower intensity. The goal is to always introduce a stimulus that stays within the dog's comfort level and that does not elicit fear, allowing the counter-conditioning of relaxation and neutral (i.e., non-fearful) behavior. A sit- or down-stay exercise also can be in-

TABLE 10.2   Stimulus Gradient for Systematic Desensitization Program (Fear of Young Unfamiliar Children)

Stimuli (exposed in neutral setting)	Dog's Typical Response
Familiar adult female	Friendly, no fear
Familiar adult male	Friendly, no fear
Familiar teenager	Friendly, no fear
Familiar 10-year-old	Friendly, no fear
Familiar 5-year-old	Indifferent, no fear
Unfamiliar adult female	Indifferent, no fear
Unfamiliar adult male	Timid
Unfamiliar teenager	Timid
Unfamiliar 10-year-old	Fearful, mild avoidance
Unfamiliar 5-year-old	Fearful, extreme avoidance

cluded as a counter-commanding technique. As the dog becomes desensitized at each level of the stimulus, the next level can be introduced, always staying within an exposure level that does not induce fear. While some owners are able to progress all the way to the highest intensity stimulus, others reach a certain point where the dog is capable of going no further. In these cases, a lessening of fear often is achieved, but the problem is not completely resolved.

The use of systematic desensitization and counter-conditioning can be a bit more complicated when treating noise phobias because these problems require that a suitable artificial stimulus be found. Recordings of thunderstorm noises are available for this purpose, but because most dogs are reacting to multiple stimuli such as changes in air pressure, blowing wind, and temperature changes, the use of these recordings frequently is not successful in completely eliminating the dog's fear. In some cases, drug therapy is advantageous during the treatment program if exposure to the eliciting stimuli cannot be prevented (for example, during a real storm). Pharmacological therapy for behavior problems in dogs should always be conducted under the direct supervision of a veterinary behaviorist.

Flooding involves exposing the animal to the fear-inducing stimulus and only removing the stimulus when the dog shows no fear (see Chapter 9). For success, it is imperative that the dog, the environment, and the stimulus are well controlled. When used, the initial stages of flooding involve presenting mild forms of the stimulus, if that is possible. The dog is prevented from escaping, and reinforcements (food treats, praise, petting) are given only when the dog stops showing fear and becomes calm. Once exposure to flooding has started, the owner must stay committed until the dog becomes calm or fearful behavior will be reinforced. Since it is not known how adversely the dog will react, there is always the risk of inadvertently reinforcing the dog's fear with this procedure. When successful, flooding is an expedient method for solving fear problems and involves much less time commitment on the part of the owner.

However, there are several serious disadvantages to this method of treatment. When the dog is very fearful, she may injure herself in attempting to escape, become aggressive, or become so highly stressed that calmness can never be reinforced. Some dogs may respond by generalizing their fear to other associated stimuli that are presented during the flooding process. These stimuli may include the owner, the setting, or the equipment used to restrain the dog. In general, fears that have been exhibited for a long duration do not respond well to flooding and may actually be exacerbated by this technique. Flooding is, therefore, more appropriate for moderate fear responses that have been exhibited for a short duration rather than for severe phobias.

Some cases of fear-related behaviors are resistant to treatment because of the degree of fear the dog shows, duration of the problem, a genetic disposition, or the owner's inability or unwillingness to commit to a complete behavior modification program. In such cases, managing the dog's environment to prevent exposure to the fearful stimuli may be the best solution. However, the owners should be aware that this simply masks the underlying problem and that fears do not usually abate over time in most dogs.

Separation-related Problems

The term separation anxiety or separation stress is used to describe problem behaviors dogs may show when they are isolated. These include destructiveness (chewing furniture and doorways, digging, scratching), vocalizations (barking, whining, howling), and inappropriate elimination (urination, defecation). Destructive and vocalization behaviors appear to represent attempts by the dog to be reunited with the owners, while defecation and urination are probably symptomatic of generalized anxiety. Because there are a number of potential causes of destructive behaviors and house soiling in dogs, a complete behavior history of the dog is essential for accurate diagnosis of separation anxiety. Treatment for destructive behaviors and house-soiling problems caused by boredom, attention-seeking, inadequate house-training, or medical problems are covered in many of the behavior books listed for Part II. The following section reviews diagnosis and treatment of these problems specifically as manifestations of separation anxiety.

Incidence: It has been estimated that separation-related problems comprise about 20 to 40 percent of the case loads of behavior consultants in the United States, with an incidence as high as 70 percent in some practices.[27,28,29] Hyperactivity and destructive behaviors are the most common signs of separation stress, with destructiveness often directed toward entry/exit areas. Although breed predilections have been reported in Labrador Retrievers, German Shepherd Dogs, and English Cocker Spaniels, these observations are primary anecdotal, and other studies of breed incidence have reported contrasting results.[30] One group found that purebred dogs were significantly more likely to be presented with separation anxiety than mixed breeds; others reported that mixed-breed dogs were more predisposed to this problem.[31,32]

Regardless of breed, the source from which the dog is obtained is significant. Dogs obtained from shelters have a higher incidence of separation anxiety than dogs obtained from other sources. While 20 to 26 percent of dogs diagnosed with separation anxiety at behavior clinics were obtained from shelters, only 8 percent of the general population of dogs attending the clinic for medical reasons had been adopted from shelters.[32] Statistical analysis of almost 500 canine behavior cases showed that dogs originating from shelters are significantly more likely to demonstrate separation anxiety signs than dogs obtained from purebred breeders, friends, pet shops, or advertisements.[28] What is not obvious from these studies is the underlying cause of this association. Are dogs abandoned or relinquished because of existing problems associated with separation, or does the environment of the shelter and the experiences of abandonment precipitate signs of separation stress? Other factors that may predispose a dog to separation-related problems include gender (males are affected more often than females), early weaning from the mother and other litter mates, multiple rehomings, and the excessive use of punishment as a training tool while young.[27,31]

Overattachment and separation anxiety: Dogs are highly social by nature and become strongly attached to their human caretakers. Attachment behaviors are essential for a social species whose survival originally depended upon cooperation between individuals and the formation of closely knit social groups. These behaviors function to keep individuals of the group together and to maintain social cohesion. Social animals engage in distress responses when separated from their companions. Distress crying and increased activity (even hyperactivity) are normal canine responses to separation from an attachment figure. Young puppies use these behaviors to communicate hunger, chilling, and loneliness. The mother reacts (and thus reinforces these behaviors) by returning to the litter and tending to the puppies. When a new puppy is brought into a home, these behaviors often are elicited when the puppy is separated from her new human pack members. It is a normal and expected response for puppies and young dogs to show some level of separation distress when isolated. As they mature, most dogs gradually become habituated to moderate periods of separation and to the normal daily routine of their owner. However, in some dogs, this habituation never occurs or a predisposition to overattachment behaviors leads to prolonged or severe signs of separation anxiety.

Signs of separation anxiety: A common circumstance reported by owners of dogs with separation anxiety is a sudden episode of separation that was preceded by a period of prolonged, relatively constant proximity to the owner. Typical scenarios include families who obtain a dog during the summer months when the children are home from school, followed by the start of the school year and sudden isolation for the dog; changes in the owner's work or travel schedule that require sudden and prolonged time periods away from home; or changes in the status of the family, such as a divorce or children leaving home for college. In some cases, separation anxiety is preceded by a stay at a boarding kennel or other enforced separation from the owner. Although many dogs adapt (i.e., habituate) to these changes with no signs of distress, dogs that are very attached to their owners may develop behavior problems when left alone.

Dogs that exhibit separation anxiety usually show other behaviors that indicate a high degree of dependency and attachment. They may greet the owner in a hyperexcitable state and are more likely to follow the owner around the home and show distress if isolated in another room. These dogs often are intolerant of confinement, and attempts to use a crate to confine the dog are met with increased anxiety and destructiveness. Some dogs with separation anxiety have been described as having "barrier frustration," a form of claustrophobia in which the dog cannot tolerate confinement to small areas or separation behind a baby gate or other type of barrier. Interestingly, many dogs with separation anxiety will tolerate confinement to the owner's car but cannot tolerate isolation in any other situation.[32] Some owners report that the dog will not willingly go outside for elimination if the owner does not accompany the dog.

Separation anxiety manifests as one or more problem behaviors, which include distress vocalizations (howling, barking, whining), destructive behaviors (chewing, digging), hyperactivity (excessive greeting behavior, constant attention-seeking), or inappropriate elimination. The most obvious feature of separation anxiety is the display of these behaviors only when the owner is not present. Typically, if the owner has had the opportunity to observe the dog, the behaviors commence within a few minutes after the owner has departed. Although some dogs are destructive or vocal for only a short period of time following the owner's departure, recent studies have found that many dogs with separation anxiety are active and destructive for several hours.[33] Signs of stress or anxiety often are displayed by the dog in response to the owner's "predeparture cues" such as putting on a coat, picking up car keys, or locking doors. Owners describe the dogs as upset and overly solicitous, often showing physical signs of stress such as trembling, salivating, and pacing.

When dogs with separation anxiety are destructive, they usually direct their effort toward a point of exit from the home or room in which the dog is kept or toward an item that carries a strong scent of the owner. For example, the dog may scratch and dig at the base of the door, doorknob, or window dressings, or may chew up a couch cushion or item of clothing. When separation anxiety is the cause of elimination in the home, the dog usually is housebroken when the owner is home, and the elimination occurs shortly after the owner leaves, regardless of whether or not the dog had eliminated outside prior to the owner's departure. Vocalization related to separation, as opposed to watchdog barking, play behaviors, or boredom, occurs primarily at the time of the owner's departure or shortly afterward and may persist at regular intervals for a few minutes or up to several hours.

Treatment program for separation anxiety: The ultimate goal for treating separation anxiety is to decrease the dog's dependency on the owner, increase her level of security when isolated, and prevent behaviors that are destructive to the owner's home or dangerous to the dog's safety. This is generally accomplished through counter-conditioning and systematic desensitization. In some cases, administering anti-anxiety medication is helpful adjunctive therapy during early stages of the behavior modification program.

The first step involves counter-conditioning the dog's anxiety response to the owner's predeparture cues. For example, a specifically designated special toy, such as a hard bone with the ends stuffed with moist treats, cheese, or peanut butter can be given to the dog while the owner engages in the predeparture cues. These toys work well because these items often occupy the dog for 30 minutes or more, thus providing a necessary time frame within which to habituate the dog to isolation. The toy is initially taken away from the dog while he or she is still very interested in it, and is only provided when the owner is engaging in the predeparture cues. Giving the dog access to a highly desirable reinforcer has the effect of strengthening its power as a counter-conditioning tool (see Chapter 9). The owner gradually desensitizes the dog to predeparture cues by repeatedly exposing the dog to the cues throughout the day but without following these cues with departure. For example, the owner may pick up the keys numerous times, counter-condition the dog using the special toy, then continue about his or her business around the house. These counter-conditioning and habituation exercises are very important components of the treatment program for separation anxiety. They serve to reduce the dog's anxiety in anticipation of the owner's absence and also begin to build a positive association between the special toy and isolation. When the dog has become desensitized to predeparture cues, a program of graduated departures can be introduced.

Graduated departures are first introduced by habituating the dog to isolation in a separate room while the owner is still at home. This can be accomplished by developing a daily schedule in which the dog is separated from the owner for gradually increasing durations. These separations are paired with one or more of the toys stuffed with food that were used to condition the dog to predeparture cues. As with the previous phase of the treatment program, these toys are only provided to the dog during the training sessions to facilitate an association between something pleasurable and the owner's absence. At the start of this phase of the program, the dog should be left alone only for periods of time that are shorter than it takes for the dog to engage in an anxiety response. If the predeparture cues have been well conditioned and the dog is given a chew toy stuffed with enticing tidbits, most dogs will tolerate absences of a few minutes. The owner simply leaves the dog in the room for a few minutes; returns; reinforces calm behavior with praise, petting, and a food treat; removes the chew toy; and releases the dog from the room. This sequence is repeated several times throughout the day.

If the dog is well conditioned to predeparture cues (i.e, the dog never experienced an anxiety response and was reliably calm to all predeparture cues), the presence of the food-stuffed toy becomes a "safety cue" for the dog. This means it can represent cues of isolation periods in which the owner is gone for a very short time and no anxiety occurred. This is why it is imperative the chew toy or bone not be provided at any other time, especially at times during the treatment program when the owner is required to be away for an extended period and there is a high probability the dog will experience anxiety. The novel toy should never be given to the dog when the owner leaves for a period longer than the dog is capable of tolerating because the item will then lose its value as a safety cue if it becomes associated with anxiety. The safety cue should always be removed when the owner returns and only be presented again to the dog prior to another departure. The owner's return should be very low-key and calm, and the toy should be quietly removed.

As the dog becomes acclimated to the room and begins to anticipate the desired toy (safety cue), the owner can progress to slowly increased durations, using variable time periods (for example, 10 minutes, 4 minutes, 12 minutes, 1 minute). Gradually, periods of 30 to 45 minutes can be included. Once a dog tolerates 45 minutes of isolation, the owner can begin to add the predeparture cues and, eventually, actually leave the house for short periods of time. When these new cues are added, however, the time period should once again be decreased to several minutes then gradually increased to 30 minutes or more. Again, a schedule of gradually increasing time periods can be devised but should be adjusted during treatment to reflect the dog's response at each level of separation.

During treatment for separation anxiety, the dog's response always determines the rate at which the owner proceeds. Since dogs differ greatly in their abilities to tolerate isolation and to counter-condition to the safety cue, the owner must use the dog's response to a previous session to determine whether or not the dog is ready to tolerate an increased time period. A written time schedule is useful as a guide, but the dog's ability to tolerate each level of separation should be the ultimate criteria in determining progress to a new level. The owner can increase the duration of separation when the dog exhibits no predeparture anxiety to the current level and the dog does not appear stressed or show exaggerated greeting behaviors when the owner returns. The most important factor is that the dog remains unanxious. If the schedule is increased too rapidly and anxiety results, the problem often is exacerbated and the usefulness of the safety cue may be lost. Ancillary recommendations during treatment for separation anxiety include providing a very regular, consistent program of exercise, training, and attention for the dog. A structured, predictable daily schedule serves to decrease overall stress.

For some dogs, drug therapy is helpful during the initial phases of treatment for separation anxiety. The two most commonly prescribed drugs are diazepam and amitriptyline. These should only be used under the supervision of a veterinary behaviorist and should be used in conjunction with a behavior modification program. Simply sedating the dog is not a solution to separation anxiety and can provide the owner with a false sense of security if used without addressing the underlying overattachment problems.

Prevention: It is known that separation distress is a normal component of all puppies' behavioral repertoire, and that these distress signals are transferred to separation from human caretakers once a puppy is placed in his new home. As they grow and develop, puppies can become habituated to short periods of isolation through regular, short periods of time during which they are kept in a separate room or in a crate. Socialization to many people and experiences coupled with regular, short periods of isolation gradually teach puppies to readily accept new experiences and to be comfortable with isolation. A safety-cue toy, such as a hollow bone stuffed with treats, can be used. Several new toys are now available that require the animal to manipulate and chew on them to receive reinforcement. These toys can be provided whenever the puppy is isolated, pairing the special toy with short periods of alone time. As the dog matures, regular periods of isolation coupled with a consistent daily routine of exercise, attention, play, and handling are essential for the prevention of separation-related problems during adulthood.

Pharmacotherapy for Behavior Problems

The treatment of some behavior problems in dogs may be augmented with pharmacotherapy. Medical problems that may cause behavior changes in dogs include endocrine imbalances (hypothyroidism, Cushing's syndrome), neurological disorders, local sources of pain, or even nutritional imbalances. A cautious approach should be taken, however, as drugs should only be used to complement a behavior modification program and should not be expected to provide a magical cure. Knowledge about the benefits of pharmacotherapy for the treatment of behavior problems in dogs has increased greatly in recent years, and there are now many veterinary behaviorists who are trained in the use of these medications. Whenever drug therapy is considered, the treatment regimen should always be prescribed under the supervision of a veterinary behaviorist.[35,36]

Conclusions

An understanding of the dog's social and developmental behavior and ways in which dogs learn are important for all professionals who work with companion animals. In addition, a thorough understanding of the cause of common behavior problems and methods for their management and prevention are integral to maintaining a strong, enduring human-dog bond. Another important component of the care and keeping of companion animals is preventive and curative medical attention. In the following section, preventive veterinary care for dogs is reviewed, and chapters are provided that examine common infectious and non-infectious diseases, internal and external parasites, and developmental skeletal disorders. The final chapter provides first aid procedures for emergency situations.

Cited References

1. Houpt, K.A., Honig, S.U., and Reisner, I.R. **Exploring the bond: Breaking the human-companion animal bond.** Journal of the American Veterinary Medical Association, 208:1653-1658. (1996)

2. Miller, D.D., Staats, S.R., and Partlo, C. **Factors associated with the decision to surrender a pet to an animal shelter.** Journal of the American Animal Hospital Association, 209:738-742. (1996)

3. Voith, V.L. and Borchelt, P.L. **Elimination behavior and related problems in dogs.** In: *Readings in Companion Animal Behavior,* Veterinary Learning Systems, Trenton, New Jersey, pp. 168-178. (1996)

4. Voith, V.L. and Borchelt, P.L. **History taking and interviewing.** In: *Readings in Companion Animal Behavior,* Veterinary Learning Systems, Trenton, New Jersey, pp. 42-47. (1996)

5. Hart, B. and Hart, L. *Canine and Feline Behavioral Therapy,* Lea and Febiger, Philadelphia, Pennsylvania. (1985)

6. Lockwood, R. **The ethology and epidemiology of canine aggression.** In: *The Domestic Dog: Its Evolution, Behavior, and Interactions with People* (J.A. Serpell, editor), Cambridge University Press, Cambridge, United Kingdom, pp. 131-138. (1995)

7. Sacks, J.J., Sattin, R.W., and Bonzo, S.E. **Dog bites: Related fatalities from 1979 through 1988.** Journal of the American Medical Association, 1489-1492. (1989)

8. Serpell, J.A. and Jagoe, J.A. **Early experience and the development of behaviour.** In: *The Domestic Dog: Its Evolution, Behavior, and Interactions with People* (J.A. Serpell, editor), Cambridge University Press, Cambridge, United Kingdom, pp. 80-102. (1995)

9. Mugford, R.A. **Behavior problems in the dog.** In: *Nutrition and Behavior in Dogs and Cats* (R.S. Anderson, editor), Pergamon Press, Oxford, United Kingdom, pp.207-215. (1984)

10. Campbell, W.E. *Behavior Problems in Dogs,* American Veterinary Publications, Inc., Santa Barbara, California. (1975)

11. Beaver, B.V. **Clinical classification of canine aggression.** Applied Animal Ethology, 10:35-43. (1983)

12. Line, S. and Voith, V.L. **Dominance aggression of dogs toward people: Behavior profile and response to treatment.** Applied Animal Behavior Science, 16:77-83. (1986)

13. Polsky, R.H. **Factors influencing aggressive behavior in dogs.** California Veterinarian, 37:12-15. (1983)

14. Borchelt, P.L. **Aggressive behavior of dogs kept as companion animals: Classification and influence of sex, reproduction status and breed.** Applied Animal Ethology, 10:45-61. (1983)

15. O'Farrell, V. and Peachey, E. **Behavioral effects of ovariohysterectomy on bitches.** Journal of Small Animal Practice, 31:595-598. (1990)

16. Jagoe, J.A. **Behaviour problems in the domestic dog: A retrospective study to identify factors influencing their development.** Unpublished Ph.D. Thesis, Cambridge University, United Kingdom. (1994)

17. Borchelt, P.L. and Voith, V.L. **Dominant aggression in dogs.** In: *Readings in Companion Animal Behavior* (V.L. Voith and P.L. Borchelt, editors), Veterinary Learning Systems, Trenton, New Jersey, pp. 230-239. (1996)

18. Borchelt, P.L. and Copopola, M.C. **Characteristics of dominance aggression in dogs.** Paper presented at Annual Meeting of the Animal Behavior Society, North Carolina, June. (1985)

19. Donaldson, J. *Culture Clash: A Revolutionary New Way of Understanding the Relationship between Humans and Domestic Dogs,* James and Kenneth Publishers, Oakland, California, 221 pp. (1996)

20. Voith, V.L. and Borchelt, P.L. **Fears and phobias in companion animals.** In: *Readings in Companion Animal Behavior,* Veterinary Learning Systems, Trenton, New Jersey, pp. 140-152. (1996)

21. Goddard, M.E. and Beilharz, R.G. **Factor analysis of fearfulness in potential guide dogs.** Applied Animal Behaviour Science, 12:253-265. (1984)

22. Tuber, D.S., Hothersall, D., and Peters, M.F. **Treatment of fears and phobias in dogs.** Veterinary Clinics of North America: Small Animal Practice, 12:607-623. (1982)

23. Thorne, F.C. **The inheritance of shyness in dogs.** Journal of Genetic Psychology, 65:275-279. (1944)

24. Clark, R.S., Heron, W., and Fetherstonhaugh, M.L. **Individual differences in dogs: preliminary report on the effects of early experience.** Canadian Journal of Psychology, 5:150-156. (1951)

25. Fox, M.W. and Stelzner, D. **Behavioural effects of differential early experience in the dog.** Animal Behaviour, 14:273-181. (1966)

26. Landsberg, G., Hunthausen, W., and Ackerman, L. **Fears and phobias.** In: *Handbook of Behaviour Problems of the Dog and Cat,* Butterworth/Heinemann, Oxford, United Kingdom, pp.119-128. (1997)

27. McCrave, E.A. **Diagnostic criteria for separation anxiety in the dog.** Veterinary Clinics of North America, Small Animal Practice, 21:247-255. (1991)

28. Voith, V.L., Goodloe, L., Chapman, B., and Marder, A.R. **Comparison of dogs presented for behavior problems by source of dog.** Paper presented at AVMA Annual Meeting, Seattle, Washington, July 18. (1993)

29. Landsberg, G. **The distribution of canine behavior cases at three behavior referral practices.** Veterinary Medicine, 86:1011-1018. (1991)

30. Mugford, R.A. **Attachment versus dominance: An alternate view of the man-dog relationship.** In: *The Human-Pet Relationship,* Vienna, Proceedings of the Institute for Interdisciplinary Research on the Human-Pet Relationship, pp. 157-165. (1985)

31. Voith, V.L. and Ganster, D. **Separation anxiety: Review of 42 cases.** An abstract. Applied Animal Behavior Science, 37:84-85. (1993)

32. Voith, V.L., and Borchelt, P.L. **Separation anxiety in dogs.** In: *The Domestic Dog: Its Evolution, Behavior, and Interactions with People,* Cambridge University Press, Cambridge, United Kingdom, pp. 124-139. (1995)

33. Tuber, D.S. **The soft exercise.** Animal Behavior Consultants Newsletter, 3:2. (1986)

34. Simpson, B.S. and Simpson, D.M. **Behavioural pharmacotherapy.** In: *Readings in Companion Animal Behavior,* Veterinary Learning Systems, Trenton, New Jersey, pp. 100-115. (1996)

35. Landsberg, G., Hunthausen, W., and Ackerman, L. **Drugs used in behavioural therapy.** In: *Handbook of Behaviour Problems of the Dog and Cat,* Butterworth/Heinemann, Oxford, United Kingdom, pp.47-64. (1997)

Part 3   Health and Disease

11 Infectious Diseases and Vaccination Programs

CARING RESPONSIBLY for dogs includes attention to health and the provision of appropriate preventive vaccinations. In Chapter 3, procedures for recognizing a normal, healthy dog were presented. Assessing body temperature, pulse rate, respiration rate, food intake, changes in weight and body condition, and skin health are all helpful in determining a dog's health and vitality. In addition to these, preventive health care measures such as regular veterinary checkups, vaccinations for viral and bacterial diseases, and dewormings are important. In this chapter, several important viral, bacterial, and fungal diseases of dogs are reviewed, and vaccination programs for immunization against disease are presented.

Viral Diseases

Viruses and related agents such as rickettsia are relatively simple microorganisms. They are very small particles composed of strands of nucleic acid (either RNA or DNA) enclosed in a protein shell called a capsid. Some include special types of enzymes that aid in their replication within host cells. Viruses cannot survive outside of a host cell and require the host for **replication**. Once a virus has gained access into a susceptible cell, it exerts control over all biochemical processes, allowing virus replication and the infection of other cells. When host cells are destroyed by the virus, the damaged tissue and the host's immune reaction to the infection result in clinical disease.

Very few viral diseases respond to antiviral medication, so the control of pathogenic viruses in dogs is achieved principally through supportive therapy and prevention of infection through vaccination. Treatment of infections consists primarily of fluid and electrolyte support, prevention of secondary bacterial or fungal infections, and **palliative** therapy for specific effects of the virus. Predominant viral diseases that occur in dogs in the United States include canine distemper, infectious canine hepatitis, rabies, canine infectious tracheobronchitis, canine parvovirus, and canine coronavirus (Table 11.1).

Canine distemper: Distemper is caused by a virus that is a member of the Paramyxoviridae family of viruses and is similar but not identical to the virus that causes measles in humans. The disease, also called Carre's disease, was first recognized early in the twentieth century. Although the distemper virus does not persist for long periods of time in the environment, it is easily transmitted between animals through aerosol contamination or direct contact

TABLE 11.1   Major Infectious Viruses of Dogs

Disease	Transmission	Body Systems Affected	Primary Signs
Canine Distemper	aerosol contamination; contact with body fluids	respiratory system, gastrointestinal system, skin and mucous membranes, nervous system	fever, nasal/ocular discharge, cough; progressing to pneumonia, diarrhea, and eventually paresis and convulsions
Infectious Canine Hepatitis	direct contact with infected animal	liver, kidney, central nervous system, vascular endothelium	fever, anorexia, liver failure, hemorrhagic diathesis; can be rapidly fatal in young puppies
Rabies	bite from or direct contact with infected animal	central nervous system, respiratory system, gastrointestinal system, salivary glands	change in temperament, hypersensitivity, photophobia, paralysis; eventually fatal
Canine Infectious Tracheobronchitis	contact with nasal or oral secretions of infected animal	upper respiratory tract	persistent cough, transient fever; can progress to pneumonia in severe cases
Canine Parvovirus	contact with feces or body tissues of infected animal; virus is extremely hardy and persists for long periods in the environment	gastrointestinal tract, lymph nodes, thymus, bone marrow, heart tissue in young puppies	fever, abdominal pain, anorexia, severe bloody diarrhea, dehydration; respiratory distress (myocarditis syndrome)
Canine Coronavirus	direct contact with feces or fluids of infected dogs	gastrointestinal tract, upper respiratory tract (infrequent)	lethargy, anorexia, vomiting, diarrhea

with body secretions. The virus has a special affinity for attacking the epithelial cells that line the conjunctival membranes of the eye, mucous membranes of the gastrointestinal (GI) tract, and parts of the nervous system. In addition to infecting the dog, canine distemper virus also infects coyotes, wolves, foxes, raccoons, skunks, and several other wild mammals.

Several strains of distemper virus with varying abilities to cause disease have been identified. Because most strains have low virulence and because there is widespread immunity in the domestic dog population, the majority of infections in adult dogs are asymptomatic or very mild in nature. When serious infections occur, they are seen most often in puppies or adolescent dogs. Puppies less than 7 weeks of age who are born to mothers that have not been vaccinated against distemper are most susceptible. Distemper in preweaned puppies takes the form of **hemorrhagic enteritis**. Signs include a low-grade fever, depression, anorexia, and sudden and severe diarrhea. Puppies do not respond to treatment and will usually die within 1 to 2 weeks after signs begin. This form of the disease occurs most often in crowded, unsanitary conditions and can cause the death of entire litters of puppies.

Older puppies and adolescent dogs that are infected typically develop distemper in two stages. Clinical signs of first-stage distemper are seen 3 to 15 days following exposure to the virus. The dog develops a fever (103 to 105 degrees F), is depressed and lethargic, has a decreased appetite, and develops a nasal and ocular discharge. Within a few days, the discharge becomes **purulent,** and the dog may begin to cough sporadically. While some dogs gradually recover from this stage over a period of several weeks, others show fluctuating health without recovery and eventually progress to second-stage distemper. Second-stage distemper is signified by infection in multiple tissues of the body. Involvement of the lungs and upper respiratory tract leads to pneumonia, infection in the small intestine causes diarrhea and dehydration, and viral spread to the integument (skin) results in a rash and **hyperkeratosis** (thickening of the skin). The term "hard pad distemper" refers to infection of the skin on the bottom of the dog's feet with the distemper virus.

Spread of the virus to the nervous system and the brain is the final manifestation of the disease and is the cause of most fatalities. Neurological involvement can be insidious because it may occur up to 6 weeks after a dog has apparently recovered from other signs of distemper. Partial paralysis (**paresis**) and **myoclonus** are first seen, and these signs eventually progress to dementia and convulsions. Dogs that recover from this form of distemper often retain neurological problems, such as mild forms of myoclonus, seizures, or balance abnormalities.

Infectious canine hepatitis: The virus that causes infectious canine hepatitis is classified as adenovirus type 1. This virus also infects foxes, coyotes, wolves, skunks, and bears but is not the same virus that causes hepatitis in humans. Transmission occurs through direct contact with infected animals. The disease is seen most commonly in unvaccinated dogs that are less than 1 year old. This prevalence indicates that many dogs develop natural immunity to the hepatitis virus by the time they are 1 to 2 years of age.

Infection with the hepatitis virus affects primarily the liver, kidneys, and lining of blood vessels (the vascular endothelium). Infected dogs may develop one of several forms of the disease. Subclinical cases are characterized by a transient fever, decreased appetite, and reddening of the mucous membranes of the mouth and eyes. Recovery often occurs without the owner becoming aware of the dog's infection. In contrast, puppies that are less than 6 weeks of age are susceptible to a severe form of hepatitis that causes death within a day or less. Puppies rapidly develop a high fever, abdominal pain, and reddening of the membranes of the mouth and conjunctiva. Death occurs despite supportive treatment. Slightly older puppies (6 to 10 weeks of age) usually show milder initial signs of the disease but also can be severely affected. While some recover, most become progressively ill and develop a bleeding syndrome called **hemorrhagic diathesis**. Liver and central nervous system involvement eventually occur and result in death. In general, prognosis improves with age, with mortality rates much lower in older puppies and adolescents.

Dog that recover from infectious canine hepatitis may develop interstitial keratitis, or "blue eye." This is seen most commonly after recovery from mild forms of hepatitis and is caused by an immunologic reaction to the invasion of the virus. This condition is usually self-limiting and disappears within a few weeks post-infection. Early vaccines for the control of hepatitis caused blue eye in some dogs as a temporary side effect. However, the development of vaccines for adenovirus type 2, which protect against both hepatitis and kennel cough do not cause this problem.

Rabies: Rabies is an invariably fatal disease that is found throughout the world, with the exception of Australia and Antarctica. Rabies can be transmitted to all warm-blooded animals. Despite effective vaccines for animals and humans, rabies remains a worldwide problem whenever outbreaks occur in populations of wild animals or in areas in which there are large numbers of unvaccinated dogs and cats. The principle reservoirs of the rabies virus in the United States are skunks, raccoons, bats, and foxes. Because of widespread vaccination programs, there is an effective immunological barrier between domestic dogs and the rabies virus in this country. In 1947, 6,949 cases of canine rabies were reported in the United States. This has been reduced to only 130 in 1993.[1] However, dogs remain a primary reservoir host for rabies and are the principal source of human exposure to the disease in some developing countries.

The rabies virus is classified within an RNA-containing family of viruses called the Rhabdoviridae. Animals that are infected secrete large amounts of virus particles in their saliva. As a result, the primary mode of transmission is a bite from an infected animal. Salivary transmission of the virus can begin as early as 2 weeks before an animal shows clinical signs of disease.

A unique aspect of infection with rabies is its variable incubation period. An incubation period refers to the time between exposure to the virus and the onset of clinical signs of disease. The incubation period for rabies varies from 1 week to 10 weeks after exposure. Cases have even been reported that developed more than 1 year after contact with an infected animal. This occurs because the virus can be retained within muscle cells for a variable period of time at the site of the bite wound. After several days to a few weeks, the virus travels to the nervous system and gains access to the spinal cord and brain. After this stage of infection, the virus begins to infect other tissues of the body, including the salivary glands, respiratory system, and digestive system.

Initial signs of rabies infection involve a change in temperament. The dog may be restless, insecure, apprehensive, or overly affectionate. Clinical manifestations of rabies have been classified into two different forms. Most animals show some signs of each of these, and the paralytic form always represents the terminal stage of disease. The excitatory or "furious" form of rabies occurs for 1 to 7 days and is characterized by restlessness, change in behavior, and inappropriate aggression. Dogs often bite or snap at any type of stimulus, even inanimate objects. As the disease progresses, the dog shows hypersensitivity to touch, light (photophobia), and occasionally to sound. Partial paralysis of the muscles of the face and throat lead to bizarre facial expressions and changes in the dog's voice. Eventually, the dog develops convulsions. While some animals die during a convulsion, most progress to the paralytic form of the disease. This stage lasts only 1 to 2 days, rapidly causing death. Initially, the dog's facial muscles become paralyzed, causing the dog's mouth to hang partially open. The dog is unable to ingest water or food because of the loss of the ability to swallow. Eventually, total paralysis and death occur.

Dogs that are suspected to have contracted rabies usually are euthanized, and brain tissue is submitted to a rabies diagnostic laboratory for diagnosis. Dogs that have bitten a person are required to be confined (quarantined) for at least 10 days following the bite and are observed for the development of signs of rabies. A dog that is vaccinated and has been bitten by an animal suspected to be rabid should be given a rabies booster immunization immediately and kept under observation for 90 days.

Canine infectious tracheobronchitis (kennel cough): The term "tracheobronchitis" refers to inflammation of the upper respiratory tract, including the **larynx, trachea**, and **bronchi**. The common term for acute infectious tracheobronchitis in dogs is "kennel cough" and is referred to as a **syndrome** because the same signs can be caused by several different viral and bacterial agents. Kennel cough occurs most commonly, though not exclusively, in dogs that are housed in kennels or shelters.

Controlled research studies have been important in identifying the major causative agents. While each of these agents is capable of producing tracheobronchitis independently, most naturally occurring cases involve infection with several agents, referred to as "mixed infections."[2] Kennel cough is highly contagious between dogs and is transmitted through nasal and oral secretions. It is seen most often in dogs that have been housed in boarding kennels or animal shelters, or dogs that are traveling on dog show circuits. Kennels often are poorly ventilated, include a dense population of dogs, and can be stressful environments for some dogs. All of these factors contribute to the spread and development of acute tracheobronchitis.

The major complex of viruses that cause kennel cough include canine parainfluenza-3, canine adenovirus type 2, and canine herpesvirus. The parainfluenza virus belongs to the same family as the virus that causes distemper in dogs. It appears to be the most common viral cause of tracheobronchitis in dogs and results in a generally mild form of kennel cough.[3] However, severe forms of the disease can occur when parainfluenza and *Bordetella bronchiseptica* infect the upper respiratory tract at the same time. Canine adenovirus type 2 is related to the virus that causes infectious canine hepatitis (adenovirus type 1). This agent is less common, but when infection occurs, it causes a relatively severe form of tracheobronchitis that may lead to pneumonia in susceptible animals. Canine herpesvirus produces a mild respiratory tract infection by itself but is most often found in mixed infections with other viruses or with *Bordetella bronchiseptica*.

The bacteria *Bordetella bronchiseptica* is considered to be the principle bacterial cause of kennel cough and can cause a severe form of kennel cough without co-infection with other microbes.[4] It is the most common cause of kennel cough in dogs housed in large kennels or animal shelters. The *Bordetella* bacteria are capable of producing chronic low-level infections because each organism has the ability to adhere to the cells lining the trachea and resists being swept away by normal movement of the cilia. *Bordetella* can survive in the dog's upper respiratory tract for several months, damaging the lining of the trachea and allowing other bacteria and viruses to invade and further complicate the original infection. Because of *Bordetella*'s ability to colonize the respiratory tract, dogs can continue to pass this organism to other dogs for several weeks after clinical signs have disappeared. Other bacteria that have been implicated as causative agents of kennel cough include *Pasteurella*, *Streptococcus* and *Staphylococcus* species. However, these microbes are usually found with other viruses or *Bordetella*, and do not seem to be singular causes of kennel cough.

All agents that cause kennel cough have relatively short incubation periods, usually between 4 and 8 days.[5] The severity of the signs that the dog develops varies, depending upon the dog's immune system, age, and the number and type of microorganisms involved. The most consistent and obvious sign is a persistent cough that has a characteristic "honking" sound. Fever, eye and nasal discharges, lethargy, or anorexia are usually *not* seen. Some dogs develop a transient low-grade fever during the first few days of infection, but this resolves quickly and usually is undetected by the owner. In most cases, the dog appears healthy but has a persistent cough. Initially, the cough is moist and productive but quickly becomes dry and harsh. Coughing often is stimulated by excitement or pressure on the dog's trachea. In most cases, the disease is self-limiting, and the cough gradually decreases in frequency over a period of 1 to 2 weeks, disappearing completely by 3 weeks. However, some dogs develop a chronic cough that persists for as long as 6 weeks. This occurs most often in young puppies or elderly dogs. In very young puppies, severe infections with kennel cough can lead to the development of pneumonia, and veterinary care should be provided.

Affected dogs should be isolated from other dogs and kept in a quiet environment. Humidifying the environment often provides some relief from the persistent cough. Many veterinarians prescribe a cough suppressant to allow the trachea to heal during the acute phase of the illness. The use of antibiotic therapy for dogs with kennel cough has been controversial. However, recent studies have shown that dogs with kennel cough recover faster with antibiotic therapy, regardless of the causative agent that is involved.[6] The two antibiotics shown to be most effective in ameliorating clinical signs were trimethoprim-sulfonamide and ampicillin (or amoxicillin). Antibiotics should always be given when there is a risk the dog will develop pneumonia.

Vaccination programs are effective in reducing a dog's risk of contracting kennel cough. However, because there are numerous causative agents, the available vaccines do not protect against all forms of the disease. In addition, natural infections are best prevented through local immunity of the respiratory tract. Local immunity is mediated by a specific type of immunoglobulin called IgA, and once stimulated is protective for only 6 months or less. Frequent re-vaccinations may be necessary in dogs that are at high risk of exposure. Keeping a clean, well-ventilated environment and reducing crowding are also effective measures for limiting the exposure and spread of kennel cough.

Canine parvovirus: This serious disease was first recognized in the United States in 1978 when a group of dogs at a large dog show in Louisville, Kentucky, became very ill. Canine parvovirus is now known to be found throughout the world as a cause of severe and sometimes fatal hemorrhagic gastrointestinal disease. The responsible virus, canine parvovirus-2b is classified with the Parvoviridae family. When it was first identified in the late 1970s, the virus was named canine parvovirus type 2. It is believed that this variant emerged from a parvovirus that causes panleukopenia in domestic cats.[7] The virus has mutated to more virulent strains on two separate occasions since 1979. They were designated canine parvovirus-2a and canine parvovirus-2b, respectively. Today, canine parvovirus-2b appears to be the cause of the majority of cases of parvovirus infections in dogs in the United States.[8] The virus is also capable of infecting coyotes and several other canid species.

Parvovirus is a highly resistant virus. It can survive most cleaning agents and disinfectants, and is capable of persisting in the environment for 6 months or longer. Only exposure to direct sunlight, formalin, or sodium hypochlorite (chlorine bleach) inactivates the virus and renders it non-infectious.[9] Moreover, infected animals secrete large numbers of virus particles in their feces, further contributing to a high rate of transmission. Contact with feces and other body tissues of infected animals is the most common route of transmission.

Once the virus gains access to a host animal, it replicates within actively dividing cells, most of which are found in the intestinal tract, bone marrow, thymus, and lymph nodes. Nondividing cells are resistant to infection with parvovirus. Young puppies and dogs less than 6 months of age are most susceptible, and transmission and disease outbreaks are highest in puppies living in overcrowded, unsanitary environments. The presence of intestinal parasites and inadequate levels of protective immunity from maternal antibodies further increase risk of infection. Certain breeds are reported to have a higher risk for infection with parvovirus. These include Rottweilers, Doberman Pinschers, and Labrador Retrievers.[10,11] It is theorized that these breeds may develop active immunity at a later age than other dogs, resulting in a longer period of susceptibility as maternally derived immunity decreases in puppies.

Parvovirus has an incubation period of 7 to 14 days and causes two primary forms of disease. The most commonly seen manifestation of infection is a severe and often hemorrhagic **enteritis**. After gaining oral access into the body, the virus infects epithelial cells lining the small intestine, begins to replicate, and eventually kills infected cells. This leads to a loss of the epithelial lining, inflammation, hemorrhagic diarrhea, and a decrease in the intestine's absorptive capacity. Clinical signs of illness include abdominal pain, depression, loss of appetite, vomiting, and severe diarrhea. Most dogs develop a high fever, between 103 and 106 degrees F. The diarrhea that is produced eventually becomes bloody and has a characteristic appearance and odor. Because of the severity of the enteritis, the dog rapidly loses fluids and electrolytes. Fluid replacement to prevent dehydration is an important component of treatment in this stage of disease. If veterinary care is not provided promptly, there is a high risk of mortality, especially in puppies.

The second and less common manifestation of parvovirus infection is a **myocarditis**. This is seen almost exclusively in puppies that are less than 2 months of age and is a result of infection in utero or shortly after birth. Heart cells reproduce rapidly in fetuses and newborns. The rate of cellular division decreases significantly after puppies are several weeks old. This change in cellular growth makes the heart tissue susceptible to infection for only a short period of time. The myocarditis syndrome is seen almost exclusively in puppies of nonvaccinated bitches. Signs occur suddenly and are nonspecific. Puppies cry persistently, gasp for breath, and show difficulty breathing. Death occurs within 24 to 48 hours. Today, the myocarditis syndrome is relatively rare, owing to improved vaccination programs for dogs. If a puppy recovers from this form of the disease, it may develop chronic congestive heart disease several months later. In cases in which entire litters are infected, a very high mortality rate is seen.

Diagnosis of parvovirus is made indirectly by eliminating other possible causes of the vomiting and bloody diarrhea, and rapidly through a laboratory test that detects and identifies the virus in a fecal sample.[12] As with other viral diseases, there is no antiviral therapy for parvovirus. Care is directed toward preventing dehydration, replacing electrolytes, and preventing the invasion of secondary bacterial infections. The primary goal is to stabilize the dog until its normal immune responses can become activated and can rid the virus from the body. Fluid therapy is the most important component of therapy for parvovirus infections because of the large amounts of fluid loss that occurs. Although fewer dogs die from parvovirus today, mortality is still relatively high for very young puppies and elderly dogs that contract the disease.

Prevention of infection involves vaccination and proper sanitation practices. Dogs that have recovered from canine parvovirus infection acquire a long-term immunity, and several types of parvovirus vaccines are available. Parvovirus is an extremely hardy virus. Once canine parvovirus has occurred in a house or kennel, the virus can persist in the environment for many months and can be carried on the shoes or clothing of people. However, parvovirus can be inactivated with a 1:30 solution of chlorine bleach. This is roughly equivalent to diluting 1 cup of bleach in 2 gallons of warm water. Proper housing and sanitation are also important components in controlling the spread of canine parvovirus.

Canine coronavirus: This virus was first isolated and identified in 1971 in Germany when an outbreak of intestinal enteritis occurred in a kennel of military dogs. It is in the same family of viruses as the virus that causes feline infectious peritonitis in cats. Because clinical signs of coronavirus are similar to those of parvovirus, it is believed that misdiagnosis of coronavirus as parvovirus occurred relatively frequently prior to the development of rapid diagnostic tests.[13] Mixed infections of coronavirus and parvovirus also are seen. Like canine parvovirus, coronavirus is highly contagious and is transmitted through direct contact with feces or materials that were contaminated with feces or fluids of infected dogs. The virus has a relatively short incubation period (1 to 4 days) and causes intestinal illness that is similar to but less severe than canine parvovirus.

Primary signs are a mild to moderately severe gastrointestinal disease and, less frequently, upper respiratory disease. Anorexia and lethargy are first seen, followed within a day by vomiting and diarrhea. Unlike parvovirus, dogs with coronavirus usually do not develop a fever. Diarrhea often is intermittent, and most dogs recover completely within 7 to 10 days. Occasionally, relapses of diarrhea occur for several weeks. Supportive therapy is provided to control the vomiting and diarrhea, and fluid replacement may be given in severe cases. Prevention is primarily through vaccination and preventing exposure to infected animals.

Bacterial Diseases

There are numerous types of bacterial infections that can infect the domestic dog. Some are natural pathogens, and others are opportunistic, only causing disease when the host has been compromised through infection with another agent. Leptospirosis is an important bacterial disease in dogs because it is one of the few zoonotic diseases of the dog. A zoonosis is a disease that is the natural host of both humans and other species and for which cross-transmission can occur. Humans can contract leptospirosis from several sources, and the bacteria can be transmitted from an infected dog to a susceptible human. Canine pyoderma is a common skin infection that is usually caused by infection with a species of *Staphylococcus*. For a thorough review of other bacterial disorders that occur in dogs, see the Part 3 list of reference books.

Leptospirosis: The causative agent of this disease is a filamentous, spiral-shaped organism called a spirochete. There are more than 170 different species of this bacterium, several of which are known to infect dogs. The two most common forms that occur in dogs are *Leptospira canicola* and *Leptospira icterohaemorrhagiae*. The spirochetes that cause leptospirosis are water-borne and can be found in water sources that have been contaminated by the urine of infected wild animals, such as rodents, and in some areas of the country, by infected cattle. Animals that have recovered from leptospirosis can continue to excrete the organisms in their urine for many months. The spirochetes can survive for long periods of time in surface waters, and dogs that are infected contract the disease through exposure to these water sources.

The majority of cases of leptospirosis in dogs are asymptomatic. Although the disease often is not fatal, severe cases can occur, and, occasionally, irreparable kidney damage results from chronic infection. *Leptospira canicola* is the most common form that infects dogs, causing acute kidney disease (**nephritis**). The kidney damage usually is short-term and reversible. Initially, the clinical signs are nonspecific and include depression, decreased appetite, and a slightly elevated body temperature. Reddening of the mucous membranes and conjunctiva may be seen. Measurement of blood urea nitrogen (an indirect indicator of kidney function) will show slightly elevated levels. In some cases, the liver also is affected, and signs of **jaundice** are seen. If not treated, leptospirosis can become chronic and lead to severe kidney and liver damage.

Although it is less common, infection with *Leptospira icterohaemorrhagiae* causes more serious illness. This organism can damage the kidney and liver and cause a generalized bleeding disorder. The most prevalent host reservoir for *Leptospira icterohaemorrhagiae* is the rat. Food sources that have been contaminated during storage by heavy rat populations are a potential mode of transmission to dogs.

Antibiotic therapy is used to treat leptospirosis and is completely successful if the disease is diagnosed during early stages of infection. If kidney disease is severe, supportive therapy and dialysis may be needed. Because there is the potential for the transmission of leptospirosis to humans, personal hygiene is important when caring for a dog with leptospirosis. Prevention through vaccination and through preventing access to potential sources of the bacterium, such as stagnant water sources or the urine of wild animals or cattle, is effective.

Canine pyoderma: Pyoderma is a general term used to describe any skin disease that is accompanied by the production of pus. In the majority of cases in dogs, this disease is caused by the bacteria *Staphylococcus intermedius*, with fewer cases caused by *Staphylococcus aureus*.[14] It appears that *Staphylococcus intermedius* is present in the skin of many healthy dogs but only causes disease in some.[15] *Staphylococci* species are widely distributed in nature and are highly resistant to drying and to household disinfectants. They are considered to be opportunistic organisms, living in small numbers in the skin and mucous membranes and only becoming pathogenic if suitable conditions arise.

Canine pyoderma can manifest in several ways. Impetigo is a common condition in puppies and young dogs and involves superficial infection of the dog's muzzle and chin. Impetigo is often self-limiting but can be treated with antibiotic therapy and antibacterial shampoos. Superficial pyoderma (also called "superficial bacterial folliculitis") is a common skin disease characterized by infectious pustules that are associated with hair follicles. These show up as crusty lesions on the dogs underside in skin folds. Although some dogs show pruritus (itchiness), others do not appear to be uncomfortable. In many dogs, the lesions are found only in folds of skin, such as the facial folds of Bulldogs, Shar Peis, and Pekinese. Infections also occur around the vulva of females and within the tail folds of dogs with curled tails.

In many cases, superficial pyoderma develops in association with flea infestation or infection with the mite *Demodex canis* (see Chapter 14). Deep pyoderma is a less common but more serious form of pyoderma. Because this problem often is seen in middle-age to older German Shepherd Dogs, it has been anecdotally referred to as "German Shepherd pyoderma." However, it also has been recognized in other breeds, including Golden Retrievers, Irish Setters, Bull Terriers, Dalmatians, and Doberman Pinschers. The infection involves deep layers of the skin, and most lesions occur over the hips and thighs. If not treated, the infection will spread to other parts of the body and can become very painful for the dog.

Topical antibiotics and steroid preparations are used to treat localized areas of pyoderma. If the dog has generalized lesions, antibacterial shampoos and systemic (oral) antibiotics are prescribed. Because *Staphylococcus intermedius* has been shown to be resistant to several antibiotics, including penicillin, ampicillin, and tetracycline, selection of an appropriate product is important.[16] If there is an associated problem such as flea infestation or infection with mites, these problems should be simultaneously treated.

Fungal Infections

Ringworm: Ringworm, or dermatophytosis, is a fungal infection of the hair follicles and is caused by several different species of fungi. The most common cause of ringworm in dogs is the organism *Microsporum canis*. Warm, humid conditions are ideal for promoting ringworm infections, and dogs that are less than 1 year of age are more susceptible to infection. Transmission is through direct contact with infected animals or with materials contaminated with their skin debris. Ringworm is a zoonotic disease and can be easily transmitted to humans and other pets.

Ringworm lesions typically are first observed around the dog's head, ears, or forelimbs and appear as patchy, circular areas of hair loss. Small lesions or bumps may be found on the outer edges of the spots with **erythema** (red areas) present in the center. These features give the lesion its characteristic "ring" appearance. Although most cases of ringworm are restricted to small areas of the body, some develop into large areas of hair loss that can cover much of the body. Most dogs show no discomfort or pruritus, so the lesions may go unnoticed by the owner. In some cases, an inflammatory skin response does occur, causing small bumps or lesions and discomfort for the dog.

Microscopic examination of hair or skin scale allows identification of the ringworm fungi. In many dogs, infections are self-limiting, and the dog is able to rid itself of the fungus without veterinary treatment. If necessary, topical medications that contain iodine or the compound chlorhexadine are used to kill the ringworm fungus. These are usually incorporated into a shampoo but may also be applied as an ointment or cream. Griseofulvin is a drug used for systemic treatment of ringworm and usually is used when several pets are infected or when recurrent infections are seen. Because ringworm is contagious to humans and other animals, the dog's environment also should be treated. All bedding should be washed using a disinfectant solution, and frequent vacuuming can be of aid in ridding the house of infective skin scales.

Vaccinations

Vaccines are administered to protect dogs from certain infectious diseases. They are composed of altered infectious agents that have the desired effect of inducing an immune response that confers complete or partial protection from the disease. Because of a lack of therapeutic antiviral agents, vaccination plays an important role in the control of many viral diseases in the domestic dog population. In addition, some vaccines are effective against infection with bacterial agents such as *Leptospira canicola*, *Leptospira icterohaemorrhagiae*, and *Bordetella bronchiseptica*. Although no vaccine is 100 percent effective, the use of vaccination programs for dogs has been instrumental in preventing widespread outbreaks of many of the debilitating and life-threatening diseases discussed in this chapter.

Types of immunity: The term "immunity" refers to an animal's capacity to resist infection with a certain disease due to adequate levels of circulating antibodies against the disease. Natural immunity is species-specific immunity and simply means that a disease that infects one species may not be infectious to another. For example, feline infectious peritonitis is caused by a type of coronavirus that is potentially fatal to cats but that does not infect dogs.

Passive immunity, also called acquired immunity, occurs when an animal receives a source of protective antibodies from another animal or another source. The most important type of passive immunity in dogs is the protection that newborn puppies receive when they consume their mother's colostrum. Colostrum is a form of milk produced by bitches during the first few days after whelping. It is specifically suited for newborns and contains **antibodies** derived from the mother's serum. By consuming the colostrum and absorbing these antibodies, the puppies passively acquire protection against any disease for which the mother is adequately protected. If the mother has been vaccinated properly (or if she has recovered from infection with a disease), she will have sufficient levels of circulating antibody to provide to her newborn puppies through her colostrum. In contrast, if the mother is not adequately protected, the puppies will not receive protective levels of antibodies in the colostrum.

Antibodies are large protein molecules. Normally, the stomach and small intestine digest protein, breaking it down to amino acids for absorption into the body (see Chapter 16). Newborn puppies, like the young of many species, have the ability to absorb these antibodies in their intact form for only a short period of time, about the first 36 hours after birth. After this time period, the cells lining the small intestine lose their ability to absorb large protein molecules, and the puppies cannot obtain further protection from the colostrum. For this reason, it is imperative that newborn puppies receive the mother's colostrum within the first few hours after birth.

The length of time a puppy will be protected by passive immunity is dependent upon the antibody level of the mother. Dams that are vaccinated immediately before they are bred usually have the highest antibody **titers** and so provide the highest concentration of antibodies in their colostrum. The higher the concentration of antibodies in the milk, the longer the protection will last for the puppy. The maximum length of maternal antibody protection in puppies is about 16 weeks. This protection is highly important because the newborn puppies' immune system is not fully functional, and puppies cannot develop active immunity until they are about 6 weeks old.

The third type of immunity is active immunity. This occurs when an animal's reticuloendothelial (immune) system is challenged by an **antigen** and responds by producing antibodies against the antigen. In the case of vaccines, the antigen is a bacteria or virus that has been altered in some way to make it nonpathogenic. When it is injected into the body, the dog's immune system responds to it in the same manner that it would to invasion with the actual pathogen. This results in the production of antibodies that will subsequently provide protection against the natural form of the organism. Active immunity decreases slowly with time. Therefore, booster vaccines must be given at regular intervals to maintain a high level of circulating antibody.

Types of vaccines: There are two major types of vaccines that currently are used in veterinary medicine. These are called modified live vaccines and inactivated (or killed) vaccines. Most vaccines are administered through subcutaneous or intramuscular injections. Vaccines that are designed to confer local immunity are administered intranasally (Table 11.2).

Modified live vaccines contain a weakened or "attenuated" form of the microorganism responsible for causing disease. After injection into the dog, the modified virus replicates in the host animal but does not cause illness. Through replication, a larger number of viral particles are produced, which serve to strengthen the dog's immune response. The immune response that develops (active immunity) is protective against the pathogenic form of the virus. Although a single dose of a modified live vaccine usually produces long-lasting immunity, a series of initial vaccines are recommended for puppies and yearly "boosters" for adults to ensure continued protection. For dogs, most vaccines for canine distemper, infectious canine hepatitis, viral forms of kennel cough, and canine parvovirus are modified live vaccines.

Inactivated vaccines contain an inactivated or "killed" form of the infectious agent. When injected into the dog, the agent cannot cause disease but is still capable of stimulating an immune response. Inactivated vaccines are more stable than modified live vaccines and have a longer shelf-life. Killed vaccines do not replicate in the host, so there is no possibility they will ever revert to a pathogenic form and cause illness. For this reason, inactivated vaccines are considered to be safer for use in pregnant females. However, because the host animal is exposed to a smaller number of antigens, more than a single dose of inactivated vaccine is required to produce a strong, enduring immunological response. Commonly used inactivated vaccines include those that protect against rabies, canine coronavirus, leptospirosis, Lyme disease, and *Bordetella bronchiseptica*.

TABLE 11.2   Types of Vaccines

Type of Vaccine	Description	Advantages	Recommended Use
Modified Live	contains a weakened form of the disease agent, which replicates in the host animal but does not cause illness	increased number of antigens stimulate strong active immunity; one dose is usually sufficient	canine distemper, infectious canine hepatitis, viral forms of kennel cough, canine parvovirus; use with puppies and adults (nonpregnant females)
Inactivated (Killed)	contains a "killed" form of the infectious agent, which cannot cause disease, but stimulates active immunity	longer shelf-life and more stable than modified live vaccines; no possibility of causing illness	rabies, canine coronavirus, leptospirosis, Lyme disease, Bordetella bronchiseptica; recommended for use in pregnant females
Intranasal	designed to stimulate local IgA immunity in the upper respiratory tract	although short-lived immunity is produced, this type of vaccine is most effective against upper respiratory infections with *Bordetella bronchiseptica*	recommended for dogs who are going to be exposed to high-risk environments for kennel cough; dogs kept in high-risk settings should be re-vaccinated every 6 months

Combined vaccines: For convenience and to help ensure that pet owners adhere to a complete vaccination program, most of the vaccines marketed for dogs will immunize against several diseases. Combined vaccines for dogs typically include agents that will immunize against canine distemper, infectious hepatitis, canine parvovirus, canine parainfluenza, canine adenovirus type 2 (which protects against both kennel cough caused by adenovirus type 2 and hepatitis caused by adenovirus type 1), leptospirosis, and coronavirus.[17] Individual parvovirus vaccines are available and often are used to immunize dogs who are at increased risk for contracting parvovirus. The vaccine for *Bordetella bronchiseptica* is an intranasal vaccine and is administered separately. Immunization for Lyme borreliosis is a separate vaccine and is recommended in areas of the country where Lyme borreliosis is prevalent (see Chapter 14). The vaccine for rabies is also provided as a separate vaccine, usually by an intramuscular injection.

Routes of administration: With the exception of rabies and the vaccine for Lyme disease, which are intramuscular vaccines, most vaccinations for dogs are administered subcutaneously. A third route of vaccine administration is intranasal. Intranasal vaccines are aimed at stimulating local immunoglobulin A (IgA) immunity in the upper respiratory tract. Although this type of immunity is relatively short-lived, it is most effective in protecting against *Bordetella bronchiseptica*, the primary bacteria that causes infectious tracheobronchitis. Dogs who are going to be exposed to high-exposure areas (i.e. boarding kennels or dog shows) should be vaccinated with an intranasal vaccine approximately 1 to 2 weeks prior to the exposure. Because local immunity is relatively short-lived, dogs that are kept in high-risk settings should be re-vaccinated every 6 months.

Vaccination failure: Vaccinations are given to puppies and adult dogs with the intent of immunizing them against common infectious diseases. However, no vaccine is considered to be 100 percent effective, and vaccine failures do occasionally occur. There are several causes for this. The most common is maternal antibody blocking in puppies. Puppies receive passive immunity through ingestion of their mother's colostrum during the first 1 to 2 days of life. These antibodies protect the puppy from disease but interfere with the stimulation of active immunity when vaccines are administered. This occurs because the antibodies the puppy received from the mother recognize the vaccine antigen as a disease and destroy it before the puppy can develop active immunity against it. This is generally not a problem during the first few weeks of life because the level of passive immunity the puppy received is capable of protecting the puppy from infection. However, the maternal antibodies the puppy has received begin to decline after 6 weeks of age and have decreased to levels not detectable by the time most puppies are 16 weeks of age. The age at which a puppy loses its maternal immunity varies according to the level of antibody that the mother possessed. For example, a mother that was not vaccinated prior to becoming pregnant might have a low circulating antibody, and her puppies will lose all of their maternal immunity by the time they are 7 to 8 weeks of age. In contrast, a mother with high levels of circulating antibody is expected to have puppies who are protected for a longer period of time.

Maternal immunity that protects puppies against natural infections disappears earlier than does maternal immunity against vaccination for the same viral agent. In other words, a critical period occurs during which maternal antibody levels are still high enough to block the puppy's active response to vaccination but are not high enough to prevent infection with disease. During this time period, the puppy is susceptible to infection. The critical period occurs sometime during the first 18 weeks of life and is affected by both the concentration of maternal antibodies the puppy received through colostrum and the maturity of the puppy's reticuloendothelial system.

Maternal antibody blocking is the principal reason young puppies receive a series of vaccinations after weaning. Ideally, vaccinations should be given at frequent intervals throughout the period when maternal immunity is diminishing, with the final vaccine provided when the puppy is capable of responding with an active immune response. First vaccines are usually administered when puppies are 6 weeks old, 1 to 2 weeks before they are weaned and placed into new homes. Vaccinating before 6 weeks is unnecessary because the puppy is still adequately protected by maternal immunity and because the immune system is not yet capable of producing active immunity. By giving a series of vaccinations at fairly short intervals, the period during which the puppy is most susceptible to natural infection is shortened. Although all infectious diseases are affected, protection against canine parvovirus is of greatest concern because of high puppy mortality to this disease and because of the prevalence of the virus in the environment.[18]

A second cause of vaccination failure in dogs occurs when vaccination takes place during the incubation period of the natural disease. In these cases, the body attempts to develop immunity, but invasion with the pathogenic organisms usually causes tissue damage and illness before active immunity is capable of fighting the disease. Owners may erroneously blame the vaccine for causing the disease, when, in fact, the dog had been exposed prior to vaccination. Because of the methods used to modify infectious agents, it is extremely rare that a vaccine causes serious illness in a dog.

A final cause of vaccine failure is improper handling or storing of the vaccine itself. Modified live vaccines have a relatively short shelf-life and, when rehydrated, must be kept cold. Mishandling or improper reconstitution may cause the vaccine to be ineffective. For this reason, it is important that owners who vaccinate their own dogs follow the manufacturer's directions for storage and handling prior to administering the vaccine.

Vaccination Schedules

Puppies: Puppies should receive their first vaccination when they are about 6 weeks of age, followed by re-vaccinations every 2 to 4 weeks until they are 16 to 18 weeks of age (Table 11.3).[19] Dogs of breeds that have an increased risk of parvovirus infection, such as Rottweilers and Dobermans, should continue the series until they are at least 20 weeks of age and should be given boosters every 6 months thereafter.[20] There is recent evidence that modified live vaccines for parvovirus are effective when given in only three doses at 6, 9, and 12 weeks of age.[21] However, owners and veterinarians should consider the puppy's level of risk and degree of exposure to disease when determining a vaccination schedule. Puppies who are socialized a great deal, are attending puppy classes, live in a kennel setting, or are going to be boarded at a commercial kennel should receive frequent vaccinations. One vaccine that may be given before puppies are 6 weeks old is the intranasal vaccine for *Bordetella bronchiseptica*. This vaccine can be given to puppies who are 2 weeks of age or older and is recommended for young puppies who are at high risk for infection.

Completion of the entire series of puppies vaccinations is of utmost importance because of the risk imposed by maternal antibody blocking. Most veterinarians report that the cases of parvovirus they see today are in "partially vaccinated dogs," meaning dogs that have begun but not completed a vaccination program or dogs that were given one vaccine as a young puppy

TABLE 11.3   Vaccination Schedules for Puppies and Adults

Age	Vaccine	Special Concerns
2 to 6 Weeks	intranasal vaccine for *Bordetella bronchiseptica*	recommend for puppies in high-risk settings
5 to 6 Weeks	distemper, hepatitis, leptospirosis, kennel cough, parvovirus, coronavirus	dogs of breeds that have an increased risk of parvovirus infection, such as Rottweilers and Dobermans, and puppies who are exposed to high-risk areas should continue the series
8 to 10 Weeks	repeat above	repeat above
12 to 14 Weeks	repeat above	repeat above
16 to 18 Weeks	repeat above	repeat above
4 to 5 months	rabies	1-year or 3-year vaccines available
Annually for Adults	distemper, hepatitis, leptospirosis, kennel cough, parvovirus, coronavirus; rabies (annual or every 3 years); intranasal vaccine for *Bordetella bronchiseptica*	dogs exposed to high risk environments and dogs of susceptible breeds may benefit from vaccination every 6 months for canine parvovirus and *Bordetella bronchiseptica*

that was not followed with a series of boosters.[22] The rabies vaccine is an exception to this and is first administered when puppies are 4 months old and again 1 year later.

Adults: The recommended schedule for adult dogs is to provide boosters for canine distemper, infectious canine hepatitis, leptospirosis, parvovirus, kennel cough, and coronavirus annually. A rabies vaccine is administered either annually or every 3 years, depending on the vaccine used and the requirements of the owner's county or state for rabies vaccination. Dogs who are exposed to a high-risk environment such as kennels or dog shows and dogs of susceptible breeds such as Rottweilers, Labrador Retrievers, and Doberman Pinschers may benefit from vaccination every 6 months for canine parvovirus and *Bordetella bronchiseptica*.[23] However, even in these cases, it is recommended that blood tests to measure antibody titers are first taken to determine whether or not frequent vaccination is necessary. This is important given recent concerns about the possible increase in immune-mediated disease in dogs as a result of overvaccination.

Conclusions

Although there are a host of infectious agents that can cause disease in the domestic dog, most of these can be controlled through vaccination programs and through providing a sanitary, well-ventilated, healthy environment for our dogs. Unfortunately, there are also a number of non-infectious disorders that occur in the domestic dog and affect the health, vitality, and longevity of a cherished pet. Several of the more common disorders and their treatments are reviewed in the following chapter.

Cited References

1. Seigal, M., editor. *University of California-Davis School of Veterinary Medicine Book of Dogs,* Harper Collins Publishers, Inc., New York, New York. (1995)

2. Thrushfield, M.V. **Canine kennel cough: A review**. Veterinary Annual, 32:1-12. (1992)

3. Ueland, K. **Serological, bacteriological and clinical observations on an outbreak of canine infectious tracheobronchitis in Norway.** Veterinary Record, 126:481-483. (1990)

4. Appel, M.J. **Canine infectious tracheobronchitis (kennel cough): a status report.** Compendium on Continuing Education for the Practicing Veterinarian, 3:70-79. (1981)

5. Thrushfield, M.V., Aitken, C.G.C., and Muirhead, R.H. **A field investigation of kennel cough: Incubation period and clinical signs.** Journal of Small Animal Practice, 32:215-220. (1991)

6. Thrushfield, M.V., Aitken, C.G.C., and Muirhead, R.H. **A field investigation of kennel cough: Efficacy of different treatments.** Journal of Small Animal Practice, 32:455-459. (1991)

7. Parrish, C.R. **Emergence, natural history and variation of canine, mink, and feline parvoviruses.** Advances in Virus Research, 38:403-450. (1990)

8. Parrish, C.R., Aquadrom, C.F., and Strassheim, M.L. **Rapid antigenic-type replacement and DNA sequence evolution on canine parvovirus.** Journal of Virology, 65:6544-6552. (1991)

9. Kennedy, M.A., Mellon, V.S., Caldwell, G., and Potgieter, L.N.D. **Virucidal efficacy of the newer quaternary ammonium compounds.** Journal of the American Animal Hospital Association, 31:254-258. (1995)

10. Brunner, C.J. and Swango, L.J. **Canine parvovirus infection: Effects on the immune system and factors that predispose to severe disease.** Compendium on Continuing Education for the Practicing Veterinarian, 7:979-989. (1985)

11. Glickman, L.T., Domanski, L.M., Patronek, G.J., and Visintainer, F. **Breed-related risk factors for canine parvovirus enteritis.** Journal of the American Veterinary Medical Association, 187:589-594. (1985)

12. Macintire, D.K. and Smith-Carr, S. **Canine parvovirus. Part II: Clinical signs, diagnosis, and treatment.** Compendium on Continuing Education for the Practicing Veterinarian, 19:291-300. (1997)

13. Evermann, J.F., McKeirnan, A.J., Eugster, A.K., Solozano, R.F., Collins, J.K., Black, J.W., and Kim, J.S. **Update on canine coronavirus infections and interactions with other enteric pathogens of the dog.** Companion Animal Practice, 19:6-12. (1989)

14. DeBoer, D.J. **Canine *Staphylococcus* pyoderma.** Veterinary Medicine Reports, 244-265. (1990)

15. Cox, U.H., Hoskins, J.D., and Newman, S.S. **Temporal study of Staphylococcal species on healthy dogs.** American Journal of Veterinary Research, 49:747-751. (1988)

16. Oluoch, A.L., Weisiger, R., Siegel, A.M., Campbell, K.L., Krawiec, D.R., and

McKiernan, B.C. **Trends of bacterial infections in dogs: Characterization of** *Staphylococcus intermedius* **isolates (1990-1992).** Canine Practice, 21:12-19. (1996)

17. Thrushfield, M.V., Aitken, C.G.C., and Muirhead, R.H. **A field investigation of kennel cough: Efficacy of vaccination**. Journal of Small Animal Practice, 30:550-560. (1989)

18. O'Brien, S.E. **Serologic response of pups to the low-passage, modified live canine parvovirus-2 component in a combination vaccine.** Journal of the American Veterinary Medical Association, 204:1207-1209. (1994)

19. Smith-Carr, S., MacIntie, D.K., and Swango, L.J. **Canine parvovirus. Part I: Pathogenesis and vaccination.** Compendium on Continuing Education for the Practicing Veterinarian, 19:125-133. (1997)

20. Swango, L., Barta, R., Fortney, W., Garnett, P., Leedy, D., and Stevenson, J. **Choosing a canine vaccine regimen. Part 3.** Canine Practice, 6:21-26. (1995)

21. Larson, L.J. and Schultz, R.D. **High titer canine parvovirus vaccine: serologic response and challenge of immunity study.** Veterinary Medicine, 91:210-218. (1996)

22. Swango, L. **Choosing a canine vaccine regimen, Part 1.** Canine Practice, 20:10-14. (1995)

23. Glickman, L.T. and Appel, M.J. **Intranasal vaccine trial for canine infectious tracheobronchitis (kennel cough).** Laboratory Animal Science, 31:397-399. (1981)

12 Common Non-Infectious Disorders

THE PREVIOUS CHAPTER reviewed common infectious diseases of the domestic dog. Proper vaccination programs along with good management and health care can prevent these diseases in most dogs. In addition to infectious diseases, there are a number of non-infectious disorders that can affect the domestic dog. Although this is not a comprehensive list, some of the more common of these diseases are reviewed in this chapter.

Canine Hip Dysplasia

Canine hip dysplasia (CHD) is a developmental disorder characterized by laxity of the hip joint (coxofemoral joint), resulting in joint instability and degenerative disease. It is the most common heritable orthopedic problem in dogs, affecting up to 40 percent to 50 percent of dogs of the large and giant breeds.[1] Although CHD occurs in all breeds, clinical signs most often are seen in dogs that have an adult weight of greater than 35 pounds. Breeds that have a high incidence of CHD include St. Bernards, Newfoundlands, Bullmastiffs, Bernese Mountain Dogs, Welsh Springer Spaniels, Kuvasz, and Bloodhounds.[2,3] It is also relatively common in several currently popular breeds, including Labrador Retrievers, German Shepherd Dogs, Rottweilers, Chow Chows, and Golden Retrievers. In contrast, large breeds of dogs that have a low incidence of CHD include most sight hound breeds such as the Borzoi, Saluki, and Afghan Hound, as well as the Siberian Husky and Belgian Sheepdog (Table 12.1).

Observed differences in breed incidence indicate that size alone is not responsible for tendency to develop CHD. It has been postulated that the ratio of a dog's pelvic muscle mass to the total mass of the body is an important factor in determining the degree of risk for developing CHD.[4] Dogs that have a high proportion of muscle mass relative to skeletal mass generally show a lower incidence of the disorder. However, this theory alone may not be adequate as it does not explain the relatively high incidence of CHD in heavily muscled dogs such as Rottweilers and Bullmastiffs.[5] Therefore, while pelvic muscle mass may be involved, other factors also appear to be important.

Development of CHD: The term dysplasia means "abnormal development." In the normal hip joint, the femoral head sits solidly and deeply within the acetabulum (Figure 12.1). Dogs with CHD develop a separation of the head of the femur from the acetabulum. This is referred to as subluxation and causes abnormal stresses and forces to be placed on the developing hip.

TABLE 12.1   Breed Prevalence of Canine Hip Dysplasia

Breeds with High Incidence	Breeds with Low Incidence
Rottweiler	Borzoi
German Shepherd Dog	Saluki
Bloodhound	Greyhound
St. Bernard	Whippet
Kuvasz	Afghan Hound
Newfoundland	Siberian Husky
Bullmastiff	Belgian Sheepdog
Great Dane	Most small breeds (<35 lbs)
Bernese Mountain Dog	
Golden Retriever	
Labrador Retriever	
Chow Chow	
Welsh Springer Spaniel	

FIGURE 12.1   Normal and dysplastic hips

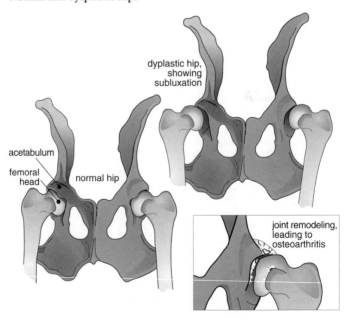

Because the hip is a major weight-bearing joint and is necessary for forward propulsion, the irregular forces caused by subluxation result in compensatory remodeling of the joint. Over time, the femoral head changes its shape, and the acetabulum becomes flattened and shallow. In the early stages of CHD, this remodeling serves to support the joint and aids in allowing normal movement. However, the abnormal shape coupled with continuing stresses result in inflammation and the development of osteoarthritis (degenerative joint disease). Most of the clinical signs of CHD, especially those in mature dogs, are caused by the degenerative joint disease that occurs and worsens as the dog ages.

Both genetics and environment influence the phenotypic expression of CHD. Survey and breeding studies have shown that CHD has a heritability coefficient between 0.2 and 0.6, depending on the population and breeds that were studied.[6,7] This means that up to 60 percent of the variability that is seen in the occurrence of CHD is due to a dog's genetic makeup. CHD is a polygenic disorder, influenced by a set of genes that affect body size, growth patterns, muscle development, pelvic muscle mass, and hip structure.[8] Because environmental factors also influence these traits, it is difficult , if not impossible, to separate genetic factors from environmental factors.

The most important environmental factor affecting the expression of CHD is rate of growth. When young dogs are fed a nutrient- and energy-dense food at a level that promotes maximal growth rate, the chance for development of CHD is increased. For example, a study of CHD-susceptible Labrador Retrievers found that puppies that were fed 25 percent fewer calories than litter mates that were fed free-choice had significant reductions in both the incidence and the severity of CHD (see Chapter 18).[9] When the dogs were 2 years old, evaluation for CHD showed that 71 percent of the limited-feed dogs had normal hips, compared to only 33 percent of the dogs that were fed free-choice. Feeding for rapid rates of growth results in earlier closure of growth plates of the acetabulum which may cause incongruity between the acetabulum and the head of the femur.[10] The larger soft tissue mass (lean and fat) that develops when a dog is growing rapidly may exert abnormal forces on the growing and immature hip. Similarly, incongruity between the stage of development of the hip's muscles and connective tissues and maturation of the skeleton during phases of rapid growth may contribute to abnormal hip structure.

While any complete and balanced diet has the potential to support maximal growth if fed in large quantities, diets that have high caloric and nutrient densities pose the greatest risk. Because these diets are usually very palatable and because complete nutrition is obtained from a relatively small volume of food, growing dogs can easily be overfed if intake is not controlled (see Chapter 19). With the exception of the diet's caloric density, other nutrients in the diet such as level of protein, fat, carbohydrate, or vitamin C have not been shown to affect the development of CHD.[11]

Trauma during growth is a second important environmental factor. Excessive weight-bearing exercise or a traumatic injury to the hip joint may predispose a dog to the development of abnormal hip structure. Trauma is often an underlying contributor to the disease when it is seen unilaterally.

Clinical signs: Pain and lameness associated with CHD are highly variable, ranging from no clinical signs in some dogs to severe lameness or even crippling in others. The most critical period for the development of CHD occurs between 3 and 8 months of age. However, only dogs that are severely affected show clinical signs at this age. The age at which dogs first show clinical signs varies from 4 months to the geriatric years. Clinically affected dogs generally fall into two groups. The first group includes dogs younger than 1 year of age who suddenly show difficulty standing, walking, running, or climbing stairs. Weight-bearing lameness in one or both rear legs is observed, and these signs are aggravated by exercise or exertion. The second group of dogs is comprised of mature dogs whose clinical signs are the result of degenerative joint disease. Signs include decreased exercise tolerance, stiffness or lameness following exercise, decreased stride length in the rear legs, and reluctance to climb stairs.

Diagnosis: Diagnosis of CHD is based on clinical signs, palpation of the hip joint, and radiographs. Palpation can effectively detect laxity of the hip joint in young dogs, but degenerative changes in older dogs preclude using degree of joint laxity as a diagnostic tool. Two methods veterinarians can use to detect joint laxity and degree of subluxation are called the Ortolani test and the Bardens' sign.[12,13] These methods are most effective in young dogs who have not yet developed degenerative joint changes. In all dogs, definitive diagnosis of CHD is made through evaluation of radiographs of the pelvis. Radiographs will indicate the degree of congruity between the head of the femur and the acetabulum, the depth and shape of the acetabulum, the presence of remodeling of the femoral head and neck, and the presence of degenerative joint disease. Several methods of radiographic evaluation can be used, some of which allow evaluation of passive hip laxity by applying stress forces while the dog is positioned for radiographing.[14,15]

Treatment: There are several approaches to the treatment of CHD. The most conservative and least invasive are weight and exercise management, and medications to decrease the dog's inflammation and pain. Buffered aspirin has historically been the drug of choice and is effective in many cases of moderate CHD. When aspirin is used, doses should be carefully monitored and care must be taken to avoid side effects of gastrointestinal upset associated with long-term use. Several prescription anti-inflammatory agents are also available and should be used under a veterinarian's supervision. In recent years, polysulfated glycosaminoglycans and related compounds have become popular for the management of degenerative joint disease in dogs. These compounds are referred to as "chondroprotective" and appear to aid in the healing of damaged cartilage within diseased joints. Clinical studies report moderate levels of success in the use of these compounds in the treatment of degenerative joint disease in dogs.[16,17,18]

Total hip replacement surgery is an appropriate method of treatment for a significant proportion of young dogs diagnosed with CHD. This surgery replaces the diseased hip with a mechanically sound prosthetic joint that provides the dog with full range of motion and the strength to use the hind legs to propel the body forward. Total hip replacement surgery for dogs was first developed in the late 1970s at Ohio State University College of Veterinary Medicine.[19] The procedure involves removing the head of the femur, removing damaged cartilage and arthritic bone spurs from the acetabulum, and replacing the damaged joint with an artificial ball-and-socket joint. A major advantage of hip replacement is that dogs will not develop degenerative disease because the joint surfaces where arthritis normally develops have been removed. Recovery time is about 2 months, during which the dog's exercise should be restricted to short walks on lead. Dogs can gradually return to normal level of activity within 3 months after the surgery.

Factors that are considered when determining if a dog is a candidate for hip replacement include the dog's age, size, and overall health. Dogs that weigh at least 50 pounds, are young adults that still have relatively good range of motion in the hip joint, and have not lost a significant amount of muscle mass are good candidates for this surgery. Although long-term prognosis is good to excellent, the cost of the surgery can be prohibitive for some owners.[20] When both hips are affected with CHD (which is true in 90 percent of the cases), the surgeries are performed separately with a recovery period of several months after the first hip is replaced.

Two other surgical procedures used to treat dogs with CHD are femoral head and neck ostectomy (FHO) and triple pelvic osteotomy (TPO). FHO involves removing the head and neck of the femur and allowing a false joint to form between the remaining femur and the pelvis. Older dogs for whom medication has not been successful and who are not good candidates of total hip replacement can benefit from this surgery. TPO involves surgical restructuring of the pelvis to create a new acetabulum for the femoral head to sit in. Young dogs that have an intact acetabular rim and minimal degenerative disease are the best candidates for this surgery.

Prevention of CHD: Selective breeding programs are the best approach for eliminating CHD from the domestic dog population. Controlled breeding studies have shown that breeding only dogs with normal hips or those dogs who had progeny with normal hips (progeny testing) significantly decreased the incidence of CHD in the tested population.[21,22] However, because of this disorder's polygenic inheritance and because there are few regulations governing breeding practices of dogs in the United States, progress has been relatively slow. The Orthopedic Foundation of Animals (OFA) is an organization that offers a central registry service for all breeds and functions to evaluate and certify radiographs of dog hips. They also monitor the incidence of CHD in registered dogs. A comparison of dogs born between 1972 and 1978 with dogs born between 1981 and 1988 found that the incidence of CHD had decreased in some breeds of dogs that were using the registry.[3] Notable decreases in CHD occurred in Golden Retrievers, Rottweilers, and Labrador Retrievers. In Golden Retrievers, the number of hips evaluated as excellent increased by 44 percent and among Rottweilers by 75 percent. The organization attributed this to increased compliance with OFA recommendations and to the exclusion of dysplastic dogs from breeding programs.

While selective breeding is important for eliminating the genotypic incidence of CHD from the dog population, the use of proper feeding and rearing practices is effective in decreasing the phenotypic expression of CHD in individual dogs. Growing puppies should be fed complete and balanced diets at levels that support normal but not maximal growth rates. As a rule of thumb, keeping puppies relatively lean as they grow and providing premeasured amounts of food contribute to optimal rates of growth and skeletal development. In addition, moderate but not excessive exercise should be provided daily. Regular exercise contributes to a lean body condition and to the development of strong muscles and connective tissues that support the skeleton as it grows.

Osteochondrosis

Osteochondrosis is a general term that describes abnormal cartilage development in growing bones. Cartilage provides the framework upon which mature bone is deposited and furnishes a smooth surface for the bones of a joint to glide across as they move. When osteochondrosis occurs, cartilage cells do not receive an adequate blood supply, leading to incomplete **ossification** and the development of a thickened layer of cartilage. Over time, the abnormal cartilage becomes weakened, resulting in inflammation and arthritic changes. The disorder is seen primarily in rapidly growing dogs of medium and large breeds. It affects the elbow and shoulder joints most often but is also seen in the hock and stifle joints.

Types: Three primary forms of osteochondrosis occur in dogs: ununited anconeal process, fragmented coronoid process, and osteochondritis dissecans (OCD). Of the three, OCD is the most common and is found primarily in the elbow or shoulder. OCD occurs when a tiny flap of cartilage separates from the underlying bone, resulting in inflammation and pain when the dog moves. Arthritic changes to the joint occur if the disorder is left untreated. Clinical signs of osteochondrosis are seen in dogs between 4 and 9 months of age and often are associated with growth spurts. About half of affected dogs have osteochondrosis bilaterally, and, in some, the problem occurs in more than one joint.[23] Dogs with OCD have a history of intermittent lameness exacerbated by exercise. Pain is elicited, and crepitus (grating) may be noted when the affected limb is palpated. Over time, the dog will begin to favor the affected leg and may stand with the leg rotated outward. Fluid buildup in the joint often occurs, making the area appear puffy and swollen. Eventually, the decreased use of the affected limb leads to muscle atrophy.

Cause: Although an exact cause of osteochondrosis is not known, several factors appear to contribute to its development. Heredity is an important factor and may affect growth rate, rate of cartilage formation, and vascularity of areas of developing bone. Other predisposing factors include rapid growth rate due to overfeeding and possible dietary supplementation with vitamins or minerals.[24]

Diagnosis: Osteochondrosis is diagnosed using clinical signs and radiographic examination of affected joints. OCD will show fragmentation of the joint cartilage or even a loose piece of cartilage (a joint mouse) floating within the joint space. Because osteochondrosis often occurs bilaterally and has the potential to affect several joints, most veterinarians take multiple radiographs to evaluate the severity with which the dog is affected. Other changes that may be seen are flattened areas or crater lines on the bone surface, arthritic changes such as bone spurs (osteophytes), and increased density of the joint surface.

Treatment: Surgery is the treatment of choice when the disease is detected before pronounced arthritic changes have occurred in the joint. The advantage of surgery is that it resolves the problem within the joint and allows the stimulation of new cartilage and bone growth. Surgery involves the removal of any pieces of loose cartilage (joint mice) or flaps, and the bone surface is curetted (scraped) to stimulate the production of new cartilage. Long-term prognosis following surgery is very good, especially when intervention occurs early in the progression of the disorder. Medical management may be desirable in very early cases or as an alternative to surgery for older dogs who have extensive arthritic changes in the joint. This therapy includes restricted exercise and the use of anti-inflammatory medications to control pain. Commonly prescribed agents include buffered aspirin, prednisone, and nonsteroidal anti-inflammatory drugs. In addition, chondroprotective agents such as glycosaminoglycans and hyaluronic acid also may be helpful.[25]

Juvenile Panosteitis (Wandering Lameness)

Juvenile panosteitis, nicknamed "wandering lameness" or "shifting leg lameness," is a condition that affects the long bones of young, growing dogs of large and giant breeds. The disease is usually self-limiting and appears to have no long-term consequences. However, it can be a difficult ordeal for owners and dogs to endure, as the disorder can cause severe pain and lameness for many months.

Clinical signs: Panosteitis is characterized by generalized inflammation of the long bones, specifically the humerus, radius, ulna, femur, and tibia. In more than half the reported cases, the disorder moves from leg to leg, eventually affecting almost all of the long bones. German Shepherd Dogs, Doberman Pinschers, St. Bernards, Great Danes, German Shorthaired Pointers, and Basset Hounds all appear to have a higher incidence of panosteitis, and male dogs are affected four times more frequently than females.[26] Affected dogs show a sudden onset of moderate to severe lameness, with no history of injury or trauma. In many cases, owners report that the dog is unusually lethargic, has a decreased appetite, and is reluctant to exercise. Muscle atrophy in the affected leg eventually occurs as a result of decreased use. Most dogs recover completely without treatment within a few months, but often the lameness progresses to other bones before eventually resolving completely. Although this can recur numerous times in different legs and bones, once an individual bone recovers, the condition usually does not return to that limb.

Diagnosis: Although panosteitis is usually self-limiting, diagnosis is important because other skeletal diseases that can cause the same signs must be ruled out. Panosteitis often is difficult to diagnose because the radiographic signs may be very slight. When changes occur, areas of increased bone density in the middle or medullary portion of the bone are seen. Because radiographic changes often lag behind clinical signs, if the radiographs do not demonstrate changes associated with panosteitis, and other causes have been ruled out, radiographs should be repeated in 1 to 2 weeks. Blood cell and blood chemistry data usually are normal, although some dogs have an elevated **eosinophil** count. For this reason, the disorder originally was called "eosinophilic panosteitis."

Treatment: Because most dogs recover spontaneously from juvenile panosteitis, treatment is directed toward the relief of pain. Buffered aspirin usually is the analgesic of choice, but other anti-inflammatory agents may be prescribed. Restricting exercise is recommended to manage pain and prevent exacerbation of the inflammation.

Gastric Dilatation Volvulus (Gastric Torsion, Bloat)

Gastric dilatation is a life-threatening condition in which the dog's stomach becomes abnormally distended as a result of the accumulation of gases, gastric secretions, or food. As the condition progresses, the stomach may twist upon itself, which is known as **volvulus.** Bloat is extremely painful to the dog and, if not treated immediately, often is fatal. When torsion occurs, the blood supply to the dog's vital organs and to the stomach is decreased or cut off completely. This rapidly leads to necrosis of these tissues and the occlusion of two major blood vessels to the heart. This is a medical emergency because the loss of blood supply to the heart rapidly leads to arrhythmia and death.

Acute gastric dilatation occurs most frequently in large, deep-chested dogs, with an extremely high incidence in certain breeds. Approximately 1 in 4 Irish Setters will suffer from bloat at some point in their lifetime. Great Danes and St. Bernards are at equal or greater risk. Other vulnerable breeds include Gordon Setters, Collies, and Standard Poodles. Although most of the dogs that are affected are large or giant breeds, the risk for developing bloat is more strongly correlated with chest conformation than with overall body size. Dogs that have high chest depth-to-width ratios have a greater risk of bloating during their lifetimes than dogs with lower ratios.[27]

The exact underlying cause of bloat is not known, and it is believed there are probably several contributing factors. These include genetic predisposition, trauma, presence of gastric **neoplasms**, overeating, and abnormalities in gastric motility or hormone secretion. Because gastric dilatation is an intestinal disorder, diet and feeding practice have naturally been targeted as potential causes. However, recent survey studies of the diets and feeding patterns of dogs with gastric dilatation found that the only significant dietary factor is the number of meals that are fed per day.[28] Specifically, feeding several small meals rather than one or two large meals correlates with a lower risk of bloat. The type of food, dietary components, and whether or not the food was soaked in water prior to feeding do not appear to affect a dog's degree of risk.

A gastrointestinal factor that may be related to the development of bloat is gastric motility. Clinical studies have provided evidence that some dogs that develop gastric dilatation have abnormal gastric contractions that may lead to delayed gastric emptying.[29] Stress and the dog's temperament may also be predisposing factors. In general, dogs that have recently experienced a stressful event or who are described by their owners as having a "fearful" or "nervous" temperament appear to be more likely to bloat. Although it has been widely believed that exercise before or after eating may predispose a dog to bloat, this relationship has not been supported by research. In fact, more than 60 percent of the dogs in the survey study were said to be sleeping or resting quietly in the late evening or middle of the night when signs developed.

Signs of acute gastric dilatation include sudden discomfort, labored breathing, panting, and restlessness. As gas accumulates and the stomach distends, the dog pants and salivates, attempts to vomit or retch, and develops severe abdominal swelling and tenderness. If untreated, the dog will quickly develop signs of circulatory collapse (shock). These signs include weakness, decreased capillary refill time and pale gums, shallow breathing, and a rapid, shallow heartbeat. Collapse and death will follow, usually as a result of cardiac arrest.

Veterinary care must be obtained immediately in cases of acute gastric dilatation. If the accumulated gas is not released and signs of shock are not treated, death occurs rapidly and postoperative losses increase dramatically. The first line of treatment consists of administering intravenous fluids to alleviate shock. Steps are then taken to decompress the stomach, either by intubation if torsion has not occurred or by direct entry into the stomach via an incision into the dog's side. If torsion has occurred, surgery is performed after decompression to reposition the stomach. During this surgery, the stomach will be sutured to the abdominal cavity (gastroplexy), a procedure that prevents future incidences of torsion. Aftercare is very important because a substantial number of dogs die postoperatively as a result of heart damage or infection. The dog is fed a largely liquid diet at first and is gradually returned to a normal diet over a period of several weeks. Any dog who has recovered from gastric dilatation should be fed 3 to 5 small meals per day for the remainder of its life, and known stressors in the dog's environment should be eliminated, if possible.

Hypothyroidism

The thyroid gland is located next to the dog's trachea and produces two primary forms of thyroid hormone: thyroxine (T_4) and triiodothyronine (T_3). Another hormone, thyroid-stimulating hormone (TSH), is secreted by the **pituitary gland** and regulates the thyroid gland's production and secretion of thyroid hormone. The major function of thyroid hormone is to regulate cellular metabolism. As a result, a lack of this hormone affects many body systems. Hypothyroidism is considered to be the most common hormonal disorder in the domestic dog. It is characterized by inadequate secretion of thyroid hormone from the thyroid gland, low levels of thyroid hormone in the blood, and the resultant clinical effects. The onset of clinical signs of hypothyroidism occur after the dog is an adult, typically between 4 and 8 years of age.

Cause: Hypothyroidism may have several underlying causes. It may be a result of an immune-mediated problem (lymphocytic thyroiditis), atrophy of the gland, decreased levels of TSH, or the presence of a cancerous growth in either gland.[30] Lymphocytic thyroiditis appears to be the most common cause of hypothyroidism. An abnormal immune response causes the body to attack the gland, eventually leading to an inability to produce thyroid hormone. Certain breeds of dogs and lines within breeds have a genetic predisposition to this problem. Golden Retrievers, Doberman Pinschers, Irish Setters, Miniature Schnauzers, Airedales, and Great Danes are at greater risk than the general population of dogs.[31] Other breeds that have been identified include Standard Poodles, Boxers, Airedales, and Old English Sheepdogs. Another common cause of hypothyroidism is idiopathic atrophy, which occurs when there is no known cause for loss of thyroid gland tissue.

Clinical signs: Because thyroid hormone controls the rate of cellular metabolism, a decline in thyroid function causes a decline in the dog's basal metabolic rate and energy needs. Owners first notice a change in the dog's energy level and a decreased interest in exercise.[32] Weight gain is common, without a corresponding increase in food intake. In mild cases, the dog's coat gradually becomes dull and sparse. As the disorder progresses, however, **alopecia** (hair loss) occurs, and the dog may develop seborrhea, hyperpigmentation, thickening of the skin, and secondary bacterial infections. In intact animals, irregular heat cycles are seen in females and atrophy of the testicles may be observed in males. Neurological signs occasionally are observed and include abnormal gait patterns, facial nerve paralysis, and intermittent seizures.[33] More than 75 percent of dogs with hypothyroidism have elevated blood cholesterol levels. Although this is not a clinical sign owners can observe, cholesterol levels are of aid in the eventual diagnosis of hypothyroidism. Some dogs with hypothyroidism also have decreased red blood cell counts and may be diagnosed as anemic.

Diagnosis: Diagnosis of hypothyroidism in dogs involves the dog's history, breed, age, clinical signs, and various blood tests for thyroid hormone. Because other diseases and certain medications can cause declines in circulating thyroid hormone levels, T_4 levels and serum cholesterol should be assessed with respect to the presence of clinical signs. Both T_4 and T_3 levels in blood can be routinely measured. However, approximately 50 percent of dogs with hypothyroidism maintain normal circulating levels of T_3. Therefore, assessment of T_4 status should always be included in the testing panel. When T_4 levels are normal or high, hypothyroidism can be ruled out. Values that are less than normal or near zero are indicative of hypothyroidism and are taken as a definitive diagnosis when clinical signs also support that diagnosis.

However, because T_4 levels can be affected by several factors, some veterinarians use additional tests of thyroid gland function to diagnose hypothyroidism.[34] These are more reliable but are more time-consuming and costly to the owner. They include measurements of thyroid-releasing hormone (TRH), TSH response, and free T_4 levels. Overall, the TSH test is most accurate and reliable in diagnosing hypothyroidism in dogs. This test often is recommended for dogs that have a difficult or complicated case. The free T_4 test provides a measurement of the biologically active form of thyroid hormone and is not easily influenced by medication or illness. A disadvantage of this test is that its interpretation requires special procedures available only at certain types of analytical laboratories. For this reason, this test is not always available to dog owners or is so costly it is not a viable alternative.

Treatment: Treatment of hypothyroidism involves hormone replacement therapy and must be given for the lifetime of the dog. However, once proper dosages are determined, the dog's long-term prognosis is excellent. The disorder is managed with a synthetic form of thyroid hormone, given orally, two times per day.[35] Many dogs will begin to shed large quantities of hair shortly after beginning replacement therapy. This is a normal response and signifies the regrowth of new hair. In most cases, complete regrowth of normal hair will take up to 6 months. If the dog had accompanying skin infections, these should be treated at the start of therapy. The dog's thyroid hormone levels should be evaluated every 6 months so replacement hormone dosage can be adjusted as necessary. When thyroid hormone replacement therapy is properly adjusted and maintained, clinical signs are resolved in the vast majority of cases and the dog can live a healthy life with a normal life span.

Cushing's Syndrome (Hyperadrenocorticism)

This disorder is also a relatively common hormonal disease and results from the overproduction of steroid hormones by the adrenal glands. The adrenal glands are small organs located above the kidneys. The outer layer of the gland, called the cortex, produces steroid hormones. Cushing's syndrome can have a number of underlying causes. Excessive production of adrenocorticotropic hormone (ACTH) by the pituitary gland can stimulate the adrenal glands to overproduce steroid hormones. This is called pituitary-dependent Cushing's. Hyperplasia (overgrowth) of the cortex of the adrenal gland or the presence of a tumor in the gland results in adrenal-dependent Cushing's. The most common cause of Cushing's syndrome in dogs, however, is the long-term administration of cortisone compounds (iatrogenic Cushing's).[36] Cortisol-containing medications that may induce Cushing's include synthetic corticosteroids that often are administered systemically for the treatment of inflammatory disorders, as well as the overuse of topical ointments, eye drops or ear medications that contain cortisol, or cortisol-like compounds. The syndrome develops gradually over a long period of time and is most commonly seen in adult dogs older than 6 years of age. Although iatrogenic Cushing's can occur in any dog that has undergone long-term treatment with corticosteroids, naturally induced Cushing's occurs more often in Dachshunds, Poodles, Boxers, and Boston Terriers.

Clinical signs: Major signs of Cushing's include polydypsia and polyuria (increased water consumption and increased urination), increased appetite, muscle weakness, lethargy, and dermatological signs such as bilateral hair loss on the body's trunk, changes in pigmentation of the skin, scaling, and delayed wound healing. The dog's skin thickens, become less elastic, and is susceptible to secondary bacterial infections (pyoderma). Changes in body shape occur because of alterations in body composition and a loss of muscle strength. The abdominal muscles weaken, and there is a redistribution of body fat, giving the dog a pot-bellied look. Owners often think their dog has become obese, but these changes often are actually accompanied by a slight loss in weight. Because the high level of corticosteroids suppresses the dog's immune system, the dog becomes more susceptible to disease. Injuries heal slowly, and infections are more likely.

Diagnosis: Cushing's syndrome is diagnosed using the dog's medical history, clinical signs, and blood or urine tests. Blood tests for glucose concentration and liver enzyme function should also be performed and assessed to determine the presence of other diseases. For example, diabetes mellitus is occasionally seen in conjunction with Cushing's syndrome. Measurement of plasma cortisol concentrations in response to ACTH administration is the primary blood test used to confirm a diagnosis of Cushing's syndrome. More recently, measuring levels of cortisol in urine relative to urine creatinine concentrations has been found to be an effective, relatively simple diagnostic tool for the diagnosis of dogs with hyperadrenocorticism.[37]

Treatment: Treatment is based on the type of Cushing's that is present. When a tumor is responsible, it usually is surgically removed, and replacement therapy with corticosteroids is necessary for the remainder of the dog's life. Pituitary-dependent Cushing's is treated with medications that selectively destroy the cells of the adrenal gland that produce and secrete cortisol. This renders the adrenal glands less able to respond to the high levels of ACTH. In these cases, proper dosages and frequent follow-up tests are necessary to keep the dog in remission. Another option is to treat the dog with medications that block the action of cortisol. Iatrogenic Cushing's is treated with the gradual decrease of the offending medication. With treatment, the long-term prognosis for dogs with most types of Cushing's syndrome is very good.

Hot Spots (Acute Moist Dermatitis)

A hot spot is the common name given to an acute, moist dermatitis that most often is seen in dogs with dense, heavy undercoats. These are warm, painful, swollen lesions in the skin that exude pus and often have a very distinctive odor.

Clinical signs: A unique characteristic of hot spots is the suddenness with which they appear. The skin lesion appears and enlarges rapidly, often within a few hours. The affected area has a yellowish center surrounded by a reddened ring of irritation, and it feels warm to the touch. The lesion can become quite painful if not treated and can grow rapidly in size or spread quickly to other areas of the body. Hot spots are more common in breeds of dogs that have a dense, woolly undercoat such as Collies, German Shepherd Dogs, and Retrievers. They are seen most commonly prior to shedding, particularly in the wet season when dead, moist hair is trapped next to the skin. Some individual dogs are particularly susceptible and may suffer from multiple, recurrent infections.

Cause: The condition is caused by some initial trauma to the skin (e.g., biting or scratching due to fleas, trauma by electric clipper blades, cat scratches, or an abrasion). Sites are often areas in which the hair is matted, poorly groomed, or damp. The initial trauma is followed by a bacterial infection and bacterial overgrowth. The lesions most commonly appear on the neck, ears, chest, back, rump, and flanks. Susceptible dogs may develop several hot spots at multiple sites simultaneously.

Treatment: Treatment is directed toward cleaning up the debris and allowing fresh air to dry the surface of the affected skin. The hair surrounding the lesion should be clipped away and the skin gently cleansed with a mild antiseptic soap to remove all exudate and crusts. If multiple areas are affected, veterinary care should be sought, and systemic antibiotics may be prescribed. Anti-inflammatory agents sometimes are administered to decrease pruritus and self-induced trauma. However, these also can delay wound healing, so they should be administered with caution. Ointments or creams are not recommended because these can prevent or delay drying of the lesion. However, some topical treatments that contain a combination of antibiotics and corticosteroids are helpful. If the dog continues to attempt to lick or bite the area, a protective collar should be used to prevent continued self-induced trauma. If an underlying cause, such as flea infestation or allergies, is identified, this problem should be treated to minimize chances of recurrence of hot spots. Long-term care involves careful attention to the care of the dog's skin and coat and immediate treatment whenever a lesion is seen.

Canine Atopic Disease (Atopy)

Atopy, also known as "inhalant allergic dermatitis" or "atopic disease," is a common skin disease in dogs that is caused by a hypersensitivity to pollens or other environmental allergens.[38] It has been estimated that approximately 10 percent to 15 percent of the canine population is affected by atopy, second in prevalence only to flea allergic dermatitis (see Chapter 14).[39,40] Observations of breed and family predilections, and results of limited breeding trials indicate that atopy has a strong heritable component in dogs.[3,41] Breeds that are at increased risk include Dalmatians, Irish Setters, Golden Retrievers, Boxers, Labrador Retrievers, Belgian Tervurens, and several terrier and toy breeds.[42,43] Symptoms occur when a susceptible dog either inhales or has skin contact with the allergen. Common allergens include the pollen, spores, or seeds of grasses, trees, weeds, or molds. In temperate climates, trees tend to pollinate in the spring, grasses in the summer, and weeds in the fall. As a result, a dog who is allergic to several types of pollens often shows intermittent signs from April until November.

Clinical signs: Clinical signs of atopic disease occur when the animal is exposed to the offending antigen, and sensitized mast cells present in the skin begin a hypersensitivity response that includes the release of inflammatory agents. Clinical signs include moderate to intense pruritus, skin lesions, and secondary bacterial infections. The dog's face, feet, and ears are most frequently affected. Excessive licking of the coat or skin leads to staining of the hair coat. Dogs often will lick the groin region and the bottoms of their feet, often resulting in hair loss, staining, and irritation in those areas of the body. Clinical signs usually first appear when dogs are between 1 and 3 years old and become progressively worse as the dog ages. Atopy is rarely seen in dogs younger than 6 months, indicating that repeated exposure to allergens is involved in the disorder.

Treatment: Treatment of atopy includes avoidance of the offending allergens and the use of medications or dietary adjustments, which decrease the dog's inflammatory response to inhaled or contact allergens. If owners are aware of the allergens to which their dog is allergic, preventing exposure by limiting the dog's access to certain parks or other outside areas that have a high concentration of allergens is helpful. In addition, frequent bathing, especially following exposure to high pollen areas, is effective in decreasing the exposure of the dog's skin (contact allergies) and opportunities to inhale pollens that may be adhering to the coat. Medicated shampoos are recommended if the dog has an accompanying pyoderma.

Medical therapy for atopy involves the use of antihistamines and anti-inflammatory agents and, if necessary, systemic treatment for secondary pyoderma. Most typically, antihistamines and different types of corticosteroids are prescribed. However, there are undesirable side effects to the chronic administration of many of these drugs, particularly the corticosteroids. In recent years, fatty acid supplements have been investigated and used as a safe, adjunctive treatment for atopic disease in dogs. The dietary manipulation of fatty acid metabolism is aimed at modifying the amount and type of inflammatory agents that are produced during an inflammatory response. Diets that include a decreased proportion of fatty acids of the omega-6 series and an increased proportion of fatty acids of the omega-3 series cause changes in the levels of these compounds in both plasma and tissues, and affect the intensity of the dog's inflammatory response.[44,45,46] Since many variables affect the effectiveness of a fatty acid supplement, dogs show varying degrees of responsiveness to omega-3 fatty acids (see Chapter 16).[47] Although a proportion of allergic dogs has been shown to require no additional therapy when provided with a dietary fatty acid supplement, many dogs still require concurrent administration of antihistamines or low dosages of corticosteroids to control pruritus.[48,49] However, since atopic disease is a disorder that is managed and not cured, the use of fatty acid therapy is a safe alternative to the long-term use of corticosteroids for many dogs.

Idiopathic Epilepsy

A recent AKC survey of breed clubs reported that canine idiopathic seizures were rated among the top five medical concerns of dog breeders.[50] Approximately 14 percent of dogs with neurological disorders exhibit seizures, and 80 percent of these are diagnosed as **idiopathic**.[51] A seizure occurs when nerve cells or neurons experience prolonged depolarization, which leads to excess electrical stimulation. Simply put, this means that the neurons are "misfiring" and sending prolonged messages to the brain and to muscles. The severity of a seizure is determined by where it starts and how many neurons it involves. Some seizures are caused by poisoning, metabolic disease, or reactions to medications. If detected in time, they often can be successfully treated. Idiopathic epilepsy refers to recurrent, periodic seizures of unknown cause. There are specific familial predispositions to this disorder. Poodles, St. Bernards, Golden Retrievers, Labrador Retrievers, and German Shepherds show a higher incidence than the general population of dogs. Pedigree analysis studies have shown that the disease has a multifactorial autosomal-recessive mode of inheritance.[52] Other contributing causes of epilepsy include recovery from the neurological stage of distemper, a high fever of long duration, or head trauma. In most cases, however, the owner is unable to trace the onset of seizures to a specific event in the dog's life.

Clinical signs: The first seizures usually are seen between the ages of 1 and 3 years. Frequency varies between every day to as infrequently as 6 months or a year. Although seizures are usually not dangerous to the dog, they can vary greatly in severity and duration. Most seizures exhibit three distinct stages. The prodromal stage is a precursor period in which the dog may become restless, frightened, or show an unusual change in behavior. In some dogs, this stage is very mild and difficult to detect. The prodromal stage is followed by the actual seizure, called the "ictus" stage, and is typified by some degree of muscular rigidity. The dog may move peculiarly, salivate, fall over on his or her side, arch her neck, or show paddling movements with her feet. Some dogs will moan or yip during a seizure and may stare blankly ahead. In severe cases, the dog may urinate or defecate. The ictus stage usually lasts only 1 or 2 minutes, rarely more than 5 minutes. Seizures that last more than several minutes should be cause for concern and may endanger the dog's life because of severe exertion and overheating. Whenever a seizure lasts for more than 5 to 7 minutes, veterinary attention should be immediately sought. Most seizures are not life threatening and dogs recover relatively quickly. The post-ictal stage follows the seizure and may last anywhere from a few minutes to a day or more. Dogs typically act disoriented and lethargic and show aberrations in eating and drinking. As with the prodromal stage, a significant number of dogs do not demonstrate an obvious post-ictal stage and rapidly return to normal behavior.

Care for a dog during a seizure involves keeping the dog safe by moving objects away and, if necessary, moving the dog away from dangerous areas such as doorways or stairs. Contrary to popular folklore, dogs do not swallow their tongues during seizures, so it is not necessary to place anything in the dog's mouth. After the seizure, if the dog is disoriented, it is helpful to confine her to a small room or crate until it has recovered completely. Staying with the dog and comforting her after a seizure often is helpful. Owners should record the date and time, duration of the seizure, and a description of the dog's behavior before and after the event.

Treatment: Mild seizures that last only a few minutes or do not occur more than once a month usually are not medically treated. Although it is still controversial when therapy for idiopathic epilepsy should be instituted, a general rule of thumb is to begin medical treatment if seizures increase in frequency to more than one per month, or if they are occurring with increasing severity. Epileptic seizures can be controlled in dogs but not cured. Treatment involves daily doses of medication, usually phenobarbital, which functions to reduce the frequency of seizures. Although it is one of the most cost-effective drugs for controlling seizures, a side effect is serious and even fatal liver damage in a small proportion of dogs. Other common side effects are lethargy, disorientation, and sedation. The drug potassium bromide often is prescribed to use in conjunction with phenobarbital. An advantage of bromide is that it is not metabolized by the liver and has a long half-life in the bloodstream, making it easier to maintain effective dosage levels. Potassium bromide has been used to treat epilepsy in people since the 1800s and has only recently been introduced in dogs. Dogs that have a relatively late onset of epilepsy and who have a relatively low number of seizures respond best to medical therapy.[53]

Conclusions

This chapter reviewed several commonly seen non-infectious disorders of the domestic dog. While some of these can be medically treated or even prevented, others are life-long disorders that involve long-term management and care. In addition to these disorders, the domestic dog is susceptible to several internal and external parasites. The occurrence of these diseases, their recognition, prevention, and treatment are examined in the following chapter.

Cited References

1. Wease, G.N. and Corley, E.A. **Control of canine hip dysplasia: current status.** KalKan Forum, 4:80-88. (1985)

2. Corley, E.A. **Role of the Orthopedic Foundation for Animals in the control of canine hip dysplasia.** Veterinary Clinics of North America: Small Animal Practice, 22:579-593. (1992)

3. Corley, E.A. **Hip dysplasia: A report from the Orthopedic Foundation for Animals.** Seminars in Veterinary Medicine and Surgery (Small Animal), 2:141-151. (1987)

4. Riser, W.H. and Shirer, J.F. **Correlation between canine hip dysplasia and pelvic muscle mass: a study of 95 dogs.** American Journal of Veterinary Research, 28:769-777. (1967)

5. Smith, G.K., Popovitch, C.A., and Gregor, T.P. **Evaluation of risk factors for degenerative joint disease associated with hip dysplasia in dogs.** Journal of the American Veterinary Medical Association, 206:642-647. (1995)

6. Hedhammer, A., Olssom, S.E., and Anderson, S.A. **Canine hip dysplasia: Study of heritability in 401 litters of German Shepherd Dogs.** Journal of the American Veterinary Medical Association, 174:1012-1019. (1979)

7. Leighton, E.A., Lin, J.M., and Willham, R.F. **A genetic study of canine hip dysplasia.** American Journal of Veterinary Research, 38:241-244. (1977)

8. Wallace, L.J. **A half century of canine hip dysplasia: Perspectives of the eighties.** Seminars in Veterinary Medicine and Surgery (Small Animal), 2:97-98. (1987)

9. Kealy, R.D., Olsson, S.E., and Monti, K.L. **Effects of limited food consumption on the incidence of hip dysplasia in growing dogs.** Journal of the American Veterinary Medical Association, 201:857-863. (1992)

10. Tomlinson, J. and McLaughlin, R. **Canine hip dysplasia: Development factors, clinical signs and initial examination steps.** Veterinary Medicine, 91:26-33. (1996)

11. Richardson, D.C. **The role of nutrition in canine hip dysplasia.** Veterinary Clinics of North America, Small Animal Practice, 22:529-540. (1992)

12. Haan, J.J., Beale, B.S., and Parker, R.B. **Diagnosis and treatment of canine hip dysplasia.** Canine Practice, 18:24-28. (1993)

13. Bardens, J.W. and Hardwick, H. **New observations on the diagnosis and cause of hip dysplasia.** Veterinary Medicine: Small Animal Clinician, 63:238-245. (1968)

14. Smith, G.K., Biery, D.N., and Gregor, T.P. **New concepts of coxofemoral joint stability and the development of a clinical stress-radiographic method for quantitating hip joint laxity in the dog.** Journal of the American Veterinary Medical Association, 196:59-70. (1990)

15. Heyman, S.J., Smith, G.K., and Cofone, M.A. **Biomechanical study of the effect of coxofemoral positioning on passive hip joint laxity in the dog.** American Journal of Veterinary Research, 54:210-215. (1993)

16. Todhunter, R.J. and Lust, G. **Polysulfated glycosaminoglycan in the treatment of osteoarthritis.** Journal of the American Veterinary Medical Association, 204:1245-1251. (1994)

17. Moore, M.G. **Promising responses to a new oral treatment for degenerative joint disorders.** Canine Practice, 21:7-11. (1996)

18. Lust, G., Williams, A.J., and Burton-Wurster, N. **Effects of intramuscular administration of glycosaminoglycan polysulfates on signs of incipient hip dysplasia in growing pups.** American Journal of Veterinary Research, 53:1836-1843. (1992)

19. Olmstead, M.L. **Total hip replacement in the dog.** Seminars in Veterinary Medical Surgery, Small Animal, 2:131-140. (1987)

20. Swift, W.B. **Getting hip to hip dysplasia.** Animals, May/June, 29-31. (1995)

21. Hutt, F.B. **Genetic selection to reduce the incidence of hip dysplasia in dogs.** Journal of the American Veterinary Medical Association, 151:1041-1048. (1967)

22. Kaman, C.H. and Grossling, H.R. **A breeding program to reduce hip dysplasia in German Shepherd Dogs.** Journal of the American Veterinary Medical Association, 151:562-571. (1967)

23. Fox, S.M. and Walker, A.M. **The etiopathogenesis of osteochondrosis.** Veterinary Medicine, February:116-122. (1993)

24. Milton, J.L. **Osteochondritis dissecans in the dog.** Veterinary Clinics of North America: Small Animal Practice, 13:117-133. (1983)

25. Harari, J. **Identifying and managing osteochondrosis in dogs.** Veterinary Medicine, June:508-509. (1997)

26. Wilford, C. **Treating shifting leg lameness.** American Kennel Club Purebred Dog Gazette, December:58-62. (1994)

27. Glickman, L., Emerick, T., Glickman, N., Glickman, S., Lantz, G., Perez, C., Schellenberg, D., Widmer, W., and Qi-long, Y. **Radiological assessment of the relationship between thoracic conformation and the risk of gastric dilatation-volvulus in dogs.** Veterinary Radiology and Ultrasound, 37:174-180. (1996)

28. Glickman, L.T., Glickman, N.W., and Perez, C.M. **Analysis of risk factors for gastric dilatation-volvulus in dogs.** Journal of the American Veterinary Medical Association, 204:1465-1471. (1996)

29. Leib, M.S., Wingfield, W.E., and Twedt, D.C. **Plasma gastrin immunoreactivity in dogs with acute gastric dilatation-volvulus.** Journal of the American Veterinary Medical Association, 185:205-208. (1984)

30. Nesbitt, G.H., Izzo, J., Peterson, L., and Wilkins, R.J. **Canine hypothyroidism: A retrospective study of 108 cases.** Journal of the American Veterinary Medical Association, 177:1117-1122. (1980)

31. Blake, S. and Lapinski, A. **Hypothyroidism in different breeds.** Canine Practice, 7:48-51. (1980)

32. Panciera, D. **Clinical manifestations of canine hypothyroidism.** Veterinary Medicine, January:44-49. (1997)

33. Jaggy, A. **Neurological manifestations of hypothyroidism: A retrospective study of 29 dogs.** Journal of Veterinary Internal Medicine, 8:328-336. (1994)

34. Panciera, D. **Thyroid-function testing: Is the future here?** Veterinary Medicine, January:50-57. (1997)

35. Panciera, D. **Treating hypothyroidism.** Veterinary Medicine, January:58-68. (1997)

36. Lorenz, M.D. **What is canine Cushing's Syndrome?** American Kennel Club Purebred Dog Gazette, April:42-46. (1985)

37. Jensen, A.L., Iveersen, L., Koch, J., Hoier, R., and Petersen, T.K. **Evaluation of the urinary cortisol: Creatinine ratio in the diagnosis of hyperadrenocorticism in dogs.** Journal of Small Animal Practice, 38:99-102. (1997)

38. Scott, D.W., Miller, W.H., Griffin, C.E. *Muller and Kirk's Small Animal Dermatology,* fifth edition, W.B. Saunders, Philadelphia, Pennsylvania, pp. 500-518. (1995)

39. Chalmers, S.A. and Medeau, L. **An update on atopic dermatitis in dogs.** Veterinary Medicine, 89:326-342. (1994)

40. Scott, D.W. and Paradis, M. **A survey of canine and feline skin disorders seen in a university practice: small animal clinic, University of Montreal, Saint-Hyacinthe, Quebec (1987-1989).** Canadian Veterinary Journal, 31:830-835. (1990)

41. Schwartzman, R.M. **Immunologic studies of progeny of atopic dogs.** American Journal of Veterinary Research, 45:375-379. (1984)

42. Reedy, L.M. and Miller, W.H., Jr. *Allergic Skin Diseases of Dogs and Cats,* W.B. Saunders Co., Philadelphia, Pennsylvania, 1989.

43. Scott, D.W. **Observations on canine atopy.** Journal of the American Animal Hospital Association, 17:91-100. (1981)

44. Savic, M.S., Yager, J.A., and Holub, B.J. **Effect of n-3 and n-6 fatty acid dietary supplementation on canine neutrophil and keratinocyte phospholipid composition.** Proceedings of the Second World Congress on Veterinary Dermatology, p. 77. (1992)

45. Campbell, K.L., Czarnecki-Maulden, G.L., and Schaeffer, D.J. **Effects of animal and soy fats and proteins in the diet on concentrations of fatty acids in the serum and skin of dogs.** American Journal of Veterinary Research, 56:1465-1472. (1995)

46. Vaughn, D.M., Reinhart, G.A., Swaim, S.F., Lauten, S.D., Garner, C.A., Boudreaux, M.K., Spano, J.S., Hoffman, C.E., and Conner, B. **Evaluation of dietary n-6 to n-3 fatty acid ratios on leukotriene B synthesis in dog skin and neutrophils.** Veterinary Dermatology, 5:163-173. (1994)

47. Scott, D.W., Miller, W.H. and Griffin, C.E. *Muller and Kirk's Small Animal Dermatology,* fifth edition, W.B. Saunders, Philadelphia, Pennsylvania, pp. 214-217. (1995)

48. Scott, D.W. and Miller, W.H. **Nonsteroidal management of canine pruritus: chlorpheniramine and a fatty acid supplement (DVM Derm Caps) in combination, and the fatty acid supplement at twice the manufacturers' recommended dosage.** Cornell Veterinarian, 80:381-387. (1991)

49. Paradis, M. and Scott, D.W. **Further investigation on the use of nonsteroidal and steroidal anti-inflammatory agents in the management of canine pruritus.** Journal of the American Animal Hospital Association, 27:44-48. (1991)

50. Smith, C.S. **Seizures.** American Kennel Club Purebred Dog Gazette, December:54-57. (1996)

51. Schwartz-Porsche, D. **Seizures.** In: *Clinical Syndromes in Veterinary Neurology,* second edition (K.G. Braund, editor), Mosby-Year Book, Inc., St. Louis, Missouri, pp. 234-251. (1994)

52. Cunningham, J.G. and Farnbach, G.C. **Inheritance of idiopathic canine epilepsy.** Journal of the American Animal Hospital Association, 24:421-424. (1988)

53. Heynold, Y., Faissler, D., Steffen, F., and Jaggy, A. **Clinical, epidemiological and treatment results of idiopathic epilepsy in 54 Labrador Retrievers: A long-term study.** Journal of Small Animal Practice, 38:7-14. (1997)

13 **Internal Parasites**

INTERNAL PARASITES, or **endoparasites,** can be found in various organs of the dog's body, where they complete part or all of their life cycle and extract nourishment from the host. By definition, parasites provide no benefit to the dog, and in many cases can cause malnourishment or illness. The primary sites inhabited by internal parasites are the gastrointestinal tract, lungs, liver, and heart. Infections typically become pathogenic when there are large numbers of worms present or when the dog is malnourished, ill, or immuno-compromised. Internal parasites are also more serious in puppies than in adult dogs. Signs of disease are caused by competition for essential nutrients, interference with nutrient absorption, destruction of cells within the gastrointestinal tract, obstruction of major blood vessels, or the production of toxins.

Common internal parasites considered to be pathogenic in the dog include several nematodes, cestodes, and protozoan parasites. An understanding of the life cycles and transmission of these parasites is important for companion animal professionals who are concerned with preventing and treating infections. Keeping a dog free of internal parasites throughout life contributes to optimal health, vitality, and longevity.

Canine Heartworm Disease

Heartworm disease is caused by infection with the nematode parasite *Dirofilaria immitis*. This parasite is distributed world-wide, wherever its mosquito vector is found. In the United States, heartworm is considered to be regionally **endemic** in all 50 states. It is most prevalent along the Atlantic and Gulf coasts and throughout the Mississippi River valley, and less common in arid regions and in states located west of the Mississippi River.[1] *Dirofilaria immitis* is classified as a filarial nematode and has a long, threadlike shape. Adults are between 6 and 12 inches in length and are found primarily in the right atrium and ventricle of the heart; the pulmonary arteries, which supply the lungs; and the venae cavae, the major veins emptying into the right atrium. Female heartworms do not lay eggs but produce motile embryos called microfilaria. These are released into the dog's bloodstream and are the form of the parasite that is ingested by a mosquito when it bites an infected dog.

Life cycle and transmission: In most areas, heartworm transmission to dogs occurs during the late spring and summer, and peaks during July and August. However, in areas of the country that have an active reproducing mosquito population throughout the year, transmission can occur during all 12 months of the year. The mosquito is an intermediate host for *Dirofilaria* *immitis,* and the heartworm relies upon this host to complete its life cycle (Figure 13.1). Initial infection of the dog occurs when a mosquito bites the dog and takes a blood meal. The mosquito deposits infective larvae onto the dog's skin. These larvae are capable of burrowing into the subcutaneous layers of the skin, where they develop near the site of the bite for approximately 2 months. After 2 months, they molt to fourth-stage larvae, migrate to the bloodstream, and eventually arrive and settle in the right side of heart and its associated arteries. By 6 months post-infection, these parasites have grown to maturity and are producing microfilaria. Adult heartworms have long life spans, and females are capable of producing microfilaria for up to 5 years.

The microfilaria that are released into the dog's bloodstream do not grow or change. They merely circulate in the bloodstream, waiting to be picked up by another mosquito. When a mosquito bites and takes a blood meal from the dog, it also ingests microfilaria. Development of the larvae in the mosquito is dependent on temperature. In warm climates, the microfilaria proceed through 3 molts to become infective within 10 to 12 days. In cooler climates, this may take as long as 21 days. The infective larvae then migrate to the mouthparts of the mosquito, where they are capable of infecting a dog when the mosquito takes a blood meal.

Clinical signs: The presence of adult parasites in the dog's right atrium and ventricle and pulmonary arteries is responsible for the clinical signs of heartworm disease. An inflammatory response to the parasites develops in the pul-

FIGURE 13.1   Life cycle of *Dirofilaria immitis*

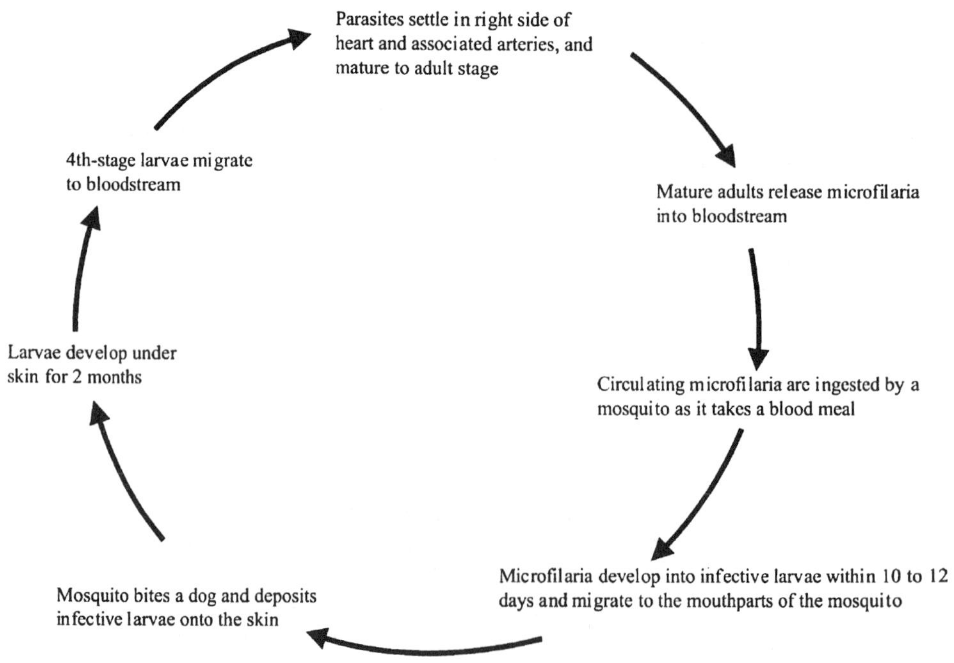

Parasites settle in right side of heart and associated arteries, and mature to adult stage

4th-stage larvae migrate to bloodstream

Mature adults release microfilaria into bloodstream

Larvae develop under skin for 2 months

Circulating microfilaria are ingested by a mosquito as it takes a blood meal

Mosquito bites a dog and deposits infective larvae onto the skin

Microfilaria develop into infective larvae within 10 to 12 days and migrate to the mouthparts of the mosquito

monary artery and its branches. This in turn leads to pulmonary hypertension, enlargement of the pulmonary artery and right side of the heart, and congestion in the liver. The physical presence of these large parasites also interferes with normal blood flow and with the ability of heart valves to function properly. These conditions all contribute to the development of congestive heart failure, which eventually can be fatal if not treated. In some dogs, kidney dysfunction develops as a consequence of the dog's immune response to the parasites and the presence of large numbers of microfilaria in renal capillaries.

A dog's clinical signs are directly related to the number of worms that are present, called the "worm burden." When only a few worms are present, the dog is usually asymptomatic. When there are fewer than 50 worms, most will be found in the pulmonary arteries. When more worms are present, they may occupy the right ventricle, right atrium, and venae cavae. A study of worm burdens in dogs in an animal shelter in Florida reported an average of 23 parasites in infected dogs.[2] It was not unusual for a heavily infected dog to have more than 200 worms. The first signs that owners typically report are listlessness, loss of stamina, and decreased exercise tolerance. If pulmonary circulation is affected, the dog will show difficulty breathing and may develop a soft, deep cough. Over time, clinical signs of congestive heart disease develop and eventually can be fatal if not treated.

Diagnosis: Definitive diagnosis of heartworm disease involves the identification of either microfilaria or heartworm antigens in the blood. The simplest test is a direct smear of fresh or concentrated blood. This is called a Knot's test or modified Knot's test and detects circulating microfilaria in a sample of the dog's blood. However, these tests are not reliable for light infections of heartworm and cannot discern cases of heartworm in which there are adult parasites in the heart but no circulating microfilaria. These are called "occult" cases of heartworm and have several possible causes. If parasites are present in the heart but are not yet sexually mature or are only of one sex, they will not be producing microfilaria but are still capable of causing disease. Certain medications can cause sterility of adult worms or kill microfilaria (for example ivermectin and milbemycin oxime). Also, dogs that develop a strong immune reaction to heartworm can produce antibodies that destroy microfilaria as soon as they are produced but do not affect the adult parasites in the heart.

Because there is evidence that a substantial portion of infected dogs do not have detectable microfilaria circulating in their bloodstream, tests that do not rely upon the presence of microfilaria are more reliable as a diagnostic tool.[3] These are called immuno-diagnostic techniques and have replaced the Knot's test for initial screening for heartworm disease in dogs. The most commonly used immuno-diagnostic tests detect circulating parasite components, or antigens, in the bloodstream. Since these components are produced by adult parasites, these tests detect all cases of infection, whether or not microfilaria are present. A number of test kits are available and have been proven to be efficacious in the detection of occult heartworm.[4,5] Antigen tests also can be used to indicate an infected dog's worm burden. This is often an important component of diagnosis because dogs with high worm burdens are at greater risk of complications associated with treatment.[6] If a positive test is found with the antigen test, dilutions of the serum can be used to provide an estimate of the number of parasites that are present.

Chest radiographs provide a final diagnostic test that provides overall assessment of cardiopulmonary disease caused by heartworms. In some cases, a diagnosis of heartworm can be made solely on the basis of thoracic radiographs. Radiography is also the best method for assessing the severity of cardiopulmonary disease caused by infection with heartworm.

Treatment: Treatment for canine heartworm involves killing the adult parasites, eliminating microfilaria from the dog's bloodstream, and providing preventive medication to protect the dog against reinfection. A pretreatment veterinary checkup is essential for all dogs undergoing treatment for heartworm because the medications used can be toxic to the liver and kidneys. Therefore, a dog who has compromised liver or kidney functioning may not be a good candidate for treatment.

Two drugs are approved for use as heartworm adulticides in veterinary medicine. These are thiacetarsamide sodium and melarsomine dihydrochloride. Melarsomine was first introduced in the 1990s and has rapidly become the medication of choice of most veterinarians.[7] Compared to thiacetarsamide, melarsomine presents a lower risk of side effects and effectively kills both immature parasites that are between 4 and 5 months of age and adults. Because melarsomine is administered intramuscularly rather than intravenously, it also is associated with fewer procedural complications. Treatment with melarsomine usually involves two stages.[8] The initial injection causes a "partial kill" and is followed by a second series of two injections 2 months later. This protocol allows gradual elimination of the adult worms from the body, which is important for decreasing health complications of heartworm treatment.

Following the administration of the adulticide, the parasites begin to die and continue to be cleared from the blood for several weeks. During this period, there is a danger of pulmonary **thromboembolism**. This occurs because the treatment that kills adult parasites located in the cardiopulmonary vasculature aggravates any existing arterial injury and increases pulmonary hypertension. In mild cases, when only a few adults are killed, mild embolism in relatively healthy areas of lung may be unnoticeable. In most cases, however, the dog is lethargic, has a slight fever and decreased appetite, and develops a cough. Severe complications of adulticide treatment may include right heart failure or liver and kidney dysfunction. Post-treatment complications can be reduced by staging the killing of adult parasites (see above) and by restricting exercise for a minimum of 1 month following administration of the adulticide.[9] However, because the agents used are highly toxic and because adult heartworms are large parasites that must be cleared from the dog's heart and circulatory system, treatment for heartworm is always associated with some level of risk. Following recovery, a follow-up assessment for the presence of adult heartworms should be performed to confirm that all of the adult heartworms have been killed and eliminated from the blood.

Treatment for the removal of microfilaria from the blood of an infected dog is started 4 weeks following successful adulticide therapy. Ivermectin and milbemycin oxime are the safest and most effective microfilaricide drugs available for veterinary use. The administration of these medications causes rapid death of large numbers of microfilaria within 4 to 8 hours. Dogs should be closely monitored during this period because side effects of vomiting, inactivity, lethargy, salivation, and tachycardia (increased heart rate) are common. Retesting for the presence of microfilaria in the blood should be conducted 7 days following treatment.

Prevention (chemoprophylaxis): The dangers of heartworm disease and the risks of treatment emphasize the importance of preventing infection in pet dogs. Luckily, keeping dogs free of heartworm is a relatively simple task for pet owners today. Several prophylactic medications that kill infective larvae before they are able to develop into the fourth larval stage and migrate to the dog's heart are available. Preventive medication should be administered throughout the duration of the heartworm transmission period in a geographical area. Because transmission is dependent on the seasonal presence of mosquito populations, this timing will vary depending on the region. Continuous chemoprophylaxis usually is not necessary in parts of the United States where transmission does not occur throughout the year. Before beginning preventive treatment, all dogs should be tested and determined to be free of both circulating heartworm antigen and microfilaria.[10]

Diethylcarbamazine citrate (DEC) is probably the most economical drug available to pet owners. However, it is rapidly eliminated from the dog's body, so it must be administered on a daily basis to be effective. Because this drug is effective against only the very earliest stages of parasite development, DEC must be consistently provided. If the owner fails to give the medication for a few days, and the dog is bitten by an infective mosquito during that time, the larvae can mature beyond the stage at which the drug is capable of killing them. For this reason and because of its inconvenience, DEC is no longer frequently prescribed as a heartworm preventive. Ivermectin and milbemycin oxime are the two most commonly prescribed prophylactic medications. Both have extended residual effects and are administered once every 30 days. In addition, milbemycin oxime is effective in controlling roundworm, hookworm, and whipworm infections in dogs. Administration of these two drugs should begin within 1 month of the start of mosquito season, and the last dose should be given within 1 month after transmission is no longer considered to be likely.

There are reports of Collies and Collie mixes that are unusually sensitive to high doses of ivermectin.[11] However, the dose of ivermectin used to kill microfilaria in heartworm-infected dogs is 50 μg/kg body weight, while the dose used prophylactically to prevent infection or reinfection with heartworm is 6-12 μg/kg. Both of these doses are well below the threshold level of ivermectin that has been shown to cause toxicity in Collies or Collie mixes.[12] Because ivermectin is manufactured and marketed at very concentrated dosages for use in livestock, these preparations should not be used as prophylactics for dogs as overdosage can occur if the medication is not properly diluted prior to use.

Roundworms (Ascarids)

Intestinal parasites are the most common type of internal parasite found in dogs. The four most commonly seen types are roundworms, hookworms, whipworms, and tapeworms (Figure 13.2). Ascarids are a nematode parasite and are among the most common type of gastrointestinal parasite in dogs. Adult parasites live and reproduce in the small intestine, and inactive encysted larvae can be found in muscle and other tissues. Adult parasites are large, between 1 to 7 inches long, and have the appearance of strands of spaghetti. The most common species to infect dogs in the United States is *Toxocara canis*. A second species, *Toxascaris leonina* is less frequently seen. It has been estimated that approximately 75 percent of puppies and young dogs in the United States are infected with *Toxocara canis*. Adult dogs develop resistance to the adult worm but can still carry the encysted larval stage of the parasite.

Life cycle and transmission: Dogs can contract ascarids from four possible routes: transplacental, transmammary, ingestion of eggs from the environment, or predation of infected animals such as birds and mice. The major routes of transmission to dogs are transplacental and the ingestion of eggs. The majority of puppies in the United States are born infected with *Toxocara canis* and begin shedding eggs of this parasite in their feces by the time they are 3 weeks old. Because female roundworms can produce up to 200,000 eggs per day and because transplacental transmission is difficult to control, fecal shedding of eggs by puppies is a major source of environmental contamination with *Toxocara canis* eggs.

FIGURE 13.2   Adult and egg phases of four common intestinal parasites

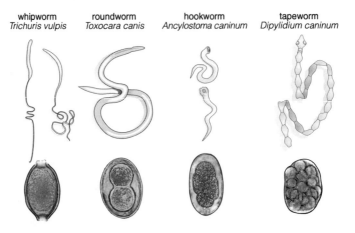

| whipworm | roundworm | hookworm | tapeworm |
| *Trichuris vulpis* | *Toxocara canis* | *Ancylostoma caninum* | *Dipylidium caninum* |

When conditions are warm and humid, eggs deposited in the environment develop (embryonate) into an infective stage in approximately 2 weeks (Figure 13.3). These eggs are relatively resistant to environmental extremes and can remain viable for several years. Dogs become infected when they consume infective eggs from the soil. The eggs larvate in the stomach and small intestine, then enter the bloodstream by penetrating the wall of the intestine. Larvae are transported first to the liver and eventually to the lungs. When they reach the lungs, the larvae become motile and crawl up the trachea, causing the dog to cough. When this occurs, larvae are expelled into the oral cavity, swallowed, and return to the small intestine. In puppies that are less than 3 months of age, the larvae develop into adults in the small intestine, begin to reproduce, and pass eggs in the feces. The entire cycle from ingested egg to intestinal adult takes only about 30 days.

Dogs that are older than 3 months develop partial immunity to ascarids, so they rarely are infected with the intestinal form of this parasite. However, when eggs are consumed from the environment, some dogs may develop a short-term infection and shed large numbers of eggs in the feces. This often occurs in lactating females when they lick the anus of their puppies or consume puppies' fecal matter when cleaning up after the litter. Another way in which adults can contract short-term, self-limiting intestinal ascarids is through ingesting infected wild animals such as rodents, birds, and some insects.

FIGURE 13.3   Life cycle of *Toxocara canis*

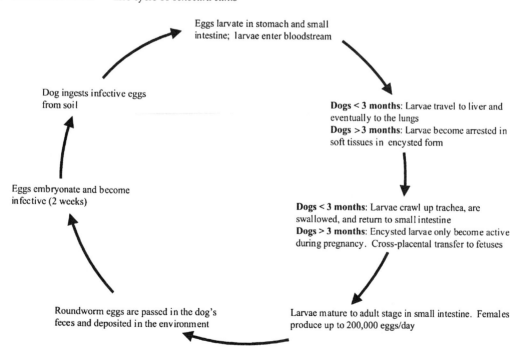

Eggs larvate in stomach and small intestine; larvae enter bloodstream

Dog ingests infective eggs from soil

Dogs < 3 months: Larvae travel to liver and eventually to the lungs
Dogs > 3 months: Larvae become arrested in soft tissues in encysted form

Eggs embryonate and become infective (2 weeks)

Dogs < 3 months: Larvae crawl up trachea, are swallowed, and return to small intestine
Dogs > 3 months: Encysted larvae only become active during pregnancy. Cross-placental transfer to fetuses

Roundworm eggs are passed in the dog's feces and deposited in the environment

Larvae mature to adult stage in small intestine. Females produce up to 200,000 eggs/day

In most cases, transmission of ascarids to dogs older than 3 months of age results in the deposition of encysted larvae in soft tissues. After traveling to the liver, larvae become arrested in muscles, kidneys, eyes, or the brain. In male dogs, spayed females, and intact females who are never bred, these encysted larvae remain dormant indefinitely and do not affect the dog's health. However, in pregnant females, these encysted larvae become reactivated around the 42nd day of gestation. They travel to the bloodstream and eventually to the placenta where they cross to the developing fetuses, infecting them before birth. The larvae are deposited in the fetal liver and immediately after birth continue their migration to the lungs. They follow the tracheal route to the intestines, where they develop into adult parasites within 3 weeks. Less commonly, encysted larvae of the mother travel to her mammary tissue and infect nursing puppies. Because most females have some arrested roundworm larvae in their tissues, almost all puppies will be born with ascarids. Most deworming medications are not effective against the encysted larvae. Therefore, a dam who has been wormed before breeding is still capable of passing ascarids to her unborn puppies.

Another species of ascarids that infects dogs is *Toxascaris leonina*. This is primarily a cold-climate parasite, and in contrast to *Toxocara canis*, the larvae of *Toxascaris leonina* do not migrate to the liver or lungs as part of their life cycle. As a result, encysted larvae are not deposited in tissues, and transmammary and transplacental routes of infection do not occur. Ingestion of eggs is the only clinically important mode of transmission of this type of roundworm to puppies and adult dogs. Although there is no age-related immunity to intestinal infection with *Toxascaris leonina*, the number of infections in dogs that are seen by veterinarians is much lower than that of *Toxocara canis*.

Clinical signs and diagnosis: Infection with ascarids is rarely a health problem in adult dogs but can be very serious in young puppies. If large numbers of larvae are passed to the fetuses transplacentally, still births and early neonatal death can occur as a result of heavy larval infection in the liver and lungs. In newborn puppies, developing adult parasites in the intestine cause malnutrition, impaired growth, and emaciation. In severe cases, ascarids can cause death within the first few weeks of life. The typical ascarid-ridden puppy has a pot-bellied appearance, with a rough hair coat and poor muscle development. Vomiting and diarrhea occur, and adult worms may be seen in the vomit or feces. Diagnosis is through the appearance of adult worms in feces or vomit and through microscopic identification of ascarid eggs in a fecal sample (see Figure 13.2).

Treatment: Several deworming agents are effective against intestinal ascarids (Table 13.1). Two that are safe for use with puppies are piperazine and pyrantel pamoate. Fenbendazole is also effective and has become a popular drug for the treatment of several types of intestinal parasites. When a single treatment series of fenbendazole is administered, it is effective against only the intestinal form of ascarids. However, recent studies have shown that administering higher dosages of this drug to gestating and lactating females starting during pregnancy and continuing until the 4th or 5th week of lactation significantly decreases transmission of roundworm to fetuses and puppies. However, because of the cost, inconvenience, and concerns over potential side effects, this has not yet become a routine practice for the control of roundworms.

Because of the high prevalence of ascarids in the environment, newborn puppies and their mothers should be dewormed at 2, 4, 6, and 8 weeks of age,

TABLE 13.1   Commonly Used Anthelmintics (Deworming Agents) for Dogs

Medication	Brand Names	Effective Against	Method of Administration	Special Concerns
Piperazine	Wormicide	roundworm; partially effective against hookworm	oral (non-prescription; several forms)	May cause vomiting within 1 hour of administration; use in puppies older than 6 weeks and adults
Pyrantel pamoate	Nemex, Evict	roundworm, hookworm	oral (non-prescription; several forms)	Causes vomiting in small percentage of dogs; safe for puppies as young as 2 weeks; highly effective anthelmintic
Mebendazole	Telmintic	roundworm, hookworm, whipworm, *Taenia* sp.	oral (powder)	Not effective against *Dipylidium* sp. of tapeworm; may result in liver toxicity in some dogs
Fenbendazole	Panacur	roundworm, hookworm, whipworm, tapeworm (*Taenia* sp.)	oral (granules)	Preferred over mebendazole; is not effective against *Dipylidium* sp. of tapeworm; may cause vomiting in some dogs but is not associated with liver toxicity
Dichlorophene	Happy Jack	tapeworm (*Taenia* sp. and *Dipylidium* sp.)	oral (non-prescription)	May cause vomiting or diarrhea within 12 hours of treatment
Praziquantel	Droncit	tapeworm (*Taenia* sp. and *Dipylidium* sp.)	oral or injectable	May cause vomiting or diarrhea in some dogs; can be used in puppies as young as 4 weeks and pregnant females
Epsiprantel	Cestex	tapeworm (*Taenia* sp. and *Dipylidium* sp.)	oral	May cause vomiting in small percentage of dogs; can be used in puppies 7 weeks or older; not accepted for use in pregnant females
Sulfadimethoxine	Albon, Bactrovet	coccidia	oral or injectable	Coccidiosatic; must be administered for minimum of 10 to 12 days
Metronidazole	Flagyl	giardia	oral	Bactericidal; may cause vomiting or diarrhea in small percentage of dogs; should not be administered to pregnant females

regardless of whether or not fecal examinations are positive for ascarid eggs. The initial treatment will kill intrauterine-acquired ascarids, and subsequent treatments will expel ascarids acquired through the bitch's milk or through ingesting eggs. This should be routine practice in a breeding program, since there is no way to know if a female is passing ascarids to her unborn puppies. Puppies in new homes should be dewormed at least twice at 2-week intervals. Long-term control of ascarids in dogs has improved significantly with the widespread use of heartworm preventives that also control ascarid and hookworm infections. Minimizing exposure of young puppies to public areas that may be heavily infested with eggs, cleaning up feces daily, and having fecal checks conducted on a regular basis are also practices that aid in decreasing infection with roundworm.

Hookworms

Adult hookworms are relatively small in size compared to heartworms and ascarids. They are white to gray in color and between 1/2 and 3/4 of an inch in length. The anterior end of the worm has a slight hook, with cutting plates for attaching to the lining of the intestine and ingesting blood. Hookworms reside primarily in the small intestine but may be found in the colon and cecum in heavily infested dogs. Several species can infect the domestic dog. These include *Ancylostoma caninum*, *Ancylostoma braziniense*, and *Unicaria stenocephala*. *Ancylostoma caninum* is by far the most important and the most pathogenic hookworm parasite that infects dogs in the United States. *Ancylostoma* species are blood-ingesting parasites and can lead to serious blood loss when large numbers occur. *Unicaria stenocephala* commonly is referred to as the "fox hookworm" because of its prevalence in that species. It infrequently infects dogs in the United States but is seen in Great Britain and northern parts of Canada. Unlike the *Ancylostoma* species, *Unicaria* species are not blood-ingesting parasites and so do not cause severe health problems in dogs.

Life cycle and transmission: In dogs, two common routes of hookworm infection are transmammary and infection with third-stage larvae from the environment (Figure 13.4). Adult females that are attached to the intestinal mucosa deposit eggs that are passed in the feces. These eggs hatch very quickly into an infective stage. If eggs are deposited in relatively humid conditions and temperatures between 70 to 88 degrees Fahrenheit (F), the eggs will hatch within 12 to 24 hours. Larvae develop for 1 week until they reach an infective stage. These larvae either can be consumed orally from the soil or can enter the dog's body by penetrating the skin on the pads of the feet. Orally ingested larvae travel to the small intestine where they mature into adults. Larvae that penetrate the skin enter the bloodstream and eventually arrive in the lungs. In young dogs, these are coughed into the mouth and esophagus, swallowed, and carried to the small intestine where they mature into adults. Adult dogs often have acquired some immunity to hookworms.

In these dogs, the penetrating larvae do not make it to the lungs but are arrested and deposited as encysted larvae in various tissues of the body. As with ascarids, these encysted forms of hookworm remain dormant indefinitely in male dogs, spayed females, and females who are never bred. However, in pregnant females, encysted hookworm larvae deposited in muscle become activated during pregnancy, travel to mammary tissue, and infect newborn puppies through the mother's milk. This is a major route of transmission of hookworm to newborn puppies. Approximately 60 percent of the larvae transmitted through milk do so during the first week of nursing. These larvae travel directly to the intestine and have matured to adult parasites by the time the puppies are 3 weeks old.

Clinical signs and diagnosis: *Ancylostoma* species cause moderate to severe blood loss through feeding and damage to the intestinal wall. Anemia occurs rapidly in young puppies and is characterized by weakness, depression, lethargy, and pale mucous membranes. Hookworms typically cause chronic diarrhea, usually containing blood and mucus. If heavily infected, newborn puppies may die as early as 8 days following exposure. As dogs grow older, most develop immunity to hookworms. However, adult dogs that have compromised immune systems, are housed in a highly contaminated environment, or are experiencing malnutrition can develop chronic hookworm infections. In these cases, mild clinical signs that include diarrhea and vomiting are seen. Diagnosis is through identification of adult hookworms in fe-

FIGURE 13.4   Life cycle of *Ancylostoma caninum*

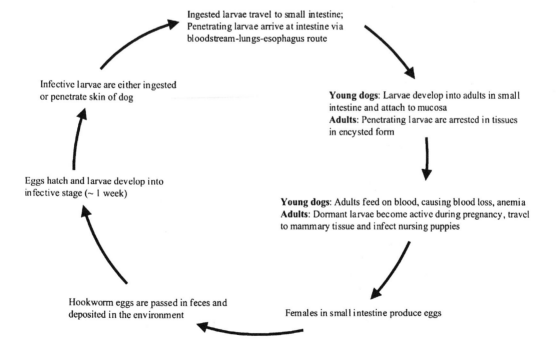

cal samples or vomit and microscopic identification of hookworm eggs in fecal samples (Figure 13.2).

Treatment: Acute cases of hookworm in young puppies should be treated as a medical emergency because puppies can rapidly die from severe blood loss. Supportive therapy in the form of fluid replacement, blood transfusions, and fast-acting anthelmintic medications are required. Because statistics show that many puppies are infected with hookworms shortly after birth, it is recommended that all puppies be dewormed for this parasite beginning when they are 2 weeks of age.[13] This allows deworming to take place before the worms have fully matured and started contaminating the environment with eggs. Due to the potential for continued infection from the bitch's milk and from infective eggs in the environment, deworming should be repeated at 2- to 3-week intervals until puppies are 10 to 12 weeks of age. Bitches should be dewormed prior to breeding and concurrently with their puppies. Conveniently, the same agents that are effective against ascarids and safe for young puppies are also effective against hookworms (Table 13.1). Environmental sanitation is important as a method for decreasing the number of infective larvae present and as an aid for controlling the number of encysted larvae that accumulate in the tissues of adult dogs.

Whipworms

Whipworm infection, called trichuriasis, is caused by nematode parasites of the genus *Trichuris*. *Trichuris vulpis* is the species that commonly infests dogs. Adult parasites are 2 to 3 inches in length, and the anterior three-quarters of the body is much thinner than the posterior quarter, giving the parasite an appearance similar to a whip (see Figure 13.2). Whipworms are blood-ingesting parasites and inhabit the cecum and colon (large intestine) of their host.

Life cycle and transmission: Adult whipworms attach firmly to the mucosa of the cecum and proximal colon where they feed on blood (Figure 13.5). The female's eggs are passed in the feces and larvate within 9 to 10 days when temperatures are between 77 and 80 degrees F. If conditions are cooler, the eggs may take as long as 35 days to larvate. Freshly deposited whipworm eggs are resistant to cold but are readily destroyed by very hot or dry conditions. Larvated parasites remain within the egg shell, are highly resistant to cold, heat, and drying, and can remain infective for very long time periods. When these larvae-containing egg packets are consumed by a dog, they hatch within 30 minutes of ingestion and are imbedded in the mucosa of the dog's small intestine within 24 hours. As they mature, the parasites migrate from the small intestine to the cecum and colon. Adult whipworms are fully mature and begin producing eggs 74 to 87 days after the dog ingests infective larvae and may live as long as 16 months.

Clinical signs and diagnosis: Clinical signs of trichuriasis vary with the numbers of parasites that are present, the individual dog's susceptibility, and the extent to which adult worms penetrate the intestinal mucosa. Adult dogs do not appear to develop immunity to this intestinal parasite as they age, so they are susceptible to repeat infections throughout life. Clinical signs include diarrhea, vomiting, and weight loss. Light infections may show no diarrhea but may be associated with gradual weight loss. Heavy infestations may be associated with chronic bloody diarrhea, dehydration, and anemia. Because infective whipworm larvae persist for very long periods in the environment, reinfection after treatment is very common. Diagnosis is typically through clinical signs, history of whipworm infection, and the identification of eggs in fecal samples. Because the number of adults to infect dogs is often quite low, adult worms are infrequently seen in fecal matter. In addition, female whipworms lay relatively low numbers of eggs compared to other intestinal parasites. Because low numbers of eggs are present, fecal samples of infected dogs do not consistently contain detectable eggs. As a result, many veterinarians recommend treating a dog for whipworms if clinical signs are seen and the area is known to be infected with larvae, even if whipworm eggs are not detected in the fecal sample.

Treatment: Whipworms are difficult to treat because reinfection from the environment is very common. Dry conditions and sunlight facilitate destruction of newly deposited eggs but the larvated form is resistant to most environmental conditions. Several anthelmintics are effective against whipworms, and follow-up treatments are recommended at 3 weeks and again 3

FIGURE 13.5   Life cycle of *Trichuris vulpis*

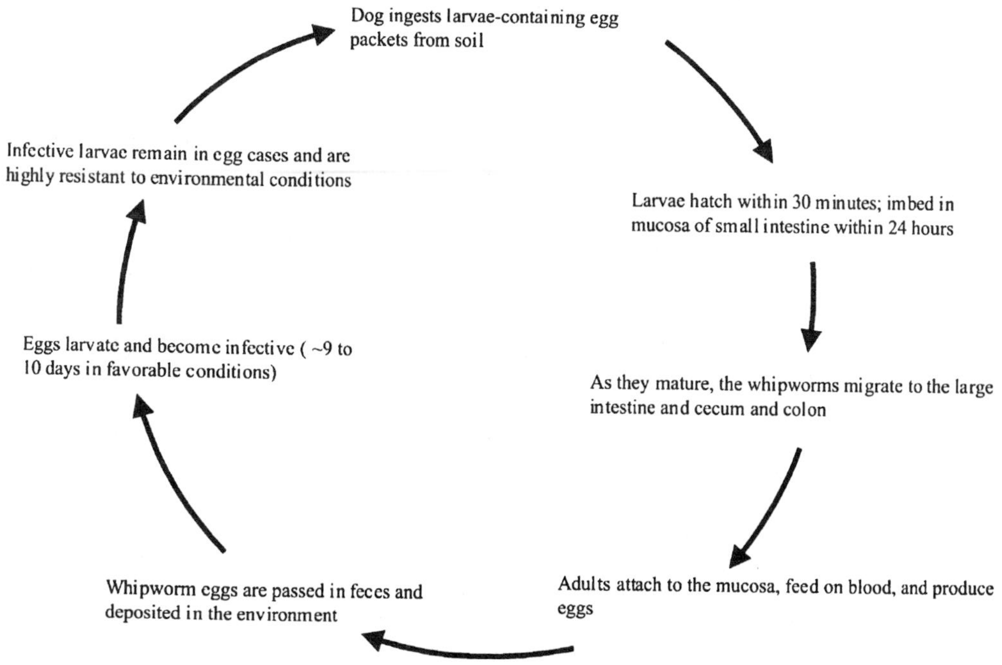

Dog ingests larvae-containing egg packets from soil

Infective larvae remain in egg cases and are highly resistant to environmental conditions

Larvae hatch within 30 minutes; imbed in mucosa of small intestine within 24 hours

Eggs larvate and become infective (~9 to 10 days in favorable conditions)

As they mature, the whipworms migrate to the large intestine and cecum and colon

Whipworm eggs are passed in feces and deposited in the environment

Adults attach to the mucosa, feed on blood, and produce eggs

months after the initial treatment is given (Table 13.1). If the dog lives in a heavily contaminated area, treatment every 2 to 3 months is sometimes necessary to control infections. The heartworm preventive, milbemycin oxime, is effective in controlling whipworm infections in dogs and is recommended in areas that are heavily contaminated with larvae. One of the most important goals for controlling recurrent whipworm infections is to prevent large numbers of infective larvae from accumulating in the dog's environment. Keeping premises dry and clean, picking up feces frequently, and limiting dogs' exposure to contaminated areas are all helpful in decreasing the transmission of whipworm.

Tapeworms (Cestodes)

Tapeworms, also known as cestodes, are highly adaptive internal parasites that can be found in all groups of vertebrate animals. At least 14 different species of tapeworm infect dogs in the United States, of which *Dipylidium caninum* and *Taenia* species are the most common. The tapeworm is a long, flattened, segmented parasite (see Figure 13.2). The body can be divided into three main regions. The **scolex** is the "head" of the organism and has hooks that attach to the mucosa of the small intestine. The neck of the tapeworm is located immediately behind the scolex and is the region from which individual tapeworm segments grow. The remainder of the body is called the **strobila** and is composed of a chain of segments called **proglottids**. Gravid proglottids refer to segments that are sexually mature and contain eggs. These segments break off and are passed in the feces. They are motile and may be seen in fecal matter or around the tail and anus of an infected dog. The entire tapeworm can vary in length from less than an inch to several feet, and a dog may have several dozen parasites in a single infection.

Life cycle and transmission: The life cycle of the tapeworm depends on the species of parasite. All tapeworms have one or more intermediate hosts. The intermediate host ingests gravid proglottids from the environment, and dogs are subsequently infected when they ingest the intermediate host. For example, the species *Dipylidium caninum* is carried by fleas and lice and will infect dogs that swallow one of these external parasites (see Chapter 14). This species of tapeworm is so prevalent that without good flea control, the control of infection with tapeworm in dogs is almost impossible. Rabbits, rats, and mice are common intermediate hosts for the *Taenia* species of tapeworm, and larvae can be found in many body tissues of these mammals. As a result, dogs that are allowed to hunt or consume carrion may become infected with *Taenia* species.

Clinical signs and diagnosis: Tapeworm infection rarely causes health problems in the dog, except in heavy infections. Over time, an infected dog may develop a dull, lusterless coat and show a decreased appetite or slight weight loss. However, most cases are asymptomatic. Diagnosis of tapeworm infection is made through the identification of gravid proglottids or eggs in feces and around the dog's tail and anal region.

Treatment: Several agents are available for treating tapeworm infection in dogs, but they may vary in their effectiveness against the *Dipylidium* species and *Taenia* species (Table 13.1). Two agents that are 100 percent effective against both *Dipylidium* and *Taenia* species are praziquantel and epsiprantel. Preventing flea infestations and the consumption of rabbits or mice is also effective in limiting a dog's exposure to tapeworm. As with all intestinal parasites, frequent fecal checks should be part of the dog's routine health care program.

Coccidiosis

Coccidiosis is a parasitic disease that is caused by a protozoan, which is a microscopic, single-celled organism. There are at least 12 species of the coccidia protozoa that can infect dogs, but the most common is *Isospora canis*. Coccidiosis is widespread throughout the domestic dog population in the United States and is particularly prevalent in the southern states. Clinical disease most often is seen in puppies and is highly contagious within litters. Infections can be serious in young puppies and can cause death from dehydration and malnourishment. Infected adult dogs often are asymptomatic or show only mild clinical signs. Adults can become carriers and will shed infective oocysts in their feces, serving as an important source of transmission to other dogs. Coccidiosis usually occurs in connection with poor sanitation or overcrowded conditions.

Life cycle and transmission: Infected dogs pass coccidia oocysts in their feces. Oocysts are the egg form of the *Isospora* organism and are easily identified through fecal flotation. In conditions of warmth and moisture, the oocysts sporulate to an infective stage within 3 to 5 days. A dog becomes infected by swallowing the infective oocysts through ingestion of contaminated soil, water, or feces. In the intestine, oocysts rupture and release sporozoites, which penetrate the epithelial cells, reproduce, and eventually destroy the cell. Alternatively, puppies can be infected with coccidia before they are born if the mother was infected with coccidia as a puppy and became a carrier. Dogs infected as puppies can harbor encysted forms in their tissues, and pregnant females can pass these to their unborn puppies.

Clinical signs and diagnosis: In puppies and young dogs, coccidiosis is characterized by severe diarrhea, which may be mucoid and bloody; dehydration; weight loss; and anemia. Some puppies also develop slight upper respiratory infections characterized by a cough, and nasal and eye discharges. Infected adults are usually asymptomatic but are capable of passing the disease onto other animals and spreading infective oocysts in the environment through fecal contamination. Diagnosis is usually through clinical signs and the identification of oocysts in fecal samples.

Treatment: Treatment of coccidiosis is aimed toward controlling diarrhea, preventing dehydration and anemia, and eliminating the infective organism. Nonprescription medications usually are used to control diarrhea. In severe cases fluid replacement may be necessary. Antimicrobial agents commonly used against bacterial infections often are prescribed. Sulfadimethoxine frequently is used and functions to inhibit the growth of coccidiosis (coccidiostatic). Treatment is continued for a minimum of 10 to 12 days to ensure that the protozoan is completely eliminated from the intestine. Coccidia can be controlled through proper sanitation and frequent fecal pickup and disposal. Cleansing of the environment with a strong ammonium hydroxide solution and the heat treatment of kennel surfaces are also recommended in kennels that have experienced coccidia outbreaks. Because the oocysts are highly resistant, it is very difficult to rid the environment of coccidia once it is present.

Giardia

Giardia is a common flagellar protozoan, using a hairlike tail (filiform) to motivate. It is found in many vertebrate hosts, and many species have been identified. The most common species to infect humans and domestic animals is *Giardia lamblia*. In the United States, many water sources are contaminated with giardia from feces of infected wild animals, domestic animals, or humans. The most common route of infection to dogs is through the ingestion of contaminated outdoor water sources. Following ingestion of the cysts, motile feeding forms of the parasite, called trophozoites, develop in the dog's intestine. This is the pathogenic stage of the organism, and infection of mucosal cells leads to clinical disease. Infection with giardia causes mild **enteritis** and chronic, intermittent diarrhea. Signs are generally more severe in puppies. Diagnosis is made through identification of infective forms of giardia that are passed in the feces. Giardia cysts often are difficult to detect, however, because cysts are shed sporadically and are very small. Antimicrobial agents are used to treat giardia (Table 13.1). A vaccination recently has been developed and is recommended in areas in which infections with giardia are common.

Conclusions

This chapter reviewed the most common internal parasites that infect dogs in the United States today. Infection with heartworm or severe infections with intestinal parasites can be life-threatening, especially to puppies or very old dogs. However, these parasites can be prevented and controlled through yearly blood checks for heartworm, administration of preventive heartworm medications, and biannual fecal checks for intestinal parasites. When parasitic infections do occur, early detection and prompt treatment can result in minimal adverse effects upon health and the complete recovery of the dog. In addition to internal parasites, there are a host of external parasites that can infest the domestic dog. The occurrence, life cycles, prevention, and treatment of these parasites are examined in the following chapter.

Cited References

1. Calvert, C.A. and Rawlings, C.A. **Treatment of heartworm disease in dogs.** Canine Practice, 18:13-28. (1993)

2. Courtney, C.H. and Zeng, Q.Y. **The structure of heartworm populations in dogs and cats in Florida.** In: *Proceedings of the Heartworm Symposium of the American Heartworm Society,* Washington, D.C., pp. 1-6. (1989)

3. Theis, J.H. **Occult rate of heartworm infected dogs in California appears to be significantly lower than that of infected dogs from Florida and Texas.** Canine Practice, 22:5-7. (1997)

4. Hoover, J.P., Campbell, G.A., and Fox, J.C. **Comparison of eight diagnostic blood tests for heartworm infection in dogs.** Canine Practice, 21:11-19. (1996)

5. McTier, T.L. **A guide to selecting adult heartworm antigen test kits.** Veterinary Medicine, 89:528-544. (1994)

6. Rawlings, C.A. **Post-adulticide changes in *Dirofilaria immitis*-infected Beagles.** American Journal of Veterinary Research, 44:8-15. (1983)

7. Rawlings, C.A. and McCall, J.W. **Melarsomine: A new heartworm adulticide.** Compendium on Continuing Education for the Practicing Veterinarian, 10:373-379. (1996)

8. Tanner, P.A., Meo, N.J., Sparer, D., Butler, S., Romano, M.N., and Keister, D.M. **Advances in the treatment of heartworm, fleas and ticks.** Canine Practice, 22:40-47. (1997)

9. Dillon, A.R., Brawner, W.R., and Hanrahan, L. **Influence of number of parasites and exercise on the severity of heartworm disease in dogs.** In: *Proceedings of the Heartworm Symposium of the American Heartworm Society,* Washington, D.C., pp. 1–13. (1995)

10. American Heartworm Society. **American Heartworm Society recommended procedures for the diagnosis, prevention, and management of heartworm (*Dirofilaria immitis*) infection in dogs.** Canine Practice, 22:8-15. (1997)

11. Pulliam, J.D. **Investigating Ivermectin toxicity in Collies.** Veterinary Medicine, 80:36-40. (1985)

12. Paul, A.J. **Evaluation of the safety of administering high doses of a chewable Ivermectin tablet to Collies.** Veterinary Medicine, 86:623-625. (1991)

13. Kern, M.S. **Deworming your dogs.** American Kennel Club Purebred Dog Gazette, July:77-80. (1992)

14 External Parasites

EXTERNAL PARASITES, or **ectoparasites,** are found on or within the skin of the host animal. While some infestations are very light and cause mild signs of discomfort, many external parasites can cause severe pruritus, skin lesions, and chronic skin disease. In addition, external parasites are carriers of a variety of infectious diseases and may transmit some of these to the host as they feed. The three most common types of external parasites that infect dogs are fleas, ticks, and mites. All of these parasites are classified as arthropods, but fleas are insects with six legs, and ticks and mites are arachnids (like spiders) and have eight legs.

Fleas

Fleas are the most common external parasite of the domestic dog. Almost 2,000 species and subspecies of flea have been identified, but the most common species seen on dogs in the United States is the cat flea, *Ctenocephalides felis.* Fleas are **endemic** in warm, humid environments but do not survive for long periods of time in extreme heat, cold, or low humidity. The adult cat flea is dark brown or black in color, has a laterally flattened body, and is between 2 and 5 mm in length (Figure 14.1). Like other insects, the flea has an exoskeleton and three pairs of jointed legs. Although the flea cannot fly, it is capable of jumping as high as 2 feet. Adult fleas feed exclusively on the blood of the host animal. They accomplish this by using syphonlike mouthparts that can cut a small laceration in the skin. Adults are found close to the dog's skin, most commonly on the abdomen, around the base of the tail, and the head. However, in very heavy infestations, fleas may be seen throughout the dog's coat and on many parts of the body.

Life cycle: Although the adult flea spends most of its time on the dog, the majority of the flea's life cycle takes place off of the host animal, in the environment. It is estimated that only 1 percent of the flea population is in the adult stage at a given time. The majority of fleas are either in the ova, larval, or pupal stages. The total length of the flea's life cycle can be as short as 16 days or as long as 21 months, depending on conditions. An ideal environment for flea development is an ambient temperature of 65 to 80 degrees Fahrenheit with humidity between 75 and 85 percent. The flea's life cycle includes four stages: adult, egg, larvae, and pupae (Figure 14.2). The adult flea is a permanent resident on its host and usually feeds once every 1 or 2 days. Newly emerged adult fleas, also called prefed adults, can live up to 1 year without food if conditions are favorable. However, after locating a host and having a blood meal, the adult becomes sexually mature, reproduces, and dies within a few weeks. A female flea lays to 20 to 50 eggs per day, and feeds more often and consumes more blood per meal than a male flea. This enables her to feed the large number of larvae that hatch from her eggs. Larvae feed on flea excrement that contains remnants of the ingested blood and organic matter found in the environment.

FIGURE 14.1   Common external parasites of the dog

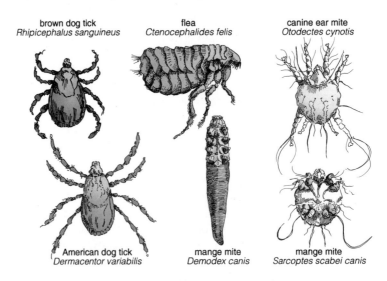

FIGURE 14.2   Life cycle of *Ctenocephalides felis* (cat flea)

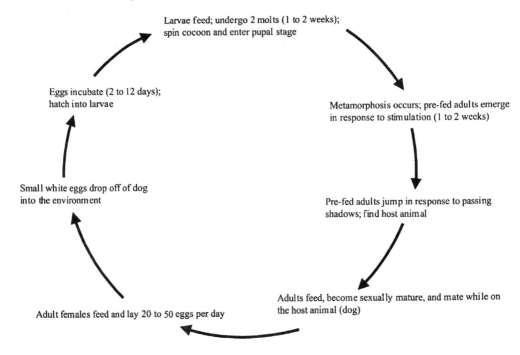

Flea eggs are small white ovals, 0.5 to 2 mm in length. They are not sticky, so they readily fall off the dog and onto carpet or grass. When temperatures are between 65 and 80 degrees and relative humidity is 70 percent or greater, the eggs will incubate for 2 to 12 days, then hatch into larvae. Flea larvae are small, slender, white parasites, with a wormlike appearance. Immediately after hatching, the larvae burrow down into rugs or the dog's bedding and begin to feed. The larvae go through two molts and grow to about 6 mm in length. In favorable conditions, the larval stage lasts about 1 to 2 weeks. When conditions are not favorable, this stage can become arrested and may last as long as 200 days. When the larvae reach the third stage of development, they spin a cocoon and enter the pupal stage. The flea cocoon appears as a small, sticky, white mass. Because of its small size and because dust, dirt, and organic matter readily stick to the cocoon, it usually is well hidden in rugs, the dog's bedding, or grass. Like other stages of the flea's life cycle, the time period the flea pupates is dependent on environmental conditions. In warm, humid environments, metamorphosis occurs rapidly, and adult fleas emerge from cocoons within 1 to 2 weeks. Less ideal conditions slow this process. Pupae are capable of remaining dormant in the cocoon for as long as a year and will rapidly develop and emerge when conditions become favorable. New adult fleas require stimulation for emergence from the cocoon. Important factors include vibration (such as a person or dog walking past), increased CO_2 pressure (produced from respiration), and warmth. Once emerged, prefed adults react to passing shadows by jumping, eventually landing upon a susceptible host.

Clinical signs: The primary clinical sign of a flea infestation is pruritus (itching). When the flea inserts its cutting mouthparts into the dog's skin to take a blood meal, it injects the site with several compounds that cause inflammation. These include a histamine-like chemical, proteolytic enzymes, and a small molecule (hapten) that attaches to **collagen** in the dog's skin. In susceptible dogs, it is this collagen-hapten complex that causes an allergic reaction to flea bites. Irritation from the flea bite and the allergic reaction that occurs in some dogs cause recurrent inflammation and pruritus. The dog's persistent scratching and biting can lead to secondary skin trauma and hair loss. Chronic flea infestations often are accompanied by pyoderma or hot spots. Because the female flea ingests large amounts of blood each day, heavy infestations also can result in significant amounts of blood loss. Over time, this causes parasitic anemia, which may be life-threatening when it occurs in young puppies. Fleas cause flea allergy dermatitis, one of the most common skin disorders seen in dogs (see below) and can transmit *Dipylidium* species of intestinal tapeworms to dogs when the dog swallows an infected flea (see Chapter 13).

Diagnosis: The presence of fleas on the dog is a definitive diagnosis for flea infestation. Other signs include the presence of flea dirt (feces) and flea eggs on the dog or in the environment. Flea dirt looks like small black flecks. If some of these are rubbed on a piece of wet white paper, the resultant smear is deep reddish brown in color. Flea eggs are small and white, and may be found on the dog's bedding or in areas where the dog spends a lot of time. When infestations are great, the owner may also notice the small flea larvae crawling on the dog's bedding or on carpet.

Flea allergy dermatitis: Flea allergy dermatitis (FAD) is the most common dermatologic disease diagnosed in dogs in the United States. It affects all breeds and ages of dogs and usually is diagnosed in dogs that are between 1 and 3 years of age. FAD is caused by a hypersensitive response to the collagen-hapten complex formed in the dog's skin after being bitten by a flea. This allergic reaction results in severe pruritus and skin inflammation. Over time, self-induced trauma exacerbates the condition and results in skin lesions, hair loss (alopecia), hyperpigmentation, and thickening of the skin.

Dogs with FAD show two types of allergic response. The immediate response to a bite occurs at the site of the bite within 15 to 20 minutes of being bitten. The dog will suddenly bite or scratch intensely at the site of the flea bite. This is followed by a delayed response that occurs within 24 hours after a bite. It is this delayed response that causes the dog the greatest amount of discomfort, because it involves inflammation and pruritus that is generalized throughout the skin over many areas of the body. Small papules (bumps) form and break open to develop into crusty scabs. This generalized response occurs in greatest intensity on the rear half of the dog, around the lower back, abdomen, and thighs. In chronic cases, the dog appears to have little or no relief from itching, and secondary skin infections are very common.

In temperate climates, FAD is seasonal. Signs occur in the summer and autumn months, corresponding to periods of time when flea populations are highest. In mild climates, signs of FAD may occur throughout the year. Dogs with FAD are diagnosed using clinical signs and the presence of fleas. Because allergic dogs do not need to be heavily infested with fleas to show extreme responses, diagnosis often is based on clinical signs and the elimination of other causes of inflammatory skin disease. Intradermal testing with purified flea allergens can be helpful in a diagnosis, but results are not always reliable.

Treatment of FAD involves the elimination of all fleas on the dog and in the dog's environment, and the prevention of re-infestation. Strict flea control is necessary because even one flea bite can cause a generalized inflammatory response in a dog with FAD. The availability of several new systemic and topical products for flea control has greatly improved the success of FAD treatment. When fleas cannot be effectively controlled, or when there is poor owner compliance, systemic glucocorticosteroids and antihistamines may be prescribed to decrease inflammation and pruritus. However, these products have undesirable side effects, are not recommended for long-term use, and function only to relieve the symptoms without affecting flea populations. In the majority of cases, flea control on the dog and in the environment is the most efficacious method of treatment.

Desensitization to flea allergens is effective as a treatment of FAD in some cases. This involves administering flea allergens on a regular basis in an attempt to achieve a state of nonreactivity. Injections that contain small doses of the allergic flea components are given intradermally and subcutaneously. Repeated and frequent exposure to these allergens results in an eventual state of nonreactivity. Most dogs require exposure to the flea allergens on a biweekly or monthly basis for the remainder of their lives. The disadvantages of this treatment are that it is time-consuming, expensive, and not always successful. For these reasons, it is not routinely recommended for the treatment of FAD.[1]

Treatment and control: Because 3 of the 4 stages of the flea's life cycle take place in the environment and not on the dog, the standard recommendation for treating flea infestations in the past has been to treat the dog and the environment simultaneously. This typically involved bathing the dog with a shampoo or dip that killed adult fleas and treating the home and yard with sprays or aerosol bombs that killed adults and contained an insect growth regulator (IGR) to inhibit the development of eggs, larvae, and pupae. However, the availability of new topical and systemic flea control products that inhibit the flea's life cycle and have extended residual effects has led to simpler and more effective approaches to flea control. The fundamental goal of a flea control program is to eliminate adult fleas from the pet and prevent subsequent generations of fleas from developing. With these products, this often can be accomplished through treatment of the dog alone. In dogs that have FAD, control of the environment with an effective IGR in combination with an adulticide may still be necessary.

Topical treatment for flea control refers to the application of an adulticide or IGR onto the dog's skin and coat. The chemical is applied as either a liquid or spray and is slowly absorbed into the **sebaceous glands** in the dog's skin. The chemical is then gradually re-released onto the skin and coat from these glands. It is this effect that provides the residual activity of these products and allows intermittent application. If the dog is bathed, goes swimming, or becomes wet, the chemical is still effective because it is constantly reapplied onto the skin from the sebaceous glands. Two chemicals currently sold as topical agents are imidacloprid (trade name Advantage™) and fipronil (trade name Frontline™). Imidacloprid is a chemical of the family of insecticides called the heterocyclic nitromethylenes. It kills adult fleas by causing impairment of the insect's nervous system. Imidacloprid is also effective as a larvicide in the environment of treated dogs.[2] Dead adult fleas and skin debris from treated dogs fall off the dog and onto bedding, carpets, and kennel flooring. The chemical that adheres to this debris effectively inhibits larvae in the environment from developing into the pupal stage.

The second chemical, fipronil, is also an adulticide. It is a member of the pyrazoles, a new class of insecticides that kill external parasites by blocking the movement of chloride ions within the central nervous system. Fipronil is effective against fleas, ticks, and spiders. Because this chemical kills insects immediately upon contact, most fleas are dead before they have had a chance to feed, and newly emerged fleas are killed before they lay eggs. This effectively breaks the flea's reproductive cycle and controls fleas on the dog and the stages in the environment. Studies of the effect of fipronil treatment on flea control on dogs and in the household environment have shown that monthly applications of fipronil to the dog's coat eliminated existing flea infestations and prevented the recurrence of infestations without the need for any other type of premise treatment.[3]

The technique used for topical application involves placing one or more drops of the liquid directly onto the skin along the top of the dog's back. In large dogs, up to four spots may be applied. Both Advantage and Frontline are available in premeasured tubes designed for monthly application to dogs based on body weight.[4] Frontline is also available in dosages that can be applied at 2- or 3-month intervals. Dogs that are bathed frequently or who swim several times per week may require more frequent applications of the chemical, usually every 3 weeks. Benefits of both imidacloprid and fipronil topical treatments are that they are extremely safe for use around animals and humans, are convenient for owners to use, and provide effective and rapid control of fleas on the dog and in the environment. Because of the large safety margins of these chemicals for use with mammals, they can be used on puppies as young as 8 weeks of age. One additional type of topical product that is available contains the adulticide permethrin (trade names Pro-Spot™ and Ex-Spot™). This flea treatment effectively kills adult fleas and has a 30-day residual effect but is not effective against other stages of the flea's life cycle.

Systemic products are adulticides or IGRs that are administered orally. The presence of the chemical in the dog's blood kills the adult flea or inhibits its ability to reproduce when the flea takes a blood meal. The product Pro-Ban™ contains the compound fenthion, which is a pyrethroid adulticide. A product introduced during the 1990s contains the IGR lufenuron (trade name Program™). Lufenuron impairs the development of viable eggs and larvae produced by adult fleas that have taken a blood meal from dogs treated with this chemical. It accomplishes this by inhibiting the flea's ability to synthesize chitin, a protective component found in the egg shells. Because systemic products are effective only after the flea has bitten the dog, they are generally not a good choice for dogs with FAD or in cases in which there is heavy infestation of fleas. A study comparing the efficacy of imidacloprid and lufenuron for environmental flea control found that topical treatment with imidacloprid reduced the number of fleas on dogs to zero on the first day of treatment.[5] In contrast, dogs treated orally with lufenuron did not begin to show a decrease in the number of fleas until 3 weeks after the start of treatment. Numbers of adult fleas on lufenuron-treated dogs then declined until the end of the study at 11 weeks but never reached zero. These results indicate that while systemic treatment with lufenuron is effective in controlling flea infestations over time, the concurrent use of conventional insecticides may be necessary when the dog lives in an environment that has an existing flea population. Like the topical treatments, the systemic products are administered every 30 days.

There are a variety of insecticides that are effective against adult fleas (adulticides) and are sold for use to control fleas in homes and in yards. These can be classified into three major chemical groups: the pyrethrins and pyrethroids, the organophosphates, and the carbamates. Pyrethrins are natural insecticides found in the flower of the chrysanthemum plant. Pyrethroids are synthetic forms of these compounds. In addition to killing adult fleas, these compounds also have some repellent effect. Organophosphates include chlorpyrifos, diclorvos, diazinon, and cuthioate. Examples of commonly used carbamates are carabyl, propoxur, and bendiocarb. Both of these types of chemicals are cholinesterase inhibitors, which means they interfere with the metabolism of neurotransmitters in the insect's nervous system. These adulticides are used less frequently since the introduction of lufenuron, fipronil, and imidacloprid.

Mange Mites

Mites spend the majority of their life cycle living on or under the surface of the dog's skin and are capable of causing mild to severe skin or ear disorders in infected dogs. The three mange mites of greatest concern to pet care professionals and dog owners are *Sarcoptes scabei canis*, *Demodex canis*, and *Otodectes cynotis*.

Sarcoptes scabei canis: This mite is responsible for causing canine scabies, also called sarcoptic mange. The mite is very host specific and can only complete its life cycle within the skin of a dog. It is highly contagious between dogs and can cause short-term infections in humans, cats, or other animals that have contact with an infected dog. *Sarcoptes scabei canis* is a very small, oval, light-colored mite (Figure 14.1). It is too small to be observed with the naked eye but can be identified microscopically in skin scrapings. Transmission occurs through direct contact with an infected dog, and signs first develop about 1 week following exposure. The primary sign of scabies is intense pruritus, which is caused by the mites burrowing into deep layers of the dog's skin.

The mite also produces toxins and allergens that cause an inflammatory response and exacerbate skin irritation. Infected dogs are restless and uncomfortable and will continually scratch, bite, and dig at affected areas of skin. Small reddened papules develop, and these form crusty scabs and eventually result in hair loss. The most commonly affected areas are the ears, face, legs, and elbows. However, in severe cases, the dog's entire body may be infected. Diagnosis of scabies is made through clinical signs and microscopic identification of the mite from skin scrapings or biopsies. However, because the female mite often burrows very deeply into the skin to lay her eggs, these mites are not always detectable in skin scraping samples. For this reason, veterinarians often will treat for scabies if clinical signs and history alone support the diagnosis.

Treatment for scabies involves isolating the dog from all other animals to prevent transmission. If exposure has already occurred, other animals should be treated simultaneously regardless of the presence of clinical signs. The hair is clipped away from affected areas of the body, and an insecticide dip or ointment is applied directly to the skin. Miticidal medications are applied every 5 to 6 days for a minimum of six total treatments. If the skin is very inflamed, short-term therapy with glucocorticosteroids may be helpful during the initial stages of treatment, and antibiotic ointments are applied to control secondary skin infections.

Demodex canis: This mite causes demodicosis in dogs, which is a noncontagious form of mange. Demodex mites are normal inhabitants of the hair follicles of many species of animals, including dogs, and can complete their entire life cycle within the hair follicle. The demodex mite is microscopic and has an elongated, cigar-shaped body that is well adapted for living within a hair follicle (Figure 14.1). In most healthy dogs, the mites maintain a small but consistent population and do not cause any clinical signs of disease. Clinical disease is seen only when the mite begins to proliferate to large numbers, usually when alterations in the normal protective mechanisms of the skin occur. It is theorized that dogs who are susceptible to demodicosis may have a type of compromised immune function that affects local immunity in the skin. However, the exact nature of this problem has not been identified. Physical trauma or exposure to stress also can precipitate proliferation of the mite. Because families of dogs often are affected, it appears there is a genetic component to susceptibility. Therefore, dogs who have recovered from clinical infections with *Demodex canis* should not be used for breeding.

Two forms of demodicosis have been identified: localized and generalized. Localized demodicosis is relatively common and is usually very mild and self-limiting. It is most often seen in young dogs between 3 and 12 months of age. The first signs are a thinning of the hair around the eyes, corners of the mouth, or on the front legs. Typically, affected areas have a "moth-eaten" appearance and will progress to patches of hair loss that are 1 to 2 inches in diameter. Reddening of the skin (erythema) and scaling are occasionally seen. However, because demodicosis does not cause pruritus and because skin lesions are often very mild, these patches may go unnoticed by the dog's owner. A substantial proportion of dogs infected with the localized form of demodicosis recovers spontaneously within 1 to 2 months. When localized demodicosis is diagnosed, treatment involves the application of an insecticidal dip to affected areas.

The generalized form of demodicosis is much more serious and typically is a localized case that progressively spreads to cover much of the dog's body. The damage the mite causes to hair follicles and skin leads to chronic inflammation, hair loss, and the development of secondary pyoderma. Diagnosis is made through clinical signs, history, and identification of the mites in skin scrapings. Because some dogs appear to be highly susceptible to *Demodex canis*, the generalized form of demodicosis can be very resistant to treatment and is considered to be incurable in some animals. Generalized demodicosis requires aggressive medical treatment in the form of applying an insecticidal dip to the entire body. This is repeated one or two times per week until skin scrapings are negative for the presence of *Demodex canis*.

Otodectes cynotis: This is a mite that infects the external and internal ear canal of the dog. It is more common in cats than dogs, and cats are a primary source of infection to dogs. The mite has a 3-week life cycle that takes place completely within and around the ear canal of the host animal. Signs of ear mites include intense pruritus around and inside the ears, causing the dog to scratch, dig, and rub. Repetitive head shaking is common and can lead to ear flap hematomas. The inside of the ear usually is filled with a dark brown or black waxy secretion, the outer canal is inflamed, and a strong odor may be noticed. In heavy infestations, the entire ear canal becomes obstructed with debris, leading to secondary infections with yeasts or bacteria. Ear mites are barely visible to the naked eye but can be seen if a cotton swab is used to clean the ear and the wax is placed on a white piece of paper under bright light. Treatment includes first thoroughly cleaning the dog's ears with a medicated cleaning solution and removing as much of the debris as possible with cotton swabs. In severe cases, the dog may require sedation for ear cleaning if the ears are heavily infected and clogged with exudate. After cleaning, the ears are treated for a minimum of 3 weeks with a miticide medication and an antibiotic preparation. In addition, the dog's bedding and other areas should be thoroughly cleaned. Other animals in the household, especially cats, should be examined for mites and treated at the same time.

Ticks

Ticks are blood-ingesting parasites that, like mites and spiders, are classified as arachnids. Heavy infestations with ticks can cause severe blood loss and anemia, toxic conditions such as tick paralysis, and tick bite allergies. Ticks are also responsible for transmitting a variety of infectious agents. Examples of diseases that can be transmitted to dogs by ticks include ehrlichiosis, Rocky Mountain spotted fever, and Lyme borreliosis.

Ticks that commonly feed on dogs include the brown dog tick, *Rhipicephalus sanguineus,* and the American dog tick, *Dermacentor variabilis.* The brown dog tick is found throughout the United States, and the American dog tick is found primarily on the east coast of North America. Both of these ticks are three-host ticks, requiring three feedings on a host animal to complete their life cycle. However, unlike other ticks, the brown dog tick is capable of feeding exclusively on the dog during all stages of its life cycle, so it can be difficult to exterminate when it infests kennels or homes.

Dogs usually become infested with ticks when they brush against grass or underbrush where the tick resides. Ticks are active during the late spring and summer months in temperate climates. After crawling onto the dog, they preferentially attach around the head, ears, or neck area. The female tick is easier to identify because she feeds for a longer period of time and her body enlarges as it fills with blood. Male ticks are smaller than females and usually can be found attached near a female. They have a flattened body shape and do not expand greatly in size as they feed.

The tick's life cycle has four stages: egg, larvae (seed tick), nymph, and adult

(Figure 14.3). The complete life cycle can take up to 2 years to complete, depending on the species of tick and the availability of host animals. The female brown dog tick mates while she is attached to a dog and feeds for about 7 days. She then drops off of the host animal and will lay up to 5,000 eggs before dying. The eggs take approximately 3 weeks to hatch, if conditions are favorable. The larvae return to the dog where they feed for 3 to 8 days before dropping off to molt into the nymph stage. Nymphs return once again to a host dog and feed for up to 11 days. After feeding, they drop into the dog's environment, develop for about 2 weeks, and molt into the adult stage.

The brown dog tick is the principle reservoir and transmitter of *Ehrlichia canis*, the rickettsia that causes canine ehrlichiosis.[6] Ticks become infected with this organism when they feed on an infected animal and can carry *Ehrlichia* organisms for several months. They infect another dog when they attach to a new host and obtain a blood meal. Although *Ehrlichia* originated in tropical areas, it has spread worldwide. In the United States, it is primarily a problem in the South, but cases have been diagnosed wherever there are active tick populations. Early signs of canine ehrlichiosis are nonspecific and include depression, decreased appetite, fever, enlarged lymph nodes, and lameness.[7] Although some dogs recover from this phase, most will progress eventually to a chronic and potentially fatal stage. Long-term infection leads to weight loss, weakness, anorexia, and anemia due to micro-hemorrhages caused by decreased platelet numbers. Over time, the organism may infect many organs, causing kidney failure, arthritis, reproductive impairment, and infec-

FIGURE 14.3   Life cycle of *Rhipicephalus sanguineus* (brown dog tick)

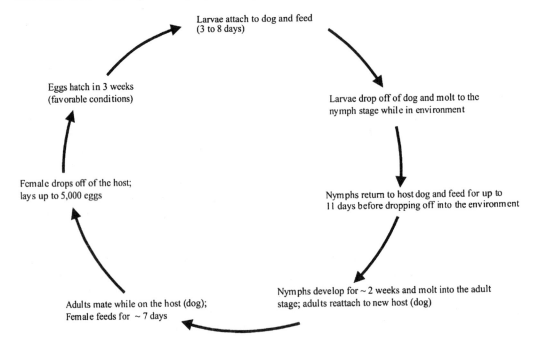

Larvae attach to dog and feed
(3 to 8 days)

Eggs hatch in 3 weeks
(favorable conditions)

Larvae drop off of dog and molt to the
nymph stage while in environment

Female drops off of the host;
lays up to 5,000 eggs

Nymphs return to host dog and feed for up to
11 days before dropping off into the environment

Adults mate while on the host (dog);
Female feeds for ~ 7 days

Nymphs develop for ~ 2 weeks and molt into the adult
stage; adults reattach to new host (dog)

tion of the central nervous system. If not treated, the chronic phase of ehrlichiosis is often fatal. Antibiotics, usually tetracycline, are used to treat canine ehrlichiosis. If diagnosed in the early stages, treatment is usually successful. However, chronic cases usually require long-term therapy, and not all dogs make a complete recovery. The dog may always suffer from long-term health problems.

The American dog tick, *Dermacentor variabilis*, is found primarily in wooded areas. Females feed on a variety of host animals. After feeding for up to 2 weeks, the female drops off the host and lays up to 6,000 eggs. The resultant larvae are extremely resistant to environmental conditions and often go through the winter without feeding. In the spring, they locate a host and feed for up to 2 weeks before dropping off to molt to the nymph stage. This stage can be prolonged for almost a year if a host animal is not found or if environmental conditions are not favorable. As nymphs, the American dog tick feeds again on a host animal, drops off, and molts to the adult stage. The dog is just one of many possible host animals (including humans) for this tick, and the nymph and adult stages are capable of transmitting disease when they feed. The American dog tick is the vector of Rocky Mountain spotted fever, a serious disease that can infect dogs and humans. This tick also causes tick paralysis, a motor paralysis caused by a neurotoxin injected by the female tick when she feeds. Some dogs are extremely susceptible to this toxin, but in most cases tick paralysis is associated with heavy tick infestation. Signs of tick paralysis include weakness and lack of coordination, leading to partial then complete paralysis. If not treated, death can occur within 2 days. The removal of all ticks during their early stages of feeding is essential for preventing and treating tick paralysis.

Another tick-borne disease that can infect humans, dogs, and a variety of other mammals is Lyme disease, or Lyme borreliosis.[8] This disorder is caused by infection with the spirochete *Borrelia burgdorferi*, which is carried primarily by ticks of the genus *Ixodes*. However there is evidence that other types of ticks are also capable of carrying and transmitting this organism. Lyme borreliosis is currently considered to be the most common tick-transmitted disease in the United States and is seen primarily in the Northeastern and mid-Atlantic regions and several Midwestern states. However, there is evidence that the disease is spreading throughout the Midwest and to several Southwestern states.[9] The small deer tick, *Ixodes scapularis* is the primary carrier of Lyme disease. Small rodents, such as the white-footed mouse, are primary hosts for the larval stage of this tick. These rodents are the primary host reservoir for *Borrelia burgdorferi* and transmit the microorganism to the feeding tick. Adult ticks generally attach to larger hosts such as deer, sheep, and dogs. The white-tailed deer are considered to be an important cause of the spread of Lyme disease, as they carry infected ticks in their migration patterns. Dogs become infested with the tick when they are running in fields or parks where the tick resides.

In dogs, infection with Lyme disease leads to chronic and often crippling arthritis. Infection in other tissues can lead to heart disease and kidney disease.[10] Initial clinical signs include depression, anorexia, swelling of lymph nodes, and fever. This progresses to lameness, joint pain, and swelling in the affected joints. Over time, lameness can become severe and lead to long-term arthritic changes to joints if the disease is not diagnosed and treated promptly. Lyme disease is diagnosed in dogs using clinical signs, history of exposure to ticks, and a blood test for increased antibody titers to *Borrelia burgdorferi*. Several antibiotics can be used to treat Lyme disease in dogs, including tetracycline and amoxicillin. Antibiotic therapy is continued for several weeks even if a response is observed in the dog after just a few days. As in the case of canine ehrlichiosis, early diagnosis and treatment are essential for full recovery. A vaccine for canine borreliosis is available and is recommended for dogs who live in high-risk areas.

Tick infestations should always be treated with care because of their potential to transmit a variety of serious diseases to humans and to dogs. An attached tick should be sprayed with an insecticide intended for use on dogs. Once it has been killed, the tick can be gently removed by pulling it off using a forceps or tweezers. A variety of products are available that will kill or repel ticks and are recommended for dogs that live in areas with high tick populations. Many of these are the same products used to prevent or treat flea infestations. Topical products that have long-term residual effects have been shown to effectively protect dogs from ticks. Fipronil, the active component in Frontline, will kill ticks for 1 month or more after a single application to a dog's coat.[11] Ticks are killed within 48 hours of contact, which is too short a time period for the transmission of most tick-borne illnesses. Another recent study has shown that ticks failed to transmit Lyme disease to fipronil-treated dogs.[12]

Conclusions

The previous chapters have provided information about infectious and noninfectious diseases and internal and external parasites that can infect the domestic dog. Routine health care procedures and responsible pet ownership and care will prevent the occurrence or limit the detrimental effects of many of these disorders. However, there are times that even the most diligent owner and well-trained dog can experience unexpected mishaps or accidents. The final chapter of this section addresses common toxins that can be found in the dog's normal environment, along with a collection of emergency care procedures that are important to have available if accidents do occur.

Cited References

1. MacDonald, J.M. **Flea control in animals with flea allergy dermatitis.** Compendium on Continuing Education for the Practicing Veterinarian, Supplement, 19:38-40. (1997)

2. Hopkins, T.J., Woodley, I., and Gyr, P. **Imidacloprid topical formulation:**

Larvicidal effect against *Ctenocephalides felis* **in the surroundings of treated dogs.** Compendium on Continuing Education for the Practicing Veterinarian, Supplement, 19:4-10. (1997)

3. Keister, D.M., Meo, N.J., and Tanner, P.A. **A comparison of flea control efficacy of Frontline™ Spray Treatment against the flea infestation prevention pack (Vet-Kem) in the dog and cat.** Proceedings of the American Association of Veterinary Parasitologists, July 20-23, Louisville, Kentucky. (1996)

4. Becker, M. **New weapons in the battle against fleas.** Compendium on Continuing Education for the Practicing Veterinarian, Supplement, 19:41-47. (1997)

5. Paul, A. and Jones, C. **Comparative evaluation of imidacloprid and lufenuron for flea control on dogs in a controlled simulated home environment.** Compendium on Continuing Education for the Practicing Veterinarian, Supplement, 19:35-37. (1997)

6. Wilford, C. **Ehrlichia: a poorly understood organism, uses ticks to spread its dangerous infection nationwide.** AKC Purebred Dog Gazette, June:48-52. (1994)

7. Font, A., Closa, J.M., and Mascort, J. **Tick-transmitted diseases: a comparative study of Lyme disease, canine ehrlichiosis and rickettsiosis in the dog.** Veterinary International, 3:3-14. (1992)

8. Appel, M.J.G. **Lyme disease in dogs and cats.** Compendium on Continuing Education for the Practicing Veterinarian, 5:617-624. (1990)

9. Levy, S.A. and Dreesen, D.W. **Lyme borreliosis in dogs.** Canine Practice, 17:5-17. (1992)

10. Magnarelli, L.A., Anderson, J.F., and Schreider, A.B. **Clinical and serologic studies of canine Borreliosis.** Journal of the American Veterinary Medical Association, 191:1089-1094. (1987)

11. Tanner, P.A., Meo, N.J., Sparer, D., Butler, S.J., Romano, M.N., and Keister, D.M. **Advances in the treatment of heartworm, fleas and ticks.** Canine Practice, 22:40-47. (1997)

12. Maupin, G. **Comparative susceptibility of nymphal** *Ixodes scapularis,* **the principal vector of Lyme disease, to Fipronil and Permethrin.** Fourth International Symposium on Ectoparasites of Pets, April 6-8, Riverside, California. (1977)

15   **First Aid Procedures**

FIRST AID INVOLVES providing immediate medical care during emergency situations with the intent of prolonging life and preventing further injury until veterinary care can be provided. Although administering first aid to a dog in need does not require a thorough knowledge of veterinary medicine, it does require a calm, reasonable demeanor and an understanding of procedures that can sustain life, prevent further injury, and minimize continued pain or trauma. A variety of situations may require first aid for dogs. Some of the most common include physical trauma that may result in bleeding, shock, cardiac arrest, respiratory arrest, and broken bones. Other emergency situations include burns, poisoning, heatstroke, and allergic reactions. Emergency first aid procedures that can be used by owners and by companion animal professionals are reviewed in this chapter.

Preparing a First Aid Kit

Although many people keep some type of first aid kit for humans, most people often don't consider starting a kit for dogs. However, in an emergency situation, owners usually need to act fast. Keeping a set of first aid supplies in a designated place may mean the difference between life and death for the dog. Like a human first aid kit, most of the supplies that are kept in a first aid box for dogs are items normally found in households. These should be kept in a safe, dry place in a covered container. Table 15.1 includes a list of first aid supplies that should be included in the kit.

Immediate Procedures

The first thing to do in all emergencies is attempt to stay calm and use common sense. First aid procedures are designed to stabilize the dog and prolong life until veterinarian care can be obtained. The owner should first obtain as much knowledge as possible about how the animal was injured. This may include the circumstances of the injury, how long the dog has been injured or ill, and, if poisoning is suspected, the quantity and substance that was consumed. A veterinarian should be contacted by telephone, and the dog should be prepared for transport to the veterinary clinic. Because some injured or ill dogs become aggressive when touched or moved, a muzzle should be applied if necessary.

The dog should be assessed for level of responsiveness. If the dog is not breathing or if there is not a heart beat, artificial respiration and cardiopulmonary resuscitation must be started immediately. If the dog is responsive, its respiration rate, pulse rate, and temperature should be taken. Methods for

TABLE 15.1   First Aid Kit Supplies

Item	Purpose
Rectal Thermometer	Measure body temperature
Scissors	Cut bandaging materials; fit material for makeshift muzzle
Syrup of Ipecac	Induce vomiting
Hydrogen Peroxide	Induce vomiting; clean wounds
Activated Charcoal	Prevent absorption of toxins
Large Syringe (without needle)	Administer oral medications and treatments
Bandages (several sizes, types, and shapes)	Stop or slow external bleeding; dress wounds; secure splints; tie a makeshift muzzle
Adhesive Tape	Secure bandages and splints
Ice Pack/Heat Pack	Treat hyperthermia; hypothermia; contusions and sprains
Stethoscope (optional)	Monitor heart rate and breathing rate
Forceps (Tweezers)	Remove insect stingers, foreign bodies
Topical Antibiotic Ointment	Treat external wounds
Antihistamines	Counteract allergic reactions
Petroleum Jelly	Lubricate thermometer
Antidiarrheal Medicine	Treat diarrhea
Laxative	Relieve constipation
Muzzle	Use for restraint only when necessary
Tourniquet Material	Use only as a last resort to stem excessive bleeding in a limb

obtaining a dog's vital signs are described in Chapter 3. Normal vital statistics for healthy dogs are shown in Table 15.2. In general, decreased respiration rate occurs with poisoning, hypothermia, and the late stages of shock. Increased respiration rate is seen during heatstroke, trauma, and the early stages of shock. A dog's pulse rate decreases to fewer than 60 beats/minute during the late stages of shock and when dogs experience hypothermia. A pulse rate that is higher than normal may indicate fever, heart failure, electric shock, snake bite, certain types of poisoning, or trauma. Elevated body temperature is caused by heatstroke or infection. A decreased body temperature is indica-

TABLE 15.2   Vital Statistics for Healthy Dogs

Skin and Coat	Normal shine, growth, and shedding pattern for breed or breed type; skin that is pliable, clean, and free from lesions
Mucous Membranes	Light pink in color (unpigmented areas); normal CRT (~ 1 second)
Food Intake and Body Weight	Normal and consistent appetite; maintenance of ideal (lean) body weight
Body Temperature	100.0 to 102.5 degrees F (average 101.5)
Pulse (Resting)	60 to 140 beats/minute
Respiration Rate	10 to 30 inhalations/minute

tive of exposure to cold weather (hypothermia). Capillary refill time can be used as a general check for functioning of a dog's circulatory system and the presence of bleeding (internal or external). If mucous membranes are pale or gray and if capillary refill time is greater than 2 seconds, this indicates shock, blood loss, or anemia. If the mucous membranes in the mouth have a bluish tinge, this can mean shock, heart failure, lung failure, or certain types of poisoning. Bright red conjunctiva may mean that the dog has been poisoned by carbon monoxide or has severe heart or lung failure.

Some emergency situations may require restraint to prevent the dog from biting or struggling. A general rule of thumb with injured or ill dogs is to use the least amount of restraint necessary for the situation. Many dogs respond positively to a calm, quiet manner and to a gentle, reassuring voice. If the dog's owner is present, he or she may be able to keep the dog calm more successfully than someone the dog does not know well. If the dog has suffered trauma and might have broken bones or internal injuries, gentle transport is imperative to prevent further injury or pain. A firm, solid surface, such as a thick plywood board, works well. If this is not available, a large towel or blanket can be used. The dog should be gently eased onto the surface and fully supported as it is moved to a car for transport to a veterinary hospital. If a muzzle is necessary, this should be applied prior to attempting to move the dog. If a dog muzzle is not available, an emergency muzzle can be made from 2 to 3 long pieces of cloth. Instructions for tying a makeshift muzzle are described in Table 15.3.

Cardiac and Respiratory Arrest

Several types of emergencies can lead to cardiac arrest, respiratory arrest, or both. These include trauma, electrocution, and some types of poisoning. Dogs in cardiac arrest will be unconscious and their gums and mucous membranes will be very pale or gray as a result of the lack of blood flow. This is an

TABLE 15.3   Tying a Makeshift Muzzle

Materials Needed	2-3 feet of strong material (gauze bandage, necktie, scarf, fabric, pantyhose)
Step 1	Tie a slipknot in the middle to make a large loop
Step 2	Pass this loop over the dog's nose, with the knot on the topside of the dog's muzzle; pull it snug
Step 3	Pull the ends of cloth under the jaw and make a second knot; pull it snug
Step 4	Tie the ends of material securely behind the dog's ears
Step 5	Contact a veterinarian, administer emergency first aid, and transport dog

extreme emergency and requires immediate action. If a pulse cannot be found, cardiopulmonary resuscitation (CPR) should be started immediately. CPR functions to manually pump the dog's heart and supply blood and oxygen to the brain, heart, and other vital organs until the heart begins to pump again independently.

To begin CPR, the dog is placed on its side. With small dogs that are less than 25 pounds, the chest can be compressed by placing the flat of each hand around the widest part of the chest, just behind the dog's elbows. The rib cage is compressed at a rate of 120 to 150 times per minute by pressing simultaneously from both sides. For medium and large dogs, the chest is compressed by placing the flat of both hands directly over the heart. This is the area on the left side of the chest, approximately where the elbow meets the rib cage. The chest is compressed by pressing downward, at a rate of about 80 to 100 compressions per minute. For all dogs, the compressions should be applied in a cough-like manner to facilitate rapid increase and decrease in chest pressure. Heart compressions should be stopped briefly every 30 to 45 seconds to check to see if a heartbeat has returned. When dogs are in cardiac arrest, artificial respiration must also be provided and coordinated with CPR. If two people are present, one should provide respiration while the other compresses the chest. When only one person is available, artificial respiration and chest compressions should be alternated by doing 10 to 15 chest compressions followed by a deep breath every 15 seconds. Another rule of thumb is to give one breath after six chest compressions for a small dog or two breaths after every 15 compressions for medium and large dogs.

If the dog has a pulse but is not breathing, artificial respiration alone must be administered. In all cases, the first step for providing artificial respiration is to assure that the dog's airway is not blocked. The dog is placed on its side with neck extended, and the mouth is opened and examined for any debris, foreign bodies, food, or vomit. These should be cleared away. Once an airway is established, the dog's muzzle is held closed and the person who is administering artificial respiration places his or her mouth over the dog's nose. A slow deep breath is administered. Enough air should be blown into the dog's air passages to expand the chest. For small dogs, 20 to 25 breaths per minute should be provided. Medium and large dogs should be given 15 to 20 respirations per minute.

Shock

Shock occurs when blood circulation is not sufficient to meet the dog's needs. This can be caused by rapid blood loss (internal or external hemorrhage), severe dehydration, overheating, or trauma. The signs of shock are all caused by a collapse of the circulatory system and insufficient blood flow and oxygen delivery to body tissues. A dog that is experiencing shock is very weak and has rapid, shallow respirations, pale mucous membranes, cool extremities, and a rapid, weak heartbeat. During the early stages of shock, capillary refill time will be slightly increased to between 2 and 3 seconds. As shock progresses, the body temperature falls below normal, the dog's pupils become dilated, and capillary refill time becomes greater than 4 seconds. Severe shock results in a loss of consciousness and is rapidly fatal if not treated. Immediate emergency care includes keeping the dog warm and quiet, and positioning the dog on its side with the head slightly lower than the rest of the body. This helps increase blood flow to the brain. Dogs in shock should not be given any medications, food, or water and should be transported immediately to a veterinarian. Veterinary treatment involves the administration of intravenous fluids and treatment for the underlying cause of circulation collapse.

Bleeding

Bleeding may be internal or external. One of the most common causes is severe trauma, such as being hit by a car. If the dog has experienced physical trauma but no blood is seen, a veterinarian should still be consulted to examine the dog for internal bleeding. The development of shock after trauma often is indicative of internal hemorrhage.

Emergency care for external bleeding may require elevation, direct pressure over the wound, or pressure over pressure points. In many cases, bleeding can be stopped or controlled by applying firm, steady pressure directly to the wound. Because the body uses the clotting action of platelets and other factors in the blood to stop bleeding, a wound should never be wiped or blotted because this may remove a clot that was beginning to form at the site. To apply direct pressure, a thick cloth or gauze dressing should be prepared. If the pad of cloth becomes soaked with blood, it should not be removed from the wound. Rather, a new pad of cloth can be placed on top of the old one and pressure reapplied. The flat of the hand should be used to press down on the pad with a firm, steady pressure.

Elevation is helpful when the dog has an open wound on a limb. The injured leg should be elevated slightly by placing a pillow or rolled up blanket between the dog's legs. Direct pressure can then be applied to the wound, and, if it is possible, the wound can be wrapped and bandaged. (Note: If there is a chance that the leg has a broken bone, it should not be elevated.) If bleeding does not subside after 1 to 2 minutes of direct pressure, pressure points can be used to help decrease bleeding. These are areas of the body at which major arteries flow close to the surface. By applying pressure at these sites, the flow of blood to a wounded area can be slowed. There are five major arterial pressure points on the dog's body that may be of aid when treating external bleeding. These are identified in Table 15.4.

A tourniquet can be used in the rare instances when a laceration involving a limb is severe enough that the bleeding cannot be stopped or slowed through pressure to the limb or to pressure points on the body. Tourniquets are very dangerous to use because of the risk of completely stopping blood flow to the limb. A tourniquet should only be applied as a last resort and with extreme care. A strip of cloth or gauze is wrapped around the leg immediately above the area of severe bleeding and is tightened by hand until bleeding is controlled. Once applied, the tourniquet should be released every 10 to 15 minutes to allow blood flow into the limb. As soon as bleeding is under control, the tourniquet should be replaced with a pressure bandage.

Choking

In dogs, choking typically is caused either by a dog attempting to eat food too quickly, attempting to swallow a large piece of food or bone, or inadvertently swallowing a toy or ball while playing. Because many puppies and adolescent dogs have a tendency to pick up any new object, they are often at higher risk for choking. A dog with something lodged in its throat will initially cough forcefully, retch, or paw frantically at its mouth. If breathing is completely obstructed, the dog will rapidly become unconscious if the object is not removed. Once unconscious, the dog may stop breathing altogether. Choking is a medical emergency, and the dog should be transported to a veterinarian

TABLE 15.4   Arterial Pressure Points

Pressure Point	Location
Front Leg (Brachial Artery)	Inside the foreleg, immediately above the elbow joint
Back Leg (Femoral Artery)	Inside the thigh at the point at which the dog's leg meets the body
Front Foot	Inside of lower leg, just above the paw
Back Foot	Front of the back leg, just above the paw
Tail (Coccygeal Artery)	Underside of the tail

as quickly as possible. First aid procedures can be conducted in the car while the dog is being transported.

If the dog is still conscious, the owner should first attempt to remove the object by opening the mouth and reaching into the throat. If the object cannot be dislodged or is not visible, the dog should be laid on its side with the hindquarters slightly elevated. A modified Heimlich maneuver is used to dislodge the object. The flat of the hand is placed just beneath the rib cage and should be pressed in and upward to compress the lungs, forcing air out of the trachea. This should force the dog to cough and will dislodge the object in many cases. If the dog becomes unconscious before the object is dislodged, a series of two Heimlich compressions should be followed by two artificial respirations. The dog's mouth should be checked after each compression for the foreign body. This cycle of two compressions and breaths should be continued until the object is dislodged or the dog resumes breathing voluntarily.

Heatstroke

When dogs are unable to rid their bodies of excess heat through normal homeostatic mechanisms, body temperature rises and rapidly can become a medical emergency. Heatstroke in dogs can be rapidly fatal, especially if the body's temperature rises above 105 to 106 degrees Fahrenheit. The degree to which a dog's temperature increases depends on environmental temperature, duration of exposure, and the dog's age and physical condition. High humidity contributes to heatstroke because dogs are unable to evaporate as much moisture from respiration under humid conditions. In general, young puppies and very old dogs have less heat tolerance and are more susceptible to heatstroke. Brachycephalic breeds also are more susceptible because they are more subject to respiratory distress when attempting to increase their rate of panting in warm conditions. Common causes of heatstroke include leaving a dog in a car on a warm day, excessive exercise, and confining the dog to an outdoor area that is exposed to direct sunlight and has no access to shade.

The first sign of heatstroke is excessive panting or rapid, frantic breathing. This may include salivation or vomiting. The dog will have an increased pulse rate and bright red gums. If untreated, heatstroke leads quickly to severe shock and loss of consciousness. The dog's body temperature is increased and may be as high as 104 to 108 degrees Fahrenheit. If the body temperature is greater than 105, immediate action is crucial. The dog should be moved to a cool, ventilated area and immersed in cold water. If this is not possible, a garden hose can be used to spray the dog with cold water. Body temperature should be closely monitored and cooling procedures should be stopped when the dog's body temperature has dropped to 103 degrees. Because the cooling can be very rapid, there is actually a danger of causing hypothermia. The dog should be treated for shock if necessary and transported to a veterinarian. Many of the serious and even fatal effects of heatstroke occur after the initial incident, so veterinary care should always be sought. In many cases, the dog requires intravenous fluids to combat dehydration and stabilize the circulatory system, and anti-inflammatory agents to reduce brain edema.

Burns

Burns can be very serious, leading to shock, sepsis, and death. Even minor burns can be very painful to the dog and should receive veterinary treatment as soon as possible. A superficial burn affects the outer layer of skin (first-degree burn). Although these burns are quite painful, they require only routine care and usually heal quickly. Second-degree burns are those that go completely through the outer layer of skin and affect the middle skin layer. The site of the burn is red and swollen, and oozes serum. These burns will heal well if infection is prevented. Third-degree burns are the most serious and involve damage to the full thickness of the dog's skin. These burns always require veterinary treatment. Infections and scarring are common, and skin grafting is necessary in some cases.

First aid for burns is simply to apply ice-cold water or a cold compress as soon as possible after the burn has occurred. If the burn has just occurred, the cold compress can be applied for 20 to 45 minutes, usually enough time to get the dog to a veterinarian. In general, applying cold is helpful for the first 2 hours after a burn occurs. Ice should not be applied directly, as this can freeze the area around the burn and cause additional tissue damage. Unlike other types of wounds, bandages should not be applied to burns. Likewise, ointments and other medications should not be used because these may be difficult to remove from damaged tissue. A dog who has been burned should be transported to a veterinarian as soon as possible for treatment.

Insect Stings and Spider Bites

Because a dog's hair coat actively protects the dog from being easily bitten or stung by insects, and because some dogs enjoy snapping at flying bugs, insect stings and bites most often are seen on the face or foot pads. Stinging insects can pose a serious threat if a dog is stung repeatedly or is allergic to the insect's venom (quite rare in dogs). The most common type of insects to sting dogs are bees, hornets, and wasps. Spider bites also are relatively common. Stings result in pain, swelling, and pruritus around the affected area. Shock may occur if the dog has been stung multiple times. If the dog is in shock, this should be treated immediately and the dog transported to the veterinarian. In less serious cases, a cold ice pack can be applied to the site, and the embedded stinger can be removed using forceps. A paste of baking soda and water or instant meat tenderizer and water can be applied to the area of the sting to help neutralize the venom.

In the United States, there are only two species of spiders considered to be highly dangerous to dogs. These are the female black widow and the brown recluse spider. The black widow is about 3/4 inch in diameter, with a black body and a red hourglass shape on its underside. The brown recluse is a small spider (about 1/2 inch), light brown in color, with a dark brown fiddle-shaped mark on its back. Most spider bites occur between April and October in temperate climates. The black widow spider's bite appears as a small red spot that is sometimes but not always associated with swelling. The site will become increasingly painful and the dog will begin to show neurological signs as the venom begins to take affect. The dog becomes weak and uncoordinated, drools, has difficulty breathing, and develops muscle spasms that lead to convulsions. The dog should be kept as still as possible. If a leg has been bitten, it should be positioned below the level of the heart to decrease the rate of transport of the venom throughout the dog's body. Although black widow spider bites are not usually fatal, they can be very serious, especially in small dogs. Brown recluse spiders are found primarily in the Midwestern and Southern states and cause a painful, fluid-filled blister at the site of the bite. Within a day, the skin around the site turns black and ulcerated. This ulcerating sore will continue to spread and cause tissue death unless treated. Veterinary treatment usually involves the surgical removal of the ulcerated area and surrounding tissue. If this is not done, the wound may take weeks or months to heal. In all cases, dogs that have been bitten by either species of spider should receive veterinary attention as soon as possible.

Snake Bites

Of all of the animals that can cause serious poisonings to dogs, snakes are responsible for the largest number of cases. It is estimated that more than 15,000 pets are bitten by poisonous snakes each year.[1] Both poisonous and nonpoisonous snakes are found throughout the United States. Bites from nonpoisonous varieties are not medical emergencies and usually appear as a small scratch or puncture. However, poisonous snake bites can be very serious and even fatal. The severity of a bite depends on the type of snake; the location of the bite; the volume of venom that was injected; and the size, age, and health of the dog. The poisonous snakes that pose the greatest threat to dogs are the pit vipers (copperheads, water moccasins, and rattlesnakes) and the coral snakes.

Most dogs are bitten on either the face or the legs as a result of suddenly startling a snake. Immediate signs are swelling, pain, and redness at the site of the bite. Two puncture marks located close together may be visible and can be used to identify a snake bite. If the dog was bitten on the face, respiration may quickly become labored and difficult. Other signs include vomiting, diarrhea, increased pulse rate, and shock. The dog should be transported immediately to a veterinarian so antivenin can be administered. If possible, a complete description of the snake should be provided to the veterinarian. This will aid in the choice of appropriate antivenin. Immediate first aid procedures include keeping the dog quiet and, if necessary, providing artificial respiration. If a leg is bitten, the dog should be positioned so the leg is below the level of the dog's heart.

There are many folk remedies for snake bites, none of which are effective or recommended. For example, an incision should not be made above or around the bite site in an attempt to remove venom. This may work in the movies but is completely contraindicated in real life and can be dangerous. Similarly, the bite area should not be packed in ice, as this will only further damage the surrounding tissue and will not prevent spread of the venom. A tourniquet should not be applied to a bitten leg because this can cause irrevocable damage to blood vessels and tissues, and may result in the loss of the limb. Because venom travels via lymph, not blood, slight pressure above the leg (by using the flat of the hand or a loosely constricting piece of cloth) may be effective in slowing its movement.

Poisoning

There are many potential poisons to dogs in the household and outdoor environment.[2] One of the cardinal rules of responsible pet ownership is to keep all potential poisonous substances in a safe and nonaccessible place. However, accidents do happen. Young dogs typically explore everything that they find with their mouths, and dogs of all ages are capable of eating a plant or household product that is toxic.

The most common substances to cause poisoning in pet dogs are antifreeze (ethylene glycol), rodenticides, human medications such as acetaminophen and ibuprofen, and poisonous plants.[3,4] A more complete list is found in Tables 15.5 and 15.6. Treatment for poisoning depends on the agent that has

TABLE 15.5   Common Household Poisons

Product	Signs of Toxicity	Emergency First Aid (In all cases, veterinary care should be sought as soon as possible)
Warfarin or Coumarin (mouse/rat poison)	Micro-hemorrhages in mucous membranes, hematomas under skin, blood in urine or feces	Induce vomiting; veterinary care involves administration of vitamin K to promote blood clotting
Strychnine (mouse/rat/ mole poison)	Decreased coordination, excitability, agitation, painful tetanic seizures (triggered by outside stimuli)	Induce vomiting; avoid loud noises or other stimuli that may induce a seizure
Metaldehyde (rat/snail/slug bait)	Decreased coordination, drooling, excitability, muscle tremors, weakness, collapse	Induce vomiting
Antifreeze (ethylene glycol)	Vomiting, abdominal pain, staggering convulsions; rapidly fatal	Induce vomiting; administer activated charcoal to prevent further absorption
Corrosives (household cleaners, drain de-cloggers, solvents)	Burns to the mouth, esophagus, and stomach; discomfort, pain, presence of ulcerations and burns	Do NOT induce vomiting If acid, give antacid (milk of magnesia); if alkali, give dilute vinegar (1:4 with water)
Lead (old paint, batteries, drapery weights)	Abdominal pain, vomiting, diarrhea, staggering, convulsions, blindness	Induce vomiting if ingestion occurred recently
Carbon monoxide gas	Depression, elevated temperature, muscle twitching, red mucous membranes	Provide artificial respiration if necessary; CPR if necessary
Petroleum products (gasoline, kerosene, turpentine)	Vomiting, difficulty breathing, tremors, convulsions	Do NOT induce vomiting; administer mineral oil or vegetable oil to delay absorption; provide artificial respiration

TABLE 15.6   Common Poisonous Plants for Dogs

Irritating Indoor Plants (rash, inflammation of mouth)	Toxic Indoor Plants (vomiting, abdominal pain, systemic toxicity)	Toxic Outdoor Plants (varying effects)
Arrowhead Vine	Amaryllis	Daffodil
Boston Ivy	Asparagus Fern	Castor Bean
Caladium	Azalea	China Berry
Chrysanthemum	Bird of Paradise	Coriaria
Dumb Cane	Creeping Charlie	Indian Turnip
Emerald Duke	Elephant Ears	Larkspur
Marble Queen	Pot Mum	Lupine
Nephthytis Ivy	Spider Mum	Nightshade
Philodendron	Umbrella Plant	Poison Hemlock
Poinsettia		Poke Weed
Red Princess		Rhubarb
		Water Hemlock
		Wisteria
		Yew (American, English, Western)

been ingested. If the dog has consumed an insecticide, rodenticide, or medication, the package should be brought to the veterinarian. Likewise, if a potentially poisonous plant has been eaten, it should be brought along.

First aid procedures for poisoning are aimed at maintaining life signs until veterinary care can be obtained. There are two major steps in the immediate first aid for poisoning. The first is to remove the source of the toxin. The second is decontamination. With some exceptions, the dog should be made to vomit. This is especially important if the dog is discovered immediately after it has ingested the poison. However, if a corrosive or caustic agent has been consumed, inducing vomiting is not advocated. Examples of caustic agents are alkalies, lye, bleach, furniture polish, floor cleaners, fertilizers, tar, and pine oil cleaners. The easiest way to induce vomiting is to give 1 or 2 teaspoons of hydrogen peroxide orally. If the dog does not vomit within 5 to 10 minutes, the dose should be repeated. The total dose should not exceed 1 teaspoon per 5 pounds of body weight. Ipecac syrup given at a dose of 1 milliliter per pound of body weight is also effective but can take up to 20 minutes to induce vomiting. If veterinary care is close at hand, the dog should be transported to the veterinarian before inducing vomiting. An injectable emesis-inducing medication can be given by the veterinarian. If the dog has ingested a corrosive agent, milk of magnesia or activated charcoal should be administered to dilute the toxin and coat the dog's stomach. Knowledge about the substance and quantity consumed is of utmost importance.

Conclusions

Most emergency situations require veterinary care. Therefore, the most important first aid procedures an owner uses are aimed at prolonging life and preventing further injury while the dog is being transported to a veterinary clinic. Knowledge of a dog's normal vital signs, methods of administering CPR and artificial respiration, and knowing how to recognize and treat signs of shock may mean the difference between life and death for an injured or severely ill dog.

Part 3 provided information about general health care, infectious and non-infectious diseases, internal and external parasites, and first aid for dogs. Part 4, "Feeding for Health and Longevity," will provide pet professionals with the diet and feeding information needed to provide optimal nutrition throughout a dog's life. Nutritional knowledge can be helpful when selecting appropriate foods for different stages of a dog's life, for determining proper feeding procedures, and for treating or managing certain diseases.

Cited References

1. Dworkin, N. **Hornets, spiders and snakes.** American Kennel Club Purebred Dog Gazette, April:46-52. (1996)

2. Owens, J.G. and Dorman, D.C. **Common household hazards for small animals.** Veterinary Medicine, February:140-148. (1997)

3. Knight, M.W. and Dorman, D.C. **Selected poisonous plant concerns in small animals.** Veterinary Medicine, March:260-272. (1997)

4. Talcott, P.A. and Dorman, D.C. **Pesticide exposures in companion animals.** Veterinary Medicine, February: 167-181. (1997)

Part 4 Nutrition: Feeding for Health and Longevity

16 Nutrient Requirements of the Dog

PROPER CARE FOR DOGS includes consistent attention to health, the administration of appropriate preventive vaccinations, and the provision of optimal nutrition throughout life. An understanding of the basic nutrients and their functions is necessary when choosing an appropriate dog food and determining the best method for feeding. Progress in the field of dog nutrition has generated an improved understanding of canine dietetics and the development of well-balanced pet foods that contribute to long-term health and aid in the prevention of chronic disease. This chapter provides an overview of the dog's requirements for the essential nutrients. Subsequent chapters in this section address pet food evaluation and selection, nutrition through the dog's life cycle, and feeding management for nutritionally responsive disorders.

Essential and Nonessential Nutrients

The term **nutrients** refers to components in the diet that have specific functions within the body and that contribute to growth, tissue maintenance, and health. **Essential nutrients** are those that cannot be produced by the body at a rate that is adequate to meet the body's needs and so must be supplied in the diet. **Nonessential nutrients** are those which can be synthesized by the body and so may be obtained either through production within the body or from the diet. For example, the dog has a physiological requirement for 22 different amino acids, which are the building blocks for protein. All of these amino acids are needed by the body for the synthesis of protein. However, only 10 of the 22 amino acids are essential amino acids that must be supplied in the diet. The 12 nonessential amino acids can be synthesized by the dog, provided adequate levels of precursor substances are present. Along with a requirement for energy, all dogs have a requirement for six major categories of nutrients: water, carbohydrates, proteins, fats, minerals, and vitamins.

Energy

Like all animals, dogs require a constant source of dietary energy in order to survive. Energy is necessary for the performance of all of the body's metabolic work, which includes maintaining and synthesizing body tissues, engaging in physical work, and regulating normal body temperature. Plants obtain energy from the sun's radiation and convert it to energy-containing nutrients. Other animals consume plants and either use them directly for energy or convert plant nutrients into other energy-containing molecules. The primary form of stored energy in plants is carbohydrate; the main form of stored energy in animals is fat. Given its importance, it is not surprising that energy is always the first requirement that is met by an animal's diet. Regardless of a dog's needs for other essential nutrients, the energy-yielding nutrients of the diet will first be used to satisfy energy needs. Once energy needs are met, nutrients are available for other metabolic functions.

Metabolizable energy (ME): In the science of animal nutrition, energy is expressed in units of **kilocalories**. A kilocalorie is the amount of heat energy necessary to raise the temperature of 1 kilogram of water from 14.5° Centigrade to 15.5° Centigrade. The caloric value of pet foods and the dog's caloric requirement is expressed as kilocalories of **metabolizable energy** (ME). Like all animals, the dog is unable to absorb all of the energy that is included in a food. The food's total chemical energy is the amount of energy that is released when the food undergoes complete oxidative combustion in a bomb calorimeter. This is called **gross energy** (GE) and is a measure of the food's total potential energy. **Digestible energy** (DE) refers to the energy that an animal is capable of digesting and absorbing from the food. DE values are measured using digestibility trials. Fecal energy represents the unabsorbed energy of the diet. This is subtracted from the food's GE to provide a measurement of DE. A food's ME is the energy that is ultimately available to the animal. It is measured by subtracting both fecal energy losses (due to indigestible matter in the diet) and urine energy losses (due to metabolism of excess amino acids and other nitrogenous compounds) from GE. Because species differ in their ability to digest and utilize different types of food, DE and ME values are functions of both the food that is being tested and the species of animal that is being fed.

Energy requirements: A dog's daily energy requirement represents the sum of the energy that is needed to support resting metabolic rate, meal-induced thermogenesis, voluntary muscular activity, and the maintenance of normal body temperature. Resting metabolic rate (RMR) is the energy per day that is needed by the cells and tissues of the body to maintain **homeostasis** during periods of rest.[1] These processes include respiration, circulation, kidney and liver function, and the production of necessary hormones, enzymes, and other essential molecules. Factors that influence RMR include the dog's age, body size, reproductive status, and body condition. For example, a young intact dog who has a relatively high proportion of lean tissue compared to fat tissue will have a higher RMR than an elderly neutered dog of the same weight who has a lower proportion of lean to fat tissue. The second component of a dog's energy requirement is voluntary activity. In moderately active dogs, activity is responsible for approximately 30 percent of the body's total energy expenditure. However, the frequency, intensity, and duration of exercise that a dog engages in will significantly affect the amount of energy expended. Meal-induced thermogenesis, also called the "thermic effect of food," represents the energy cost of digesting, absorbing, and utilizing nutrients. When a meal containing a mixture of carbohydrate, protein, and fat is consumed, meal-induced thermogenesis uses approximately 10 percent of the ingested calories. Adult dogs who are in a state of maintenance and moderately active only require enough energy to support activity and maintain the body's normal metabolic processes and tissue stores. On the other hand, dogs that are growing, reproducing, or working have increased energy requirements because of increased energy needs for tissue growth or work.

Formulating an exact equation to estimate energy requirements for dogs is a difficult task because of the wide variation in body size and weight. Adult dogs of different breeds vary in weight from several pounds to more than 150 pounds. Because the amount of energy that is used by the body is related to an animal's total body surface area, rather than actual weight, the relationship between body weight and energy requirement cannot be described using a simple linear equation. For example, when expressed on a per weight basis (kcal/kg body weight), a small dog's energy requirement is significantly higher than a large dog's requirement. A solution to this problem is to express body weight in terms of its total surface area. This is called **metabolic body weight**, and can be calculated by raising the dog's weight in kilograms to a specified power. Metabolic body weight accounts for differences in body surface area between animals of varying sizes. The most commonly used value for dogs is 0.67.[2] The equation: **ME requirement = K × Wkg$^{0.67}$** provides an accurate estimate of daily energy requirements for different sizes of adult dogs. The value for *K* is assigned according to the dog's estimated level of activity. An example of the application of this equation to determine energy requirements for dogs of different sizes and activity levels is shown in Table 16.1.

The daily caloric requirements that are predicted by the energy equation are specific for adult dogs during various levels of activity. Stages of life that result in increased energy requirements include growth, gestation, lactation, periods of recovery from illness or trauma, and exposure to extreme environmental conditions. To obtain an energy requirement estimate for these con-

TABLE 16.1   Calculations of the Daily Energy Requirement of Adult Dogs

20-lb Dog (9 kg) Boston Terrier	60-lb Dog (27 kg) Labrador Retriever
ME Requirement = 132 × (9 kg)$^{0.67}$ = 575.3 kcal/day	ME Requirement = 132 × (27 kg)$^{0.67}$ = 1,201.1 kcal/day
ME Requirement = 145 × (9 kg)$^{0.67}$ = 632 kcal/day	ME Requirement = 145 × (27 kg)$^{0.67}$ = 1,319.4 kcal/day
ME Requirement = 200 × (9 kg)$^{0.67}$ = 871.7 kcal/day	ME Requirement = 200 × (27 kg)$^{0.67}$ = 1,819.9 kcal/day
ME Requirement = 300 × (9 kg)$^{0.67}$ = 1,307.6 kcal/day	ME Requirement = 300 × (27 kg)$^{0.67}$ = 2,729.8 kcal/day

K = 132   Inactive
K = 145   Active
K = 200   Very Active
K = 300   Endurance Performance

ditions, the dog's maintenance requirement is calculated and then multiplied by the appropriate factor to account for increased needs. For example, if the female Labrador Retriever in the example in Table 16.1 was determined to be active (K = 145), her estimated daily energy requirement would be about 1,319 kcal of ME per day. If she was bred and became pregnant, her energy requirement at the end of gestation would be expected to increase to approximately 1,978 kcal per day. This estimate is obtained by multiplying 1,319 by 1.5 (Table 16.2). Ultimately, the calculated daily energy requirement of a dog provides a starting point to estimate the daily energy requirement of a particular animal. This estimate can then be adjusted according to the dog's long-term response to feeding.

Energy intake: Like all animals, dogs are capable of regulating their energy intake to accurately meet their daily caloric requirements. When allowed free access to a balanced, moderately palatable diet, most dogs will consume enough food to meet, but not exceed, their daily energy needs.[2,3] Contrary to popular belief, animals are unable to self-regulate their intake of other essential nutrients. Dogs that are deficient in a particular vitamin, mineral, or essential amino acid will not seek foods that contain the nutrient or preferentially select a diet that is abundant in the deficient nutrient. In contrast, dogs readily increase or decrease the intake of food in response to an energy imbalance.

While all dogs are capable of self-regulating energy intake, the internal control mechanisms that govern food intake may be overridden by external factors such as diet palatability or caloric density, inadequate exercise, illness, or even boredom. The development of pet foods that are highly palatable and are calorically dense may cause some dogs to readily over-consume calories if allowed to eat on an **ad libitum** basis. In addition, some dogs lead very sedentary lives and as a result have very low energy needs. These factors can lead to the over consumption of food and weight gain. As a result, although all dogs are capable of self-regulating their energy intake, in most cases, portion controlled feeding is preferable as a method of monitoring and controlling caloric intake (see Chapter 18).

Energy imbalance occurs when dogs' daily energy intake is either greater or

TABLE 16.2   Daily Energy Requirements for Different Stages of Life

Stage	Change in Energy Requirement
Early Growth (8 weeks to ~ 4 months)	2 × Adult Maintenance (calculated for adult dog the same weight)
Adolescence (~ 4 months to ~ 7 months)	1.6 × Adult Maintenance (calculated for adult dog the same weight)
Late Growth (~ 7 months to adult size)	1.2 × Adult Maintenance (calculated for adult dog the same weight)
Mid to Late Gestation (after 5 weeks)	1.25 to 1.5 × Adult Maintenance
Peak Lactation (~ 4 weeks)	3 to 3.5 × Adult Maintenance (affected by litter size)
Recovery from Illness or Trauma	1.25 to 2.0 × Adult Maintenance
Exposure to Cold Weather	1.2 to 1.8 × Adult Maintenance

less than their daily requirements, leading to changes in growth rate, body weight, and body composition. Today, excess energy intake is much more common in American pets than is energy deficiency. During growth, over-consumption of energy has been shown to have several detrimental effects on dogs, especially those of the large and giant breeds. When an excess amount of a balanced, high-energy pet food is fed to growing puppies, maximal growth rate and weight gain can be achieved. However, studies with growing dogs have indicated that maximal growth rate is not compatible with healthy bone growth and development.[4,5] In fact, current research supports the theory that feeding growing puppies to attain maximal growth rate appears to be a significant contributing factor in the development of skeletal disorders such as osteochondrosis and hip dysplasia[6] (see Chapter 19). In adult dogs, the long-term intake of excess calories leads to conditions of overweight and obesity. As in humans, obesity is associated with numerous health risks. These can involve the respiratory, circulatory, skeletal, and locomotor systems. In addition, the diminished ability to exercise, play, or lead an active life can negatively affect a dog's quality of life (see Chapter 19).

Energy density and caloric distribution: The three nutrients that provide energy in an animal's diet are carbohydrate, fat, and protein. Other nutrients, though necessary for health, do not supply energy. In commercial diets that are fed to dogs, average ME values for protein and carbohydrate are 3.5 kcal ME per gram.[7] Fat is much more energy dense than protein or carbohydrate and supplies approximately 8.5 kcal/gram. The **energy density** of a pet food refers to the number of calories provided by the food in a given weight or volume. Energy density is most commonly expressed as kilocalories of ME per kilogram (kg) or pound (lb) of food. For example, a typical dry dog food formulated for adult maintenance has approximately 3,500 kcal ME/kg, or 1,590 kcal/lb.

There is an inverse relationship between a dog food's energy density and the volume of food that must be consumed to meet the dog's daily energy requirement. As a food's energy density increases, the total volume of food that is consumed decreases. An example is a very active, 70-pound dog with a daily energy requirement of 2,000 kcal. If this dog is fed a performance diet that has an energy density of 420 Kcal per cup, he will require 4 3/4 cups of food per day. If, on the other hand, he is fed a dog food that was formulated for adult maintenance and contains 340 kcal/cup of food, he will need 6 cups of food per day. Energy density is one of the most important concepts in pet nutrition because it is the principle factor that determines the amount of food that a dog requires each day and also because it directly affects the amount of all other essential nutrients that the dog ingests. A pet food must be formulated to provide optimal quantities of all essential nutrients when an amount of food that meets the dog's daily energy requirement is consumed.

Caloric distribution refers to the proportions of total metabolizable energy in a dog food that are contributed by protein, carbohydrate and fat. When considered with energy density, caloric distribution of a food provides important information for the selection of a dog food. In addition, dog foods that are formulated for different stages of life and for different activity levels can be compared. For example, a dog food that is formulated for weight reduction in adult dogs has a lower proportion of its calories supplied as fat, compared with a diet formulated for adult maintenance. Conversely, a dog food that is formulated for hard-working dogs has an increased proportion of dietary fat, necessary to supply the energy needed for work (Figure 16.1). Energy density and caloric distribution should always be considered together when selecting a dog food for a particular age, activity level and stage of life.

Water

Water is the most important essential nutrient for all animals. Animals can survive for extended periods of time without other nutrients, but will die within a few days when deprived of water. Approximately 70 percent of lean adult body weight is water, and many tissues in the body are composed of between 70 percent and 90 percent water. Within the body, water functions as a solvent that allows the occurrence of all cellular reactions and provides a

FIGURE 16.1   Caloric distributions of dog foods for different life stages

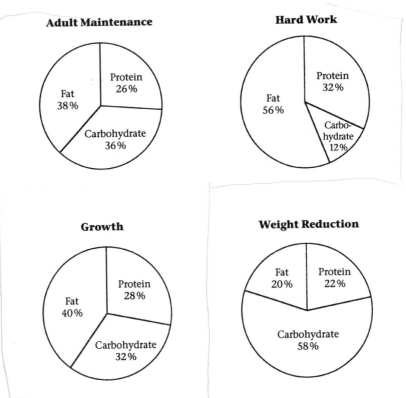

transport medium for nutrients and waste products. Water also absorbs the heat that is generated by the body's metabolic processes, allowing for the maintenance of normal body temperature. An aqueous environment is essential for the digestion and absorption of nutrients because it allows mixing of stomach and intestinal contents with digestive enzymes and is essential for the process of **hydrolysis**. Elimination of waste products from the kidneys also requires a large amount of water, which acts as both a carrier medium for waste and as a solvent for toxic metabolites.

Dogs require a constant source of water to replace losses that occur through urine, feces, and respiration. In dogs, the water losses due to respiration are important in the regulation of normal body temperature during hot weather. Panting is a specialized form of breathing that involves very rapid and shallow inhalations and exhalations, resulting in substantial increases in respiratory water and heat losses. Because of the use of panting to maintain body temperature and because dogs lack other efficient means of ridding their bodies of excess heat, water losses from respiration and evaporation during hot weather can be very high.

An animal's total daily water intake comes from three possible sources: water present in food, drinking water, and metabolic water that is produced from the assimilation of food. The quantity of water present in the food depends on the type of diet. Commercial dry dog foods contain 7 percent to 12 percent water, while canned rations contain up to 78 percent water.[8] Not surprisingly, when dogs are fed only a canned ration, their voluntary water intake is often very low.[9] In contrast, dogs fed dry diets require frequent access to fresh drinking water. Metabolic water is the water that is produced during oxidation of the energy-containing nutrients in the body. The metabolism of fat produces the greatest amount of metabolic water on a weight basis, and protein catabolism produces the least amount. In general, metabolic water is fairly insignificant because it accounts for only 5 percent to 10 percent of the total daily water intake of most animals. The last source of water intake is voluntary drinking. Factors affecting a pet's voluntary water consumption include the environmental temperature, the type of diet that is fed, and the dog's activity level, age, physiological state, and health. Water intake increases with both increasing environmental temperature and increasing exercise because more evaporative water is lost as a result of the body's cooling mechanisms. A lactating female will also have increased water requirements due to the fluid necessary for milk production. Last, the amount of calories that are consumed also affects voluntary water consumption. As energy intake increases, more metabolic waste products are produced and the heat produced by nutrient metabolism increases. In these circumstances, the body requires more water to excrete waste products in the urine and to contribute to thermoregulation.[10]

An average adult dog's daily water requirement can be estimated to be approximately equal to 1 ounce of water per pound of body weight. For example, a 60-lb dog will require approximately 60 oz, or about 2 quarts of water per day. Healthy dogs readily self-regulate water intake and should always have access to fresh, clean drinking water. When conditions are hot or dry, or during periods of strenuous exercise, dogs should be provided with frequent opportunities to drink and their water supply should be replenished often.

Carbohydrate

Carbohydrates are the major energy-containing constituents of plants, making up between 60 percent and 90 percent of plant dry matter weight. Carbohydrates are composed of carbon, hydrogen and oxygen and can be classified as **monosaccharides**, **disaccharides** or **polysaccharides**.

Monosaccharides: The monosaccharides are also called the "simple sugars" and are composed of a single unit containing between 3 and 7 carbon atoms. The three hexoses (6-carbon monosaccharides) that are most important nutritionally and metabolically are glucose, fructose, and galactose. Glucose is the chief end-product of starch digestion and glycogen hydrolysis in the body. It is the form of carbohydrate that is found circulating in the bloodstream of animals and is the primary form of carbohydrate that is used by the body's cells for energy. Fructose is found in honey, ripe fruits, and some vegetables. Galactose is not found free-form in foods. However, it makes up 50 percent of the disaccharide lactose, which is present in the milk of all species.

Disaccharides: Disaccharides are made up of two monosaccharide units linked together. Lactose is the sugar found in the milk of all mammals and contains a molecule of glucose and a molecule of galactose. Puppies consume lactose as a carbohydrate source through their mother's milk prior to weaning. However, after they have been weaned, lactose is negligible in the diet. The intestinal enzyme that is needed to digest lactose is called lactase. Like other mammals, dogs show a loss of lactase activity with age. As a result, feeding adult dogs large amounts of milk or other dairy products can result in maldigestion. Small quantities of these foods can be digested by most dogs, but large quantities cause diarrhea because of the osmotic effect of the sugar that escapes digestion and the end products that are produced by bacterial fermentation in the large intestine. A second important disaccharide is sucrose, which is comprised of a molecule of glucose linked to a molecule of fructose. Sucrose is commonly recognized as table sugar and is found in sugar cane, sugar beets, and maple syrup. Although it has not been demonstrated in dogs, data in other species indicate that very young animals have low levels of sucrase activity during the first few weeks of life. For this reason, sucrose solutions should not be used as energy sources for very young or orphaned puppies.

Polysaccharides: Polysaccharides are carbohydrates that are composed of many single monosaccharide units, linked together in long and complex chains. Starch and dietary fiber are the two types of polysaccharide that are of interest to pet nutrition. Starch is the primary carbohydrate source that is present in most commercial pet foods and is a highly digestible and available energy source. Cereal grains are the major ingredients that provide starch in the dog's diet. These include the whole grains of corn, rice, oats, barley, and wheat. Dietary fiber is plant material that consists primarily of several forms of carbohydrate, all of which cannot be digested by the enzymes of the dog's digestive tract. This means that dietary fiber cannot be broken down to monosaccharide units for absorption in the small intestine. However, fiber is fermented by intestinal microbes to varying degrees in the large intestine. Recent research has shown that the inclusion of dietary fiber in the diets of dogs is beneficial because of its effects upon the gastrointestinal tract.[11] Specifically, optimal levels of dietary fiber stimulates normal peristalsis, provides bulk to intestinal contents, and reduces gastrointestinal transit time. The end products of fiber fermentation in the large intestine, called short-chain fatty acids, are also important for the health and maintenance of the cells lining the intestine (see Chapter 19).

Functions of carbohydrate in the body: Within the body, carbohydrate is an essential and efficiently used source of energy. The monosaccharide, glucose, is an important energy source for many tissues. A constant supply of glucose is necessary for the proper functioning of the central nervous system. In all animals, only a limited amount of carbohydrate can be stored in the body, in the form of glycogen. The glycogen that is present in heart muscle is an important emergency source of energy for the heart, while liver and muscle glycogen is hydrolyzed to supply additional glucose to cells when circulating glucose is low. When dietary carbohydrate is consumed in excess of the body's energy needs, most is converted to body fat for energy storage, leading to increased body fat and obesity. Therefore, overfeeding a low fat or reducing diet can still lead to increased body fat and weight gain.

Carbohydrate requirement: All animals have a metabolic requirement for glucose. This requirement can be supplied either through **endogenous** synthesis (production within the body) or from dietary sources of carbohydrate. Metabolic pathways in the liver and kidney use other nutrients to produce glucose, which is released into the bloodstream to be carried to the body's tissues. There is convincing evidence in the dog that a source of dietary carbohydrate is not necessary if dietary levels of protein and fat are high enough to provide the needed precursors of glucose.[12] However, the need for an exogenous source of carbohydrate during the metabolically stressful periods of gestation and lactation has been debated. During gestation the bitch's needs increase because glucose is a major energy source for fetal development. Similarly, during lactation, additional glucose is needed for the synthesis of lactose, the disaccharide that is present in milk. While studies have shown that carbohydrate-free diets fed to dogs during reproduction have adverse effects, these effects do not occur if protein level in the diet is sufficiently high.[13] This information indicates that although carbohydrate is physiologically essential for the dog, it is not an indispensable component of the diet, even during the metabolically demanding stages of gestation and lactation.

The fact that dogs and cats do not require carbohydrate in their diets is usually immaterial because the nutrient content of most commercial foods includes at least a moderate level of this nutrient, most often in the form of starch (see Chapter 17). Although raw starch is poorly digested, cooked starch is efficiently digested and absorbed by dogs. The digestibility and availability of starch is significantly affected by the heat treatment that is used and by the size of the starch granules in the product.[14] Sufficient heating, such as that used in the extrusion process of dry pet foods, greatly increases digestibility, and finely ground starch is more digestible than coarsely ground granules.

Although dietary fiber is not a required nutrient per se, the inclusion of optimal amounts of fiber in the diets of companion animals is necessary for the normal functioning of the gastrointestinal tract. Insoluble fiber functions to increase the bulk of the diet, contributes to satiety, and maintains normal intestinal transit time and gastrointestinal tract motility. Soluble fiber delays gastric emptying, and when fermented by colonic bacteria, produces short-chain fatty acids that are important energy sources for colonocytes. Including a moderately fermentable fiber source such as beet pulp or rice bran provides a non-fermentable component for bulk and a fermentable component for the generation of beneficial short-chain fatty acids. Optimal levels of fiber in a dog's diet are 3 percent to 7 percent of the diet dry matter.[15] Common sources of dietary fiber in pet foods include wheat middlings, rice bran, beet pulp, and the hulls of soybeans and peanuts.

Fat

Dietary fat is part of a heterogeneous group of compounds known as the lipids. Although there are several forms of fat, triglyceride is the type of fat that is most important in the diets of dogs. Triglycerides are made up of three fatty acid molecules linked to one molecule of glycerol. Fatty acids are typically classified according to the number of double bonds contained in their carbon chain. Saturated fatty acids contain no double bonds between carbon atoms, monounsaturated fatty acids have one double bond, and polyunsaturated fatty acids contain two or more double bonds. In general, the triglycerides found in animal fat contain a higher proportion of saturated fatty acids than do those in most types of vegetable fat.

Triglycerides are the body's primary form of stored energy. In dogs, major depots of fat occur under the skin as subcutaneous fat, around the vital organs, and in the membranes surrounding the intestines. Fat depots have an extensive blood and nerve supply and are in a constant state of flux, serving to provide energy in times of need and storage in times of energy surplus. Body fat also serves as an insulator to protect the body from heat loss, and as a protective layer that guards against physical injury to the vital organs. Many different forms of lipid exist in the body and are important metabolically and structurally. Some are structural components of cell membranes, precursors for various hormones, and components of the skin that prevent water loss and provide protection.

Functions of dietary fat: Within the diet, fat has two primary roles: to provide a source of energy, and to supply essential fatty acids. Dogs, like most mammals, have a physiologic requirement for three fatty acids. These are called the essential fatty acids (EFAs) and include linoleic, gamma-linolenic and arachidonic acid. These three fatty acids all belong to a group of fatty acids called the omega-6 (n-6) fatty acid family. In most animals, including the dog, gamma-linolenic acid and arachidonic acid can be synthesized from linoleic acid. Therefore, if adequate linoleic acid is provided in the diet, there is no dietary requirement for gamma-linolenic acid or arachidonic acid. Only linoleic acid must be supplied in the diet. It is possible that the dog also has a requirement for one other fatty acid, called alpha-linolenic acid. Alpha-linolenic acid belongs to the omega-3 (n-3) fatty acid family and appears to have essential fatty acid properties in several animals. However, while omega-3 fatty acids have been shown to have some therapeutic value, the exact role of this fatty acid in the nutrition of healthy dogs is still not completely understood (see Chapter 19). Sources of linoleic acid in pet foods include vegetable oils such as corn, soybean, and safflower oils. Saturated animals fats generally contain low amounts of linoleic acid. In contrast, arachidonic acid is found only in animal fats. Whole-fat flax is a source of alpha-linolenic acid that is often included in pet foods.

Fat is an important energy source for dogs and is the most concentrated energy source of the energy-containing nutrients present in the diet. While the carbohydrate and protein in dog foods provides approximately 3.5 kcal ME/g, fat provides more than twice this amount, 8.5 kcal ME/g. In addition to its higher energy content, dietary fat is also, on average, more digestible than protein or carbohydrate.[16] Because of these properties, increasing the level of fat in a dog's diet appreciably increases its energy density. Dogs are able to maintain health when consuming diets that contain wide ranges of fat content, if other essential nutrients are adjusted to account for the changes in energy density. Dietary fat also makes dog food very palatable and imparts an acceptable texture to foods.

Dietary fat requirement: A dog's requirement for dietary fat depends on the need for essential fatty acids and for a calorically dense diet. The EFA requirement of the dog is usually expressed in terms of linoleic acid content because the dog's physiological requirement for EFAs can be met by sufficient dietary linoleic acid. Current recommendations for EFA concentration and percent fat in the diets of dogs that are fed for adult maintenance are a minimum of 1 percent of the dry weight as linoleic acid and a minimum of 5 percent of dry weight total fat.[7,17] As a proportion of energy, this corresponds to 12 percent of ME calories in a food containing 3,500 kcal ME/gram. This level should be increased to 8 percent total fat during periods of growth and reproduction (or 19.5 percent of ME calories).

In dogs, times of high energy demand occur during growth, gestation, lactation, and prolonged periods of physical exercise. Feeding an energy-dense, high-fat diet during these life stages allows a dog to consume adequate calories without having to ingest an excessive volume of food. In addition, dogs who are working strenuously have been shown to efficiently and preferentially utilize fatty acids for energy.[18] Most dry dog foods that are marketed for adult maintenance contain between 5 percent and 15 percent fat (dry matter basis). In comparison, the fat content of dry dog foods that are formulated for gestation, lactation, or performance may be 20 percent or greater.

Low amounts of fat in the diet can lead to deficiencies in total energy and EFAs. Because low-fat diets are not palatable to dogs and may not be accepted, their potential for causing an energy or EFA deficiency is further exacerbated by causing decreased food intake. In dogs, signs of an EFA deficiency are hair loss, and the development of a dry, dull coat, skin lesions and infections. However, EFA deficiencies are not common in dogs. When they do occur, they are usually associated with feeding a diet that was either poorly formulated or was improperly stored. EFA deficiency in dogs can also occur as a complication of other diseases, such as pancreatitis, biliary disease, hepatic disease, or malabsorption.[19]

Although dogs are capable of digesting and assimilating relatively high amounts of fat, providing more fat than the gastrointestinal tract can effectively digest and absorb will cause diarrhea. This problem is most commonly observed when dogs are fed high-fat table scraps or treats. Feeding a diet that is formulated for performance and which is relatively high in fat content to some dogs may lead to weight gain and obesity because of the high palatability and energy density of the diet. Regardless of the fat content of the diet, energy balance must be maintained to prevent excessively high rates of growth, unwanted weight gain, or obesity.

Protein

Like carbohydrates and fats, protein contains carbon, hydrogen, and oxygen. In addition, protein also contains nitrogen, and small amounts of sulfur. Amino acids are the basic units of proteins and are linked together by peptide bonds. Proteins range in size from just a few amino acids to very long amino acid chains which form complex molecules. During digestion, dietary protein is hydrolyzed to its constituent amino acids (and some dipeptides) and these are absorbed into the body across the lining of the small intestine. There are 22 amino acids found in protein. Twelve of these can be synthesized by the dog and so are not required in the diet. The remaining 10 are called the essential amino acids and cannot be made by the body at rates sufficient to meet the body's needs. These must be supplied in the dog's diet (Table 16.3). Dietary protein is required by the body for two major purposes: to provide essential amino acids that will be used for protein synthesis, and to supply nitrogen for the synthesis of the nonessential amino acids and other nitrogen-containing compounds. Protein has numerous functions in the body. It is the major structural component of hair, skin, nails and connective tissue. All enzymes are comprised of protein, as are many hormones. Proteins found in the blood act as important carrier substances and contribute to the regulation of acid-base balance. The body's immune system and musculoskeletal system

TABLE 16.3   Essential and Nonessential Amino Acids for the Dog

Essential Amino Acids	Nonessential Amino Acids
Arginine	Alanine
Histidine	Asparagine
Isoleucine	Aspartate
Leucine	Cysteine
Lysine	Glutamate
Methionine	Glutamine
Phenylalanine	Glycine
Tryptophan	Hydroxylysine
Threonine	Hydroxyproline
Valine	Proline
	Serine
	Tyrosine

also rely upon protein substances for normal functioning. All proteins in the body are in a constant state of flux involving **degradation** and synthesis. Although tissues vary greatly in their rate of turnover, all protein molecules in the body are eventually catabolized and replaced. The body has the ability to synthesize new proteins from amino acids, provided that all of the necessary amino acids are available.

Because amino acids, not intact protein, are absorbed into the body, animals do not have a dietary requirement for protein per se. Rather they require the essential amino acids and a certain level of nitrogen. This is commonly expressed as a protein requirement because amino acids and nitrogen are most typically supplied in the diet in the form of intact protein. Adult dogs require dietary protein for the replacement of protein losses in skin, hair, digestive enzymes, and mucosal cells, and from losses due to normal cellular protein catabolism. This is referred to as a "maintenance" protein requirement. Young animals and reproducing females have these same maintenance requirements plus an added requirement for the growth of new tissue or the production of milk. Dogs that are working hard may need slightly more protein to maintain and build muscle. In addition, an animal's activity level, physiological state, and prior nutritional status all influence an individual's dietary protein requirement.

Protein quality: The quality of protein that is included in a dog food significantly influences the amount of protein that must be fed to meet dogs' requirements. Because protein quality in pet foods varies a great deal, this is an important factor to consider when determining a dog's protein requirement and when selecting a pet food (see Chapter 17). Simply put, an animal's protein requirement varies inversely with the protein source's digestibility and with its ability to provide correct amounts of the essential amino acids. As protein digestibility and quality increase, the level (percentage) of protein that must be included in the diet to meet the animal's needs will decrease. The digestibilities of proteins that are included in high-quality, commercial dog foods range between 80 percent and 90 percent.[20] This can be compared to low-quality, commercial pet foods that have protein digestibilities as low as 70 to 75 percent. When poorly digestible protein is included in a diet, a high percentage (by weight) is required to ensure that dogs absorb adequate levels of essential amino acids to meet their requirements.

The amino acid content of the protein in a dog food similarly impacts the amount of protein that must be included. Most practical sources of protein contain excesses of some amino acids and slight or severe deficiencies of others, relative to the dog's requirement. It is for this reason that commercial pet foods usually include a mixture of protein sources. Including proteins that have complimentary profiles of essential amino acids results in the provision of a balanced profile of amino acids. If balanced optimally, a lower proportion of protein will need to be included in the diet to meet requirements, and fewer excess amino acids will be absorbed and metabolized for energy or converted to fat for storage (see below).

Protein requirements of dogs: Dietary protein serves several important functions. It provides the essential amino acids, which are used for protein synthesis in the growth and repair of tissue, and it is the body's principal source of nitrogen. Nitrogen is essential for the synthesis of the nonessential amino acids and of other nitrogen-containing molecules. Examples of these are nucleic acids, purines, pyrimidines, and certain neurotransmitter substances. Amino acids supplied by dietary protein can also be metabolized for energy. The GE of amino acids is 5.65 kcal ME/g. When fecal and urinary losses are accounted for, the ME of protein in dog diets is approximately 3.5 kcal/g, the same amount of energy that is supplied by dietary carbohydrate. Animals are unable to store excess amino acids. Surplus amino acids (such as those supplied by an imbalanced protein) are used either directly for energy or are converted to glycogen or fat for energy storage. An ancillary function of the protein in dog food is to provide a source of flavor. Different flavors are created when food proteins are cooked in the presence of carbohydrate and fat.[21]

The minimum protein requirement of the dogs fed a practical diet containing ingredients of moderate quality is 18 percent protein on a dry matter basis for adult maintenance, and 22 percent for growth and reproduction. These values assume a ME content in the dog food of approximately 3,500 kcal/kg of dry weight. If the energy density of the diet is higher, appropriate increases in protein content must be made. For example, a dog food with an energy density of 4,000 kcal/kg should contain a minimum percent protein of 20.5 percent for adult maintenance or 25 percent for growth and reproduction. In all cases, these values correspond to 18 percent of ME calories for maintenance and 22 percent of ME calories for growth.

If protein is deficient in the diet, adult dogs will experience a loss of body weight and lean body tissue (muscle). Puppies and growing dogs will show decreased weight gain or even weight loss, and impaired growth and development. Protein deficiency is uncommon in companion animals that are fed balanced, commercial pet foods. This is because the majority of commercial foods contain more protein than is needed to meet the minimum requirement.[22] When protein deficiency does occur, it is usually because owners are attempting to economize by feeding low-quality, poorly formulated rations during periods of high nutrient need, such as pregnancy, lactation, or strenuous work.

Vitamins

Vitamins are organic molecules that are needed in minute amounts to function in many of the body's metabolic processes. Although they are organic molecules, vitamins are not used as energy sources or as structural compounds. With a few exceptions, most vitamins cannot be synthesized by the body and must be supplied in the food. A general classification scheme for vitamins divides them into two groups: the fat-soluble vitamins and the water-soluble vitamins. The fat-soluble vitamins are A, D, E, and K; the water-soluble group includes members of the B-complex vitamins and vitamin C. The essential fat-soluble and water-soluble vitamins, their functions in the body, and signs of deficiency and excess are summarized in Table 16.4. Vitamin deficiencies are very rare today because of the widespread feeding of commercially prepared dog foods. When imbalances do occur, they are usually caused by improper feeding practices, or as a secondary effect of an underlying disease. These specific cases are reviewed in Chapter 19.

Minerals

Minerals are inorganic elements that are essential for normal growth, development and maintenance of the body. Although only about 4 percent of an animal's total body weight is composed of mineral matter, these elements are essential for life. A general classification scheme divides minerals into two groups, macrominerals and microminerals. Macrominerals are those that occur in appreciable amounts in the body and account for most of the body's mineral content. They include calcium, phosphorus, magnesium, sulfur, and the electrolytes sodium, potassium, and chloride. Microminerals include minerals that are present in the body in very small amounts and are required in very low concentrations amounts in the diet. The microminerals are iron, zinc, copper, manganese, iodine, selenium and cobalt.

Minerals have numerous functions in the body. Macrominerals, such as calcium, phosphorus and magnesium are major components of the skeleton and of certain transport proteins and hormones. Minerals also activate enzymatically catalyzed reactions, aid in nerve transmission and muscle contractions, and function in water and electrolyte balance. The major functions of minerals and signs of imbalance are summarized in Table 16.5. As with vitamins, mineral deficiencies are rare in dogs in the United States. When problems with minerals occur, they are usually a result of improper feeding prac-

TABLE 16.4   Vitamins: Functions and Signs of Imbalance

	Functions in the Body	Imbalances
Vitamin A (Retinol)	Component of visual pigments of the eye; necessary for proper vision; involved in normal cell differentiation and maintenance; necessary for normal skin health, and bone and teeth development	**Deficiency:** Impaired growth and reproduction; skin lesions/infections **Excess:** Liver damage; bone disease
Vitamin D	Necessary for normal calcium absorption and metabolism and for calcium resorption from bone; active form of vitamin D is synthesized from lipid compounds in the skin	**Deficiency:** Rare; if seen, is caused by concomitant imbalances in calcium and phosphorus. Rickets in young dogs and osteomalacia in adults **Excess:** Elevated blood calcium leading to calcification of soft tissues
Vitamin E	Physiological antioxidant; protects cells and tissues from oxidative damage	**Deficiency:** Reproductive failure, impaired immune function **Excess:** Not observed
Vitamin K	Involved in normal blood clotting; provided by bacteria of large intestine	**Deficiency:** Increased clotting time **Excess:** Not observed
Thiamin (B_1)	Involved in carbohydrate metabolism; requirement is influenced by the level of carbohydrate in the diet	**Deficiency:** Anorexia; neurological disorders **Excess:** Not observed
Riboflavin (B_2)	Essential for normal oxidative reactions and cellular metabolism of nutrients	**Deficiency:** Skin lesions; neurological disorders **Excess:** Not observed
Niacin	Required for oxidation and reduction reactions, and metabolism of nutrients	**Deficiency:** Black tongue disease **Excess:** Not observed
Pyridoxine	Necessary for enzyme systems involved in the metabolism of protein and amino acids	**Deficiency:** Anemia; anorexia; weight loss **Excess:** Not observed
Pantothenic Acid	Constituent of co-enzyme-A needed for carbohydrate, fat, and amino acid metabolism	**Deficiency:** Anorexia; weight loss; impaired growth **Excess:** Not observed
Biotin	Necessary for the metabolism of fats and amino acids; necessary for skin and hair health	**Deficiency:** Skin lesions; dermatitis **Excess:** Not observed
Folic Acid	Necessary for normal red blood cell development and DNA synthesis	**Deficiency:** Anemia; leucopenia **Excess:** Not observed
Cobalamin (B_{12})	Function linked with folic acid	**Deficiency:** Pernicious anemia **Excess:** Not observed
Choline	Constituent of phospholipids in cell membranes; precursor of the neurotransmitter acetylcholine	**Deficiency:** Neurological disorders; fatty liver **Excess:** Not observed
Vitamin C (Ascorbic Acid)	Necessary for formation of the structural protein collagen. NOTE: Dogs synthesize adequate levels of ascorbic acid	Dietary source not required by dogs

TABLE 16.5   Minerals: Functions and Signs of Imbalance

	Functions in the Body	Imbalances
Calcium	Along with phosphorus is a major component of bones and teeth; essential for blood clotting, and nerve and muscle function	**Deficiency:** Rickets (growing dogs); osteomalacia (adults) **Excess:** Impaired skeletal development; interferes with absorption of zinc (can lead to zinc deficiency)
Phosphorus	Component of bones and teeth; responsible for storage and transfer of energy in the body (component of "high energy bonds" found in ATP, ADP, and other compounds)	**Deficiency:** Same as calcium deficiency **Excess:** Interferes with calcium absorption and metabolism
Magnesium	Component of skeleton; necessary for muscle contraction and nervous impulse transmission; involved in energy metabolism and protein synthesis	**Deficiency:** Calcification of soft tissue; neuromuscular abnormalities **Excess**: Dietary excess is unlikely due to regulation of absorption
Iron	Component of hemoglobin and myoglobin (oxygen-carrying proteins of blood and muscle); component of enzymes involved in cellular respiration	**Deficiency:** Anemia; fatigue; weakness **Excess:** Dietary excess is unlikely due to regulation of absorption
Copper	Necessary for formation and activity of red blood cells; co-factor in many enzymatic reactions; necessary for normal pigmentation of skin and hair	**Deficiency**: Anemia; impaired bone growth **Excess:** Inherited disorder of copper metabolism in some breeds leads to toxicity (liver disease)
Zinc	Essential component of many enzyme systems, including those involved in protein and carbohydrate metabolism; necessary for maintaining healthy skin and coat	**Deficiency:** Impaired growth; reproductive failure; skin lesions; depigmentation of hair **Excess:** Rare; can interfere with calcium and copper absorption and metabolism
Sulfur	Needed for synthesis of chondroitin-sulfate in cartilage, insulin, and heparin; component of glutathione	**Deficiency:** Not observed due to high amounts in amino acids methionine and cysteine **Excess:** Not observed
Manganese	Component of enzymatic systems involved in carbohydrate and lipid metabolism; formation of cartilage	**Deficiency:** Impaired growth; reproductive failure **Excess:** Not observed
Iodine	Essential component of thyroid hormones (involved in regulating the body's metabolic rate)	**Deficiency:** Rare; goiter (enlarged thyroid gland) **Excess:** Rare; goiter
Selenium	Component of glutathione peroxidase, which acts as a cell membrane antioxidant; action is closely interrelated to that of vitamin E	**Deficiency:** Unlikely in dogs **Excess:** Unlikely in dogs
Cobalt	Component of vitamin B_{12}	**Deficiency:** Unlikely in dogs **Excess:** Not observed
Electrolytes (Sodium, Potassium and Chloride)	Acid-base balance and osmoregulation of body fluids; nerve and muscle functioning; energy metabolism	**Deficiency:** Unlikely in dogs **Excess:** Unlikely in dogs

tices, nutrient imbalances, or are secondary to other underlying illnesses. Practical cases of mineral imbalance are discussed in Chapter 19.

Digestion and Absorption in Dogs

In all species, the role of the digestive system is to break down the large complex forms of nutrients in foods into simple forms that can be absorbed into the body, circulated to tissues and used by cells. For example, most of the fat in food is hydrolyzed to glycerol, free fatty acids, and some monoglycerides and diglycerides before absorption takes place. Complex carbohydrates are broken down to the simple sugars, glucose, galactose, and fructose. Protein molecules are hydrolyzed to single amino acid units and some dipeptides. The portions of the dog's digestive tract that are important in this process are the mouth, esophagus, stomach, small intestine and large intestine. In addition, secretions of the pancreas and liver are released into the small intestine and are necessary for the proper mixing and digestion of food. The dog has monogastric (single stomach) gastrointestinal system that is adapted to an omnivorous diet containing a high proportion of animal tissue (Figure 16.2).

Mouth: When a dog begins to eat, the smell and presence of food stimulates the production of saliva by the salivary glands. Saliva functions to aid with mixing of food and to lubricate food prior to swallowing. Many dogs bolt their food with minimal chewing. However, if the food is tough or in large

FIGURE 16.2   Gastrointestinal system of the dog

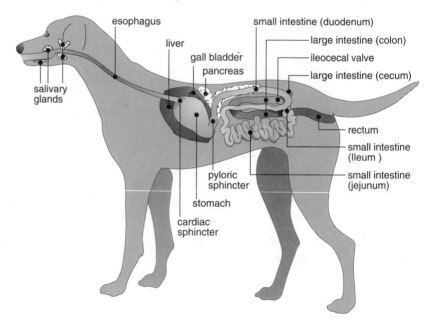

pieces, the molars and pre-molars of the dog are well suited for grinding and chewing.

Esophagus: Swallowing transfers food from the mouth to the esophagus. The esophagus is the hollow, muscular tube leading to the stomach. The cells lining the esophagus produce more mucus to aid in the passage of food. The cardiac sphincter is located at the base of the stomach and it relaxes to allow food to enter from the esophagus into the stomach. It then immediately constricts after food has passed to prevent reflux of the stomach contents back into the lower esophagus.

Stomach: The stomach is a reservoir for food. It initiates the chemical digestion of protein, further mixes the food, and regulates the flow of food into the small intestine. Thorough mixing of food in the antral or lower portion of the stomach results in the production of a semifluid mass of food called chyme. Chyme passes into the small intestine via the pyloric sphincter. Like the cardiac sphincter, the pyloric sphincter is a ring of muscle that is usually in a constricted state. This ring relaxes in response to peristaltic contractions of the stomach, and controls the rate of passage of food from the stomach into the small intestine. At this stage of digestion, carbohydrates and fats are almost unchanged in chemical composition, but the protein in the food has been partially hydrolyzed to smaller polypeptides while in the stomach.

Small intestine: Chemical digestion of food and absorption of nutrients into the body occur primarily in the small intestine. As chyme enters the small intestine, further mechanical digestion occurs through continued peristalsis. The pancreas and glands that are located in the mucosa of the intestine secrete enzymes into the intestinal lumen that chemically digest fat, carbohydrate, and protein. Bile, produced by the liver and stored in the gall bladder, is also released into the lumen in response to the entry of chyme. Bile functions to emulsify dietary fat and activate certain enzymes that are important for fat digestion. During digestion in the small intestine, protein, carbohydrate, and fat are hydrolyzed to amino acids, dipeptides, monosaccharides, glycerol, free fatty acids, and monoglycerides and diglycerides. As these small units are produced, they are absorbed across the intestinal wall into the body along with dietary vitamins and minerals. Intestinal villi are small finger-like projections lining the small intestine which function to greatly increase the surface area that is available for nutrient absorption. Absorption involves the transfer of digested nutrients from the intestinal lumen to the blood or lymphatic system for delivery to tissues throughout the body.

Large intestine (colon): The contents of the small intestine enter the large intestine through the ileocecal valve. A chief function of the large intestine in dogs is the absorption of water and certain electrolytes. Along with a large volume of water, sodium is absorbed from the large intestine. A second important function of the large intestine is the fermentation of dietary fiber. The normal bacterial colonies that are present in the colon are capable of digesting some of the indigestible fiber in the diet and other nutrients that have escaped digestion in the small intestine. The products of this bacterial fermentation can provide energy to cells that line the large intestine.

Undigested food residues, sloughed cells, bacteria, and unabsorbed endogenous secretions make up the fecal matter that eventually reaches the rectum and is excreted from the body. Fecal characteristics in dogs are significantly affected by the quantity and type of indigestible matter that is present in the diet. Bacterial fermentation of these materials produces various gases, short-chain fatty acids, and other by-products. When protein reaches the large intestine in an undigested state, bacterial degradation results in the production of compounds called indole and skatole, and of hydrogen sulfide gas. Hydrogen sulfide gas, indole, and skatole impart strong odors to fecal matter and intestinal gas. Certain types of carbohydrates found in legumes, such as soy beans, are resistant to digestion by the endogenous enzymes of the small intestine. These carbohydrates reach the colon and are attacked by bacteria, with the resultant production of intestinal gas (flatulence). The degree to which flatulence and strong fecal odors occur in dogs that are fed poorly digested materials varies with the amounts and types that are fed and with the intestinal flora that is present in the colon of individual animals.

Conclusions

Like humans, dogs have requirements for essential amino acids, fatty acids, vitamins, minerals, water and energy in their diets. Energy is the first requirement that is satisfied, and is supplied by dietary fat, carbohydrate and protein. An optimal diet for dogs will supply needed energy and essential nutrients in a volume of food that satisfies the dog's hunger. Today, most dog owners in the United States provide nutrition to their dogs by feeding commercial pet foods. The following chapter provides an overview of diets that are available, and methods for evaluating and choosing an appropriate dog food.

Cited References

1. Danforth, E. and Landsberg, L. **Energy expenditure and its regulation.** In: *Obesity—Contemporary issues in clinical nutrition* (M.R.C. Greenwood, editor), Churchill Livingstone, New York, New York, pp. 103–121. (1983)

2. Durrer, J.L. and Hannon, J.P. **Seasonal variations in caloric intake of dogs living in an arctic environment.** American Journal of Physiology, 202:375–384. (1962)

3. Romsos, D.R., Hornshus, M.J., and Leveille, G.A. **Influence of dietary fat and carbohydrate on food intake, body weight and body fat of adult dogs.** Proceedings of the Society of Experimental Biology and Medicine, 157:278–281. (1978)

4. Kealy, R.D., Olsson, S.E., and Monti, K.L. **Effects of limited food consumption on the incidence of hip dysplasia in growing dogs.** Journal of the American Veterinary Medical Association, 201:857-863. (1992)

5. Hedhammer, A., Wu, F.M., and Krook, L. **Overnutrition and skeletal disease: an experimental study in growing Great Dane dogs.** Cornell Veterinarian, 64(suppl. 5):1–160. (1974)

6. Richardson, D.C. **The role of nutrition in canine hip dysplasia.** Veterinary Clinics of North America: Small Animal Practice, 22:529-540. (1992)

7. National Research Council. *Nutrient Requirements of Dogs.* National Academy of Sciences, National Academy Press, Washington, D.C. (1985)

8. Anderson, R.S. **Water content in the diet of the dog.** Veterinary Annual, 21:171–178. (1981)

9. Anderson, R.S. **Water balance in the dog and cat.** Journal of Small Animal Practice, 23:588–598. (1982)

10. Hinchcliff, K.W. and Reinhart, G.A. **Energy metabolism and water turnover in Alaskan sled dogs during running.** *Recent Advances in Canine and Feline Nutritional Research: Proceedings of the Iams International Nutrition Symposium* (April 18-21, 1996). Orange Frazer Press, Wilmington, Ohio, pp. 199-206.

11. Bartges, J. and Anderson, W.H. **Dietary fiber.** Veterinary Clinical Nutrition, 4:25-28. (1997)

12. Blaza, S.E. and Burger, I.H. **Is carbohydrate essential for pregnancy and lactation in dogs?** In: *Nutrition of the Cat and Dog* (I.H. Burger and J.P.W. Rivers, editors), Cambridge University Press, New York, New York, pp. 229–242. (1989)

13. Kienzle, E. and Meyer, H. **The effects of carbohydrate-free diets containing different levels of protein on reproduction in the bitch.** In: *Nutrition of the Cat and Dog* (I. H. Burger and J. P. W. Rivers, editors), Cambridge University Press, New York, New York, pp 113–132. (1989)

14. Bisset, S.A., Guilford, W.G., Lawoko, C.R., and Sunvold, G.D. **Effect of food particle size on carbohydrate assimilation assessed by breath hydrogen testing in dogs.** Veterinary Clinical Nutrition, 4:82-88. (1997)

15. Reinhart, G. **Fiber nutrition and intestinal function critical for recovery.** DVM News Magazine, June, 1993.

16. Huber, T.L., Wilson, R.C., and McGarity, S.A. **Variations in digestibility of dry dog foods with identical label guaranteed analysis.** Journal of the American Animal Hospital Association, 22:571–575. (1986)

17. Association of American Feed Control Officials. *Pet Food Regulations* Official Publication, AAFCO, Atlanta Georgia. (1998)

18. Reynolds, A.J., Fuhrer, H.L., and Dunlap, M.D. **Lipid metabolite responses to diet and training in sled dogs.** Journal of Nutrition, 124:2754S-2759S. (1994)

19. Codner, E.C. and Thatcher, C.D. **The role of nutrition in the management of dermatoses.** Seminars in Veterinary Medicine and Surgery (Small Animal), 5:167–177. (1990)

20. Case, L.P. and Czarnecki-Maulden, G.L. **Protein requirements of growing pups fed practical dry-type diets containing mixed-protein sources.** American Journal of Veterinary Research, 51:808–812. (1990)

21. Brown, R.G. **Protein in dog foods.** Canadian Veterinary Journal, 30:528-531. (1989)

22. Kallfelz, F.A. **Evaluation and use of pet foods: General considerations in using pet foods for adult maintenance.** Veterinary Clinics of North America: Small Animal Practice, 19:387-403. (1989)

17 Diets: Evaluation and Selection

BECAUSE OF THE LARGE VARIETY of pet food that is available to pet owners today, selecting the best food for a dog can be a confusing process. In the United States, the majority of dog owners feed their dogs commercial dog food, and the most common type of commercial food that is fed is the dry (expanded) product.[1] Even within food categories, there are many choices to be made regarding the stage of life that the food targets, the ingredients it includes, and its level of quality. This chapter provides an overview of the types of pet food, advantages and disadvantages of each, and methods for evaluating and selecting an appropriate dog food for a particular stage of life or lifestyle.

Types of Commercial Dog Food

In general, commercial products can be categorized according to their processing method, preservation method, and moisture content. The three major types are dry, canned, and semimoist pet food and treats.

Dry-type dog food: Dry pet food includes kibbles, biscuits, meals, and expanded products, all of which contain between 6 percent and 12 percent moisture.[2] Kibbled foods are baked products made by creating a dough from all the ingredients. This is spread onto large sheets and baked. After the baked product cools, the sheets of food are broken into bite-size pieces and packaged. Dog biscuits are prepared in much the same manner, except the dough is formed or cut into the desired shapes, and the individual biscuits are baked much like cookies. Dry meals are prepared by mixing together a number of dried, flaked, or granular ingredients. Although these were very popular during the early 1960s, they have been almost completely replaced with expanded products.

Expanded (extruded) dry dog food is the most common type of dog food fed today. Extrusion refers to a cooking process in which the raw mixture of ingredients is rapidly cooked under conditions of high heat and pressure. Immediately after cooking, the material, which is still somewhat soft, is forced through a small opening called a "dye" that shapes the food into desired shapes and sizes. Extrusion technology revolutionized the pet food industry in the 1950s because this process completely cooks the starches within the product, resulting in significantly increased digestibility and palatability. As a result, dry pet food provides a substantial proportion of energy in the form of highly digestible carbohydrate. After the expanded pieces of dog food have cooled, a coating of fat or other palatable material usually is sprayed on the outside of the expanded pellets. This process is called "enrobing" and functions to increase both the palatability of the food and its caloric density. Hot-air drying reduces the total moisture content of the product to 12 percent or less.

The caloric density of dry dog food ranges between 3,000 and 4,500 kilocalories of metabolizable energy (kcal of ME) per kilogram (kg) or between 1,300 and 2,000 kcal per pound on a dry-weight basis. The energy density of these products is somewhat limited by the processing and packaging methods that are used. However, the majority of dry pet food can fully supply the energy needs of the majority of companion animals. Products that are formulated for adult maintenance may be too low in caloric density for hard-working or stressed dogs that have very high energy requirements. In these cases, "performance" pet food has been developed to meet the energy requirements of working dogs. Depending on the purpose of the food, the dry-matter content of dry dog food contains between 8 percent and 22 percent fat and between 18 percent and 32 percent protein (Table 17.1).

Ingredients commonly used in dry pet food include cereal grains, meat, poultry or fish products, some milk products, and vitamin and mineral supplements. A certain level of starch must be included in expanded products to allow proper processing of the product. In addition, the high-heat processing involved in producing the food can cause the loss of certain vitamins. As a re-

TABLE 17.1   Nutrient Content of Commercial Dog Food

	Dry	Semimoist	Canned
	Percentage	Percentage	Percentage
As-Fed Basis			
Moisture	6–12	15–35	70–78
Protein	16–30	17–22	7–13
Fat	6–20	7–12	4–9
Carbohydrate	40–70	35–60	4–13
Fiber	3–7	3–5	0.5–1
Ash	6–9	5–8	1–3
ME (kcal/kg)	2,800–4,200	2,500–2,800	850–1,250
Dry-Matter Basis*			
Protein	18–32	20–30	28–50
Fat	8–22	8–16	20–32
Carbohydrate	45–75	55–75	18–55
Fiber	3–8	3.5–7.5	2–5
Ash	6.5–10	6–10	6–10
ME (kcal/kg)	3,000–4,500	3,000–4,000	3,500–5,000

*Calculation of Dry-Matter Basis = (% of Nutrient [as fed] / % of Dry Matter in Diet) × 100

sult, reputable pet food manufacturers ensure optimal amounts of these nutrients in their products by accounting for these losses when the pet food is formulated and by conducting adequate testing of their products.

The quality of dry dog food that is available to consumers varies significantly. Harsh or improper drying or extruding of the ingredients can cause a reduction in nutrient availability, a loss of nutrients, and changes to proteins that make them less digestible. As a result, poor-quality dry food will have very low digestibilities and nutrient availabilities. From the pet owners' point of view, the most obvious effects of this are large stool volumes, poor stool quality, high frequency of defecation, and long-term changes in coat condition, health, and vitality. By contrast, companies that manufacture high-quality, premium products will use only properly treated ingredients to ensure that the digestibilities of their products remain high after processing.

There are several advantages to feeding a dry dog food. In general, these products are more economical to feed than semimoist and canned food, and they store for long periods of time because of their low moisture content. Most dry products sold today have a "best used by" date that is 12 months after the date of manufacturing. Dry food often can be fed ad libitum (free-choice) without worry of rapid spoilage. Although some dogs can be fed in this manner and will not overconsume, others will still consume too much food and gain weight. Dry pet food may also offer some dental hygiene advantages. The chewing and grinding that accompanies eating dry biscuits or pet food may aid in the prevention of plaque and calculus accumulation on teeth.[3]

Canned dog food: Canned pet food is produced by blending all of the ingredients together and adding premeasured amounts of water. The entire mixture is heated and transported along a canning conveyor line. The mixture is put into cans, which are sealed, washed, and labeled. Pressure sterilization involves cooking the cans at high temperatures for about 60 minutes. After exiting the retort (cooker), the cans are cooled under controlled conditions to ensure sterility. Paper labels that designate the product are applied during the final step of production. Three types of canned dog food are produced. These types are designated as loaf, chunks or chunks in gravy, and a chunk-in-loaf combination. Depending on the ingredients used, these products can vary greatly in their nutrient content and level of digestibility.

In general, canned food is very palatable because it contains relatively high amounts of fat and protein (Table 17.1). The high heat and pressure involved in processing canned food kills harmful bacteria and causes some nutrient losses. As with dry products, manufacturers of high-quality canned dog food conduct the research necessary to determine the extent of these losses, then adjust their formulations to compensate for them. However, some companies may not properly consider the nutrient losses that occur during the canning process. In these cases, suboptimal levels of nutrients may be present in the product. When compared on a per-meal basis, canned food usually is more expensive to feed than dry dog food. It is important to make price comparisons on either a dry-weight basis or a caloric-density basis because canned food contains a very large proportion of water. In the United States, the moisture content of pet food can be as high as 78 percent, or equal to the natural moisture content of the ingredients that are used, whichever is greater.[4] On the average, canned pet food contains about 75 percent water—substantially more than that found in dry products.

Some advantages of canned pet food include its extremely long shelf life and high acceptability to dogs. The sterilization and sealing of the cans allow these products to be kept for long time periods before opening, without the need for special storage considerations. Also, canned food usually is very palatable to most dogs. As a result, it is not unusual for dog owners to supplement a dry ration with 1 or 2 tablespoons of canned food each day. A disadvantage of this is that the high energy density of canned food may lead to weight gain in dogs who have moderate to low energy requirements. If fed ad libitum, the high palatability and fat content of canned food may override the dog's inherent tendency to just eat to meet its caloric requirements, resulting in the overconsumption of energy.

Semimoist dog food: The moisture content of semimoist pet food lies between that of dry and canned products, usually between 15 percent and 35 percent moisture. These products include fresh or frozen animal tissues, cereal grains, fats, and simple sugars as their principal ingredients. Semimoist food is soft in texture, a characteristic that contributes to its acceptability and palatability. Most semimoist dog food and treats contain high amounts of simple sugars or corn syrup, which serve as a preservative because of their capacity to bind water and make it unavailable to microbes. This high simple sugar content contributes to the palatability and digestibility of these products. The ME content of semimoist food ranges between 3,000 and 4,000 kcal/kg on a dry-weight basis, or about 1,400 to 1,800 kcal/lb. Semimoist food contains between 20 percent and 28 percent protein and between 8 percent and 14 percent fat on a dry-weight basis. The proportion of carbohydrate in semimoist food is similar to that of dry food (Table 17.1). However, by contrast, the carbohydrate in semimoist pet food is largely in the form of simple carbohydrates with a relatively small proportion of starch.

Semimoist dog food makes up a very small proportion of the dog food market today. Rather, most semimoist products are sold as pet snacks and treats. These are available in a large variety of shapes, textures, and flavors. Although these different forms do not reflect nutrient content or palatability for the pet, they do appeal to the preferences of many pet owners. Semimoist food does not require refrigeration before opening and has a relatively long shelf life. The cost of semimoist treats is substantially higher than dog food, a reflection of their purpose as a specialty item.

Snacks and treats: Snacks and treats have become increasingly popular with pet owners in recent years. Within the past 30 years, almost every major pet food company has added one or more dog treat or snack to the market.[5] This increase possibly reflects the changing roles of dogs in society within the last few decades (see Chapter 6). Owners purchase treats not because of their nutritional value but as a way of showing love and nurturance toward their pets. Pet owners also give their dogs treats and snacks as training aids to reinforce desired behaviors, at times of arrival or departure, as a means of providing variety in the pet's diet, and as an aid to proper dental health.

When treats and snacks were introduced, they all were in the form of baked biscuits. Over time, different shapes, sizes, and flavors of these biscuits were developed and marketed. Because treats are usually impulse buys, owners are more likely to try a new flavor or type of treat than they are to completely switch dog food. To capitalize on this, manufacturers have continued to develop new types of dog snacks. Today, treats can be categorized into four basic types: semimoist, biscuits, jerky, and rawhide products. Many treats are made to resemble food humans normally eat, such as hamburgers, sausage, bacon, cheese, and even ice cream. Examples of several popular treat concepts include snacks made with all-natural ingredients, ones that promote dental health, or ones that are made from livestock body parts such as ears, hooves, or even noses.

Sources and Quality of Pet Food

Selecting an optimal dog food requires being able to discern between the quality of the foods that are available. In general, the best rule of thumb when it comes to dog food is that "you get what you pay for." Because the ingredients in dog food and the processing methods can vary greatly, there are wide ranges of quality available to dogs today. Discriminating pet owners and dog professionals will become aware of these differences and use information available to consumers to select the best product for their dogs.

Commercial products can be divided into the popular, premium, and generic brands. The popular brands include food that is marketed nationally or regionally and sold in grocery store chains. Premium brands are developed with the purpose of providing optimal nutrition during targeted life stages or activity levels and are sold only through veterinarians, pet specialty stores, and some feed stores. Generic dog food is comprised of products that do not carry a brand name. They usually are produced and marketed locally or regionally on a least-cost basis. Most private label or "price brands" are generic products that have been labeled with a chain store's name brand. An alternative to purchasing a commercially prepared dog food is to prepare a homemade diet. Although this takes considerably more time and effort than feeding a commercial diet, optimal nutrition can be provided if a recipe that has been thoroughly tested and evaluated for long-term feeding is used.

Popular brands: The companies that produce popular brands of pet food devote a substantial amount of energy and finances to advertising, which results in high name recognition of their products. Most popular brands contain ingredients of moderate quality that are formulated to be highly palatable to dogs, thus ensuring acceptability to pet owners. Some nationally marketed brands carry label claims verified through the Association of American Feed Control Officials (AAFCO) feeding trials. However, smaller manufacturers that only produce and sell food regionally often use a less reliable calculation method to validate label claims. In general, popular brands of pet food have lower digestibilities than most premium brands of food, but they contain higher-quality ingredients and have higher digestibilities than the generic and private label pet foods. The major advantages of these foods are the convenience of being able to purchase dog food at a grocery store and the high degree of consumer confidence due to the large amount of advertising in popular media.

Premium brands: The manufacturers of premium pet food formulate and market their products for different stages of life, activity levels, and lifestyles. For example, dog food has been developed for hardworking dogs (performance diets), adult dogs during maintenance, growing dogs of large and small breeds, and bitches during lactation and gestation. The companies that produce these products also provide educational materials to pet owners and professionals about companion animal nutrition and feeding. Ingredients in premium products are of higher quality and digestibility than those in popular or generic brands. Immediate results of this benefit that owners notice are lower stool volume and better stool quality. Premium pet food usually is more costly on a per-weight basis because of the higher-quality ingredients used and the level of testing conducted on the products. However, because these products usually are very digestible and nutrient dense, smaller amounts need to be fed, and the cost per serving often is comparable to many popular brands of pet food.

Generic or private label: Generic products represent the least expensive and the poorest quality of pet food commercially available to pet owners. The most important consideration of the manufacturers of generic food is producing a low-cost product. For this reason, cheap, poor-quality ingredients are used, and few, if any, feeding tests are conducted. Although the low cost may be appealing to some pet owners, there are several problems that may occur with generic and private label pet food. Some generic dog food has not been formulated to be nutritionally complete and so will not even carry a label claim. Also, controlled feeding studies with dogs have shown that generic products have significantly lower digestibilities and nutrient availabilities than popular brands of food and that long-term feeding can lead to nutrient imbalances and impaired growth.[6,7] In addition, because poor-quality ingredients often result in low palatability, this food is unacceptable to some dogs. Private label pet food carries the house name of the grocery store chain or other store in which it is sold. Like generic pet food, these products usually are produced on a least-cost basis. The only difference is that private label food is produced (or simply packaged and labeled) under a contract with the grocery store whose name they carry. Most is produced by the same companies that make generic products and usually is similar in quality to generic pet food.

Homemade dog food: Although the majority of pet owners in the United States enjoy the convenience, economy, and reliability of commercially produced pet food, some owners still prefer to prepare homemade diets for their pets. If a homemade diet is going to be fed, the recipe used must be guaranteed to produce a ration that is complete and balanced. One of the problems with preparing homemade pet food is that many of the available recipes have not been adequately tested for nutrient content and availability. Once an adequate recipe is found, the ingredients that are purchased should conform as closely as possible to the recipe and should be consistent between batches of food. Most recipes allow the owner to prepare a relatively large volume at one time and freeze small portions for extended use. Ingredients should never be substituted or eliminated because of the danger of imbalancing the ration. Pet owners also should be aware of the dangers of feeding single food items in lieu of a prepared diet. Food that owners enjoy is not necessarily the most nutritious food to feed to their pets. Homemade diets can provide adequate nutrition to companion animals provided that a properly formulated recipe is used, the correct ingredients are included, and the recipe is strictly adhered to on a long-term basis.

Evaluation and Selection of an Appropriate Dog Food

Several factors must be considered when choosing a dog food. When fed in proper amounts, the food should provide adequate energy and optimal levels of all of the essential nutrients. The food also must be palatable and acceptable to the dog. Other factors to consider are quality of ingredients, cost and convenience, and the reputation of the manufacturer. The current pet food label provides some, but not all, of this information to the consumer. Additional information provided by some pet food manufacturers also can be used when evaluating and selecting pet food.

Provision of energy and nutrients: Commercially marketed pet food is governed by several agencies. The most influential of these is the AAFCO. AAFCO pet food regulations ensure that nationally marketed pet food is uniformly labeled and nutritionally adequate. A large proportion of AAFCO regulations describe the information that is allowed or prohibited on the pet food label. Although a majority of the states follow AAFCO regulations for pet food, not all states have a mechanism for inspection and enforcement of the regulations. Because of this, buying a pet food that is nationally marketed and sold will ensure that it meets AAFCO labeling regulations.

One of the most important sections of the AAFCO regulations is the Dog Food Nutrient Profile. The profile provides minimum nutrient levels for pet foods that are formulated for growth and reproduction or adult maintenance. Maximum levels are suggested for nutrients that have been shown to have the potential for toxicity or when overuse is a concern. Manufacturers use this profile when formulating pet food to meet the nutritional needs of dogs during various stages of life. The AAFCO profiles are an important starting point when formulating pet food to meet a dog's energy and essential nutrient requirements for different life stages.

Much of the dog food marketed today contains a claim of "complete and balanced nutrition" for either adult maintenance or, most commonly, for all life stages. The phrase "complete and balanced" means that a food contains all of the essential nutrients plus energy at levels that meet the dog's requirements. Essentially, this claim tells pet owners that the food, when fed exclusively, will provide complete nutrition to the dog during all life stages (or for the designated life stage). Because of its importance, AAFCO regulations require that manufacturers substantiate a "complete and balanced" claim by one of two possible methods.

Option one requires that the pet food be successfully evaluated through a series of AAFCO-sanctioned feeding trials. In these cases, the pet food manufacturer will first formulate the food to meet the AAFCO Dog Food Nutrient Profile. Once the food has been manufactured, chemical analysis and feeding trials are used to ensure that the food still meets the needs of dogs. This is the most thorough and desirable method of substantiation. Option two requires only that the food is formulated to meet the minimum and maximum levels of essential nutrients as established in the nutrient profile. Feeding trials are not required when manufacturers choose to use this method. The significance of this difference is that a pet food that has been formulated only to meet AAFCO nutrient profiles (option two) may not actually be complete and balanced when fed. This can occur due to variations in the digestibility and quality of ingredients, and as a result of the loss of nutrients during processing.

In addition, because diets tested in this manner are not fed to dogs, the nutrient profile method cannot assess the palatability or acceptability of the dog food.[8] Therefore, feeding trials with dogs currently are considered to be the most thorough, reliable method for determining nutrient availability in dog food.[9] Consumers can use this information because pet food manufacturers are required to include on the pet food label the method of substantiation that was used. If a statement that AAFCO feeding trials were conducted is included, this means the food was adequately tested through feeding trials with dogs. However, if the statement merely claims that the food meets AAFCO Nutrient Profiles, this signifies that AAFCO feeding tests were not conducted.[10] In all cases, a pet food with a nutrient content that has been substantiated through feeding trials is superior to one that was simply formulated to meet the nutrient profiles.

A dog food's energy density should be considered because it will directly affect the quantity of food that must be fed, and it impacts the ease of maintaining proper growth rates or body condition. Current AAFCO regulations allow, but do not require, pet food manufacturers to include ME values on their labels. As a result, premium products include this information, while many popular brands and generic brands do not. In addition to knowing the caloric density of the pet food, it is also helpful for pet owners to know the relative energy contributions provided by carbohydrate, protein, and fat in the diet. The dietary proportion of fat should be higher for hardworking animals and lower for sedentary adult or elderly animals. Similarly, the proportion of calories supplied by carbohydrate should be increased in diets intended for adult maintenance or for elderly animals.

Digestibility and ingredient quality: Once owners have established that the dog food contains complete nutrition, provides the needed levels of energy, and has been thoroughly tested, other concerns are ingredient quality and the digestibility of the product. The digestibility of a dog food is an important criterion because it directly measures the proportion of nutrients in the food that are available for absorption. Studies of popular brands of dog food reported that the average digestibility coefficients for crude protein, crude fat, and carbohydrate were 81 percent, 85 percent, and 79 percent, respectively.[11] Premium pet food usually has slightly higher digestibility coefficients than these values, and generic products have substantially lower digestibilities.[12] Digestibilities as high as 89 percent, 95 percent, and 88 percent for crude protein, crude fat, and carbohydrate, respectively, can occur in dry-type premium pet food. In general, the ingredients used in pet food are lower in digestibility than they are in most food consumed by humans. As the quality of ingredients included in the food increases, so will the food's dry matter and nutrient digestibility.

A pet food that is low in digestibility contains a high proportion of ingredients that cannot be digested by the enzymes of the gastrointestinal tract. These components pass through to the large intestine, where they are partially or completely fermented by colonic bacteria. Rapid or excessive bacterial fermentation leads to the production of gas (flatulence), loose stools, and, occasionally, diarrhea. In addition to these side effects, a greater quantity of a poorly digested food must be fed to the dog because it is absorbing a smaller proportion of nutrients. As the quantity of food consumed increases, the rate of passage through the gastrointestinal tract also increases. The more rapid passage of food through the intestines further contributes to poor digestibility, high stool volume, and gas production. A pet food's digestibility is decreased by the presence of high levels of dietary fiber, ash, phytate, and poor-quality protein. Improper processing or excessive heat treatment also can adversely affect the digestibility of the diet. In contrast, pet food digestibility is increased by the inclusion of high-quality ingredients, increased levels of fat, and the use of proper processing techniques.

Commercial dog food varies significantly in digestibility and ingredient quality, and it often is difficult for consumers to differentiate between high-quality and moderate- or low-quality ingredients. The labels of two products may have the same ingredient lists and guaranteed analysis panels but, when they are fed, may have substantially different digestibilities. Currently, AAFCO regulations do not allow pet food manufacturers to include quantitative or comparative digestibility claims on their labels. This information can only be obtained by actually feeding the food. Some pet food companies include digestibility data with the literature they provide about their food. However, most popular brands of pet food sold through grocery store chains do not provide information regarding digestibility. If digestibility information is not readily available, this information can be obtained by writing or calling the company directly. Consumers should choose food that has a dry-matter digestibility of 80 percent or greater and should reject any food that has digestibilities lower than 75 percent.

Buying a package of pet food and actually feeding it to a pet also can provide valuable information about a food's digestibility. A highly digestible product will produce low stool volumes and well-formed, firm feces. In addition, the fecal matter will not contain mucus, blood, or any recognizable components of the pet food. Defecation frequency should be relatively low, and bowel movements should be regular and consistent. Normal growth rates and body weight should be easily maintained by the food without the need to feed excessive quantities, and long-term feeding should result in a healthy skin and hair coat. Although these observations do not provide quantitative information about digestibility, they are a reasonably accurate measure of a diet's ability to supply absorbable nutrients to a companion animal.

Palatability and acceptability: All dog owners consider the food's palatability and acceptability because these factors determine whether or not the dog is going to eat the chosen product. Simply put, a dog must be willing to eat an adequate amount of the food to receive the required amount of calories and level of essential nutrients each day. An unpalatable food will be rejected, regardless of the level or balance of nutrients it contains. Similarly, a diet can be palatable but still not contain adequate levels of some nutrients. Contrary to popular belief, dogs are not capable of detecting nutrient deficiencies or imbalances in their diets. They will continue to consume an imbalanced diet until the physiological effects of nutrient deficiencies or excesses cause illness or a reduction in food intake. Because of the marketing value of highly palatable food, most of the products currently sold are highly acceptable to dogs. In fact, problems of overconsumption and weight gain are much more common than are problems of diet rejection. Although palatability is important, it should never be used as the sole criterion when evaluating a food and should not be considered an indication of the food's nutritional adequacy.

Feeding cost: As stated previously, a good rule of thumb when buying a dog food is that "you get what you pay for." Because higher-quality ingredients are more costly than poor-quality ingredients, the price per unit weight of a premium pet food usually is higher than the price of a popular or generic brand. When making price comparisons between foods, the cost of actually feeding the food should be considered rather than the cost per unit weight. The cost per serving of a high-quality product often is equal to or lower than that of an inferior product because a smaller quantity of the high-quality pet food is fed. When evaluating a food for the first time, owners should record the purchase date and the price of the food. When the package is empty, dividing the cost of the product by the number of days the bag lasted will provide the cost per day to feed that particular food. A second product with the same net weight can then be compared in the same manner. An alternate solution is to calculate the cost of feeding the food each day based on the quantity that is fed (Table 17.2).

TABLE 17.2   Calculating the Cost/Day of Feeding

	# Cups/Day		# Oz/Cup		Total Oz/Day	Price/Lb	Cost/Day
Dog Food # 1	4	×	3.5	=	14.0	35¢	30¢
Dog Food # 2	3	×	3.0	=	9.0	55¢	31¢

Reputation of the manufacturer: The reputation of the pet food manufacturer should always be considered when selecting a pet food. Companies that have a national reputation for producing consistent, high-quality products and devoting resources to consumer education about proper nutrition for companion animals should be selected. The inclusion of a toll-free phone number on the product's package indicates a company that welcomes inquiries about its products. In addition, the manufacturer's response to all inquiries should be timely, thorough, and direct. A pet food manufacturer should be expected to readily supply information about the pet food's level of testing, digestibility data, ME content, and nutrient content. Pet food manufacturers that produce quality products are concerned with their reputations and with serving the needs and concerns of the pet owners who buy their pet food. This concern will be evidenced by the company's accessibility to consumers and its response to questions about its products.

The overall best judge of a commercial pet food is the animal itself. Once a pet food has been evaluated and selected, pet owners should feed the product for a minimum of 2 months before evaluating its total effect on their dog's health. A diet that provides good nutrition and adequate energy will support normal weight gain or weight maintenance, healthy skin, a shiny and healthy coat, normal fecal volume and consistency, and overall vitality in the pet. Signs of a poor diet include weight loss or poor growth, poor coat quality, the development of skin problems, and a lack of vigor. Whenever any of these signs are observed, a thorough examination by a veterinarian should be conducted. Although changing the diet may be warranted, other medical causes of these problems should always be investigated.

Conclusions

A large variety of dog food is available to pet owners today. Consumers first must select from either dry, semimoist, canned, or homemade food. Commercial pet food can be further evaluated according to the level of testing that has been conducted, the type of ingredients that are included, and the food's digestibility, palatability, and cost. Choosing an appropriate dog food is also dependent on the dog's age, stage of life, and activity level. The following chapter examines nutritional needs of dogs during different stages of life and activity levels, and provides information for selecting appropriate food for dogs throughout their lives.

Cited References

1. Harlow, J. **U.S. pet food trends.** Proceedings of the Pet Food Forum, Watts Publishing, Chicago, Illinois, pp.355-364. (1997)

2. Lewis, L.D., Morris, M.L., and Hand, M.S. **Pet foods.** In: *Small Animal Clinical Nutrition,* third edition, Mark Morris Associates, Topeka, Kansas, pp. 2-1 to 2-28. (1987)

3. Samuelson, A.C. and Cutter, G.R. **Dog biscuits: An aid in canine tartar control.** Journal of Nutrition, 121:S162. (1991)

4. Association of American Feed Control Officials. **Pet Food Regulations.** In: AAFCO Official Publication, The Association of Feed Control Officials, Atlanta, Georgia. (1998)

5. Morgan, T. **Treat trends.** Petfood Industry, September/October, pp. 32-37. (1997)

6. Sousa, C.A., Stannard, A.A., and Ihrke, P.J. **Dermatosis associated with feeding generic dog food: 13 cases (1981–1982).** Journal of the American Veterinary Medical Association, 192:676–680. (1988)

7. Huber, T.L., Wilson, R.C., and McGarity, S.A. **Variations in digestibility of dry dog foods with identical label guaranteed analysis.** Journal of the American Animal Hospital Association, 22:571–575. (1986)

8. Dzanis, D.A. **Complete and balanced? Substantiating the nutritional adequacy of pet foods: Past, present and future.** Petfood Industry, July/August, pp. 22-27. (1997)

9. Deshmukh, A.R. **Regulatory aspects of pet foods.** Veterinary Clinical Nutrition, 3:4-9. (1996)

10. Morris, J.G. and Rogers, Q.R. **Evaluation of commercial pet foods.** Tijdschrehund Diergeneesk, 1:67S–70S. (1991)

11. Kendall, P.T., Holme, D.W., and Smith, P.M. **Methods of prediction of the digestible energy content of dog foods from gross energy value, proximate analysis and digestible nutrient content.** Journal of Science and Food Agriculture, 3:823–828. (1982)

12. Kallfelz, F.A. **Evaluation and use of pet foods: General considerations in using pet foods for adult maintenance.** Veterinary Clinics of North America: Small Animal Practice, 19:387–403. (1989)

18 Feeding Management throughout the Life Cycle

THE PREVIOUS CHAPTERS in Part 4 examined the nutrient and energy requirements of dogs and the types of pet food that are available to pet owners. In addition, practical feeding information is necessary to provide optimal nutrition and aid in the selection of pet food for various stages during a dog's life. This chapter reviews several methods of feeding and provides guidelines for feeding healthy dogs throughout the life stages of growth, adult maintenance, reproduction, periods of hard work, and old age.

Feeding Behavior

The dog has inherited its eating proclivities and behaviors from its wild relative *Canis lupus* (see Chapter 1). Most wolf sub-species live as cooperative hunters, obtaining their food by working together as a pack. Cooperative hunting behaviors allow wolves to prey on large game that would be unavailable to an animal hunting alone. This type of hunting leads to intermittent eating patterns in which wolves gorge themselves immediately after a kill then do not eat again for an extended period. Competition between members of the pack at the site of a kill also contributes to rapid food consumption, called **social facilitation**. When a large kill is made, wolves hoard pieces of food in caches for consumption later. The domestic dog, *Canis familiaris*, has inherited the wolves' eating behaviors. Like wolves, most dogs eat rapidly and consume more food in the presence of another dog or when fed as a group. Some dogs also develop the habit of burying or hiding pieces of food in the home or yard. Although many dogs never return to these caches, it is believed that this behavior has its origins in the hoarding behaviors of wolves.

For most dogs, rapid eating is not a problem. It is not unusual or abnormal for a dog to consume an entire meal within a few minutes. Gorging behavior should only be considered a problem if it presents a danger of choking, if large amounts of air are swallowed, or if the dog repeatedly overconsumes. Feeding a diet that consists primarily of canned food occasionally leads to rapid eating because of the palatability and texture of a food. Switching to a dry food often solves this problem. If a dog repeatedly attempts to eat dry food too quickly, adding water to the diet immediately before feeding decreases the rate of eating and minimizes the chance of swallowing large amounts of air. Dogs often overconsume food if they are fed in the presence of other dogs in the household. This social facilitation can easily be controlled by feeding dogs in separate areas, training dogs not to eat out of each other's bowls, or feeding dogs at different times.

Feeding Regimens

Several types of feeding regimens are appropriate for dogs. The method that is used often depends on the owner's daily schedule, the dog's life stage, and the acceptability of the regimen to the dog. Meal feeding involves limiting either the quantity of food offered at each meal or the amount of time the dog is allowed access to food. Free-choice feeding (also called ad libitum feeding) involves providing a continual supply of food and allowing the dog to self-regulate the amount it consumes each day.

Meal feeding: Meal feeding using controlled portion sizes is the preferred method to use when owners wish to carefully monitor the amount of food their dog receives each day. This is most important during growth, periods of hard work, and gestation and lactation. One or more meals is provided per day, and portions are premeasured to meet the dog's daily energy needs. Although some adult dogs can be maintained on one meal per day, most adjust best to two or three meals. This reduces hunger between meals and minimizes food-associated behavior problems such as begging and stealing food. A distinct advantage of portion-controlled feeding is the owner can control the pet's food consumption and will immediately observe any changes in food intake or eating behavior. The dog's growth and weight can be strictly controlled by adjusting either the amount of food or the type of food that is fed. As a result, conditions of underweight, overweight, or inappropriate growth rate can be easily prevented. In most households, the dog is fed one meal in the morning and a second meal in the early evening. Owners can initially use the guidelines for feeding that are provided on the pet food label to determine amounts to feed. Ultimately, however, the dog's growth rate, weight, and body condition are the best guides to use when determining the quantity to provide at each meal.

Time-controlled feeding is a form of meal feeding that relies on the dog's ability to self-regulate daily energy intake. At designated meal times, a surplus of food is provided and the dog is allowed to eat for a predetermined period of time. Most adult dogs who are in a state of maintenance and are not working hard will consume enough food to meet their daily needs within 10 to 20 minutes. As with portion-controlled feeding, one meal per day can be sufficient for feeding some adult dogs, but providing two meals per day is healthier and more satisfying for the dog. While time-controlled feeding is more convenient, this regimen is not recommended for growing dogs (especially those of the large and giant breeds) or for dogs who have a tendency to overconsume. A dog who eats voraciously throughout the allotted time period, apparently learning to "beat the clock," is obviously a better candidate for portion-controlled meal feeding. At the other end of the spectrum are dogs who are very slow eaters or "nibblers" and who will not consume enough food within the allotted time period. For these dogs, free-choice feeding is often the best regimen to use.

Free-choice feeding: Free-choice feeding relies upon a dog's ability to self-regulate food intake so that energy and nutrient needs are met every day. Lactating females, dogs who are working hard, and dogs who are slow or poor eaters often can be fed free-choice. Dogs who are fed free-choice usually eat several small meals throughout the day. This tendency can be a distinct advantage for dogs who do not readily eat enough to meet their energy needs when fed only one or two meals per day. In contrast, a free-choice regimen is not a good method for growing dogs or for dogs who have a tendency to over-consume and gain weight. Dry pet food is most suitable for this feeding regimen because expanded foods do not spoil as quickly as canned products. Whatever type of food is fed, the food bowl or dispenser should be cleaned and refilled with fresh food daily.

Compared with meal feeding, free-choice feeding requires the least amount of work and knowledge on the part of the owner. The food and water supply is replenished only one time per day, and it is not necessary to determine the exact volume to feed. Free-choice feeding can be beneficial in kennel settings because it minimizes the noise associated with meal time, helps relieve boredom, and may help minimize undesirable behaviors such as coprophagy and excessive barking. However, at the same time, problems such as anorexia or overconsumption can go undetected in dogs who are fed ad libitum. If a dog is sick, a change in feed intake may not be noticed until the dog has lost substantial weight. The opposite situation, overconsumption and the development of obesity, is fairly common in pets who are fed free-choice. Although almost all animals are capable of eating to meet their caloric needs, the regulatory mechanisms that control food intake can be overridden if an animal is leading a relatively sedentary lifestyle and if a highly palatable, energy-dense pet food is fed. In these cases, portion-controlled meal feeding or the selection of a less energy-dense food is warranted.

What to Feed (Overview)

Methods for selecting and evaluating dog foods are discussed in detail in Chapter 17. Owners have a choice of feeding a commercially prepared food or a homemade formula. Most pet owners prefer the convenience, cost-effectiveness, and reliability of feeding a commercial dog food. The decision of whether to feed a canned, semimoist, or dry commercial pet food can be made with an understanding of the advantages and disadvantages of each type of food. If a homemade diet is fed, care must be taken to ensure that a complete and balanced ration is prepared and that there is consistency of ingredients between batches of food. Important factors to consider when selecting a commercial dog food include the dog's age, stage of life, lifestyle, and activity level. Factors about the food that are important include its nutrient content and quality of ingredients, energy density, palatability, and reputation of the manufacturer. The food should support normal gastrointestinal tract functioning and should produce regular, firm, and well-formed stools. Most important, the long-term effects of feeding the food should support vitality and health, good coat quality, healthy skin condition, and proper body physique and muscle tone (Table 18.1).

TABLE 18.1   Factors to Consider When Selecting a Dog Food

Dog's Characteristics	Food Attributes
Age (puppy, adult, working adult, geriatric)	**Nutritional Adequacy** (feeding trials vs. nutrient profiles)
Stage of Life (growth, maintenance, gestating, lactating)	**Ingredients** (meat-based or plant-based, quality, digestibility)
Lifestyle (indoor dog, kennel dog, lives with other dogs)	**Energy Density** (ME content; caloric distribution)
Activity Level (sedentary, low activity, moderate activity, hard work)	**Palatability and Acceptablity**
	Reputation of the Manufacturer
Health (allergies, presence of chronic disease)	**Cost and Availability**

How Much to Feed?

The best determinant of the amount of food to feed is the dog itself. As discussed previously, food intake in all animals is governed principally by energy requirements. When dogs are successfully fed free-choice, the underlying control over the amount of food consumed is primarily the need for energy. When dogs are fed on a portion-controlled basis, owners should select a quantity of food based primarily on the pet's weight and body condition. If the dog gains too much weight (energy surplus), the amount fed should be decreased. Conversely, if weight is lost, an increased amount of food is provided. Commercial pet food that is formulated for particular life stages or lifestyles also is formulated to contain the proper amount of essential nutrients when a quantity is fed that meets the dog's energy requirements. Balancing energy density with nutrient content ensures that when a dog's caloric needs are met, its needs for all other essential nutrients will be

TABLE 18.2   Determining the Amount to Feed

20-lb Dog (9 kg) Active Boston Terrier	60-lb Dog (27 kg) Very Active Labrador Retriever
ME Requirement = $145 \times (9 \text{ kg})^{0.67}$ = **632 kcal/day**	ME Requirement = $200 \times (27 \text{ kg})^{0.67}$ = **1,820 kcal/day**
Feeding: Adult Maintenance Diet **(ME = 3,500 kcal/kg)**	Feeding: Performance Diet **(ME = 4,200 kcal/kg)**
Kg per Day: 632/3,500 = **180 g (6.4 oz)**	Kg per Day: 1,820/4,200 = **433 g (15.25 oz)**
1 Cup of Food = **3.0 oz**	1 Cup of Food = **3.5 oz**
Amount to Feed: 6.4/3.0 = **2.1 cups**	Amount to Feed: 15.25/3.5 = **4.4 cups**
This dog should receive approximately 2 cups of the adult maintenance diet each day.	**This dog should receive approximately 4½ cups of the performance diet each day.**

met by the same quantity of food. Therefore, the best way to determine how much to feed a particular animal is to first estimate the animal's energy needs then calculate the amount of an appropriate dog food that must be fed to meet that need (Table 18.2).

A number of factors affects a dog's energy requirement. These factors include age, reproductive status, body condition, level of activity, breed, temperament, and environmental conditions (see Chapter 6). When determining energy requirement, these factors are accounted for by adding or subtracting calories from the calculated maintenance energy requirement. The guidelines that are included on the commercial pet food label also can be used as an initial starting point when estimating a volume to feed. All pet foods that carry the complete and balanced claim are required to include feeding instructions on the product label. These guidelines usually provide estimates of the quantity to feed for several different ranges in body size. However, dog owners must keep in mind that pet food companies are in the business of selling dog food. In general, package guidelines tend to overestimate the needs of most dogs. Adjustments in these estimates should be made based on calculated energy requirements and on the dog's response to feeding.

Feeding during Growth

Puppies should be fully weaned and ready to be placed in their new home when they are between 7 and 8 weeks of age (see Chapter 7). This is an ideal time for puppies to enter their new home because this age is still within primary socialization (5 to 12 weeks). Proper feeding and nutrition are essential during this time period because puppies experience rapid growth and development during the first 6 months of life. By the time a dog reaches maturity, birth weight has increased forty- to fiftyfold. The rate at which dogs grow and the age they reach maturity is dependent on their breed and adult size. Large and giant breeds attain mature size when they are between 12 and 18 months of age, while small and toy breeds reach adult size at a younger age, usually between 7 and 12 months.[1] The enormous amount of growth and development that occurs during a relatively short period of time translates to high energy requirements in growing dogs. From weaning until about 6 months of age, the energy needs of growing puppies are approximately twice those of an adult dog of the same weight. After 6 months of age, energy requirements begin to decrease as the rate of growth declines. A general guideline suggests that a young dog's energy intake should be approximately two times its maintenance level until 40 percent of adult weight has been reached. At this point, intake should be decreased to approximately 1.6 times maintenance level, and further decreased to 1.2 times maintenance level when the dog has reached 80 percent of its adult size (Table 18.3).[2,3]

When expressed on a percent basis, the protein requirement of growing puppies is only slightly higher than the protein requirement of adults. This increase is caused by the need for protein to build new tissues associated with

TABLE 18.3   Feeding a Growing Dog (Labrador Retriever)

Puppy (10 Weeks: 15 lb)	Adolescent (5 months: 36 lb)	Young Adult (8½ months: 55 lb)	Adult (active: 70 lb)
Needs: 2 × Maintenance	Needs: 1.6 × Maintenance	Needs: 1.2 × Maintenance	Needs: 1 × Maintenance
ME Requirement = $145 \times (6.82 \text{ kg})^{0.67}$ = **525 kcal/day**	ME Requirement = $145 \times (16.4 \text{ kg})^{0.67}$ = **945 kcal/day**	ME Requirement = $145 \times (25 \text{ kg})^{0.67}$ = **1,253 kcal/day**	ME Requirement = $145 \times (31.8 \text{ kg})^{0.67}$ = **1,472 kcal/day**
2×525 = **1,049 kcal/day**	1.6×945 = **1,512 kcal/day**	$1.2 \times 1,253$ = **1,504 kcal/day**	**1,472 kcal/day**
Diet ME = 4,000 kcal/kg	Diet ME = 4,000 kcal/kg	Diet ME = 4,000 kcal/kg	Diet ME = 4,000 kcal/kg
Kg per Day: 1,049/4,000 = **262 g (9.2 oz)**	Kg per Day: 1,512/4,000 = **378 g (13.4 oz)**	Kg per Day: 1,504/4,000 = **376 g (13.2 oz)**	Kg per Day: 1,472/4,000 = **368 g (12.9 oz)**
1 Cup of Food = 3.5 oz	1 Cup of Food = 3.5 oz	1 Cup of Food = 3.5 oz	1 Cup of Food = 3.5 oz
Amount to Feed: 9.2/3.5 = ~ 2½ **cups**	Amount to Feed: 13.4/3.5 = ~ 4 **cups**	Amount to Feed: 13.2/3.5 = ~ 3¾ **cups**	Amount to Feed: 13.2/3.5 = ~ 3½ **cups**

growth. Because young dogs consume higher amounts of energy and thus higher total quantities of food than adults, they concomitantly consume the needed amounts of extra protein. This is why the actual proportion of the diet provided by protein is only slightly higher for puppies than adult dogs. (This relationship is true for other essential nutrients as well.) The protein included in puppy foods should be of high quality and very digestible. This ensures that sufficient levels of all the essential amino acids will be absorbed for use in growth and development. The minimum proportion of energy that should be supplied by protein in the diet for a growing dog is 22 percent of the ME kilocalories.[4] This corresponds to 22 percent by weight of a food containing 3,500 kcal/kg or 25 percent protein in a food containing 4,000 kcal/kg. Typical high-quality commercial puppy food contains between 26 percent and 30 percent protein and 3,700 and 4,200 kcal/kg.

Because of the important role of calcium and phosphorus in skeletal development, these minerals are often a focus of concern to owners and professionals. However, contrary to popular belief, diets containing high levels of calcium and phosphorus should not be fed to growing dogs, nor should growing dogs be supplemented with either of these nutrients.[5] The Association of American Feed Control Officials (AAFCO) Nutrient Profiles recommend that dog food formulated for growth contains a minimum of 1.0 percent calcium and 0.8 percent phosphorus on a dry-matter basis.[4] Many commercially available pet foods contain slightly more than these levels and so will supply more than adequate amounts of calcium and phosphorus to growing pets.[6] Feeding excessive amounts of calcium through either diet or supplementation is unnecessary and may contribute to the development of certain skeletal disorders in large and giant breeds of dogs.[7]

Young puppies should be fed a pet food guaranteed to be nutritionally adequate for growth or for all stages of life that has been proved by the AAFCO feeding trials (see Chapter 17). Because most of the growing dog's additional nutrient needs are readily supplied by the increased quantity of food the animal consumes, the proportion of most essential nutrients in the diet need not be much higher than those found in diets formulated for adult maintenance. However, because growing dogs need to consume higher quantities of food, the diet's digestibility and energy density are important considerations. Puppies and growing dogs have less digestive capacity, smaller mouths, and smaller and fewer teeth than adults. As a result, they are limited in the amount of food that can be consumed and digested in a single meal. If the diet is poorly digestible or has low energy and nutrient density, a larger quantity must be consumed. In this situation, the limits of the dog's stomach may be reached before adequate nutrients and energy have been consumed. The long-term result can be compromised growth and impaired muscle and skeletal development. Young dogs benefit from eating a food that is energy- and nutrient-dense because the volume of food intake need not be excessive and intake will not be limited by the size of the animal's stomach.

Growing dogs should be fed amounts of food that will support normal muscle and skeletal development and a typical rate of growth for the dog's particular breed. Feeding for a "plump" body condition or for maximal growth rate should be avoided. Providing too many calories early in life can lead to increased number of fat cells and may predispose to obesity later in life.[8] Growing dogs should be lean and well muscled, with their ribs easily felt but not seen. Growing dogs also should be fed to attain a growth rate that is average, rather than maximal, for the dog's particular breed. Rapid growth rates have been shown to be incompatible with optimal skeletal development and may predispose dogs to skeletal diseases such as canine hip dysplasia or osteochondrosis (see Chapter 12). This is of special concern in large and giant breeds of dogs, which generally exhibit a higher incidence of developmental bone disorders. Feeding growing dogs moderately restricted levels of a well-balanced diet does not affect final body size and will positively impact skeletal and muscular development.[9]

These feeding goals are best achieved through portion-controlled feeding and the frequent assessment of weight gain and body condition. Three to four premeasured meals per day should be provided until dogs are 5 to 6 months of age, after which two meals per day should be fed. As adults, dogs can be fed one or two meals per day. However, most dogs, especially the large breeds, adapt best to two meals per day.

Feeding for Adult Maintenance

Mature adult dogs who are not working hard or reproducing are said to be in a state of maintenance. This category includes most dogs who are kept as companions in the United States today. Primary nutritional concerns for feeding dogs during maintenance are providing optimal nutrition to promote health and longevity, and feeding to prevent overweight and obese conditions. Adult dogs should be fed a high-quality food formulated for maintenance or for all life stages of adults that has been proved nutritionally adequate through AAFCO feeding trials. Although canned, semimoist, or dry food can be fed, dry food often is preferred for this stage of life. Dry dog food is slightly less energy-dense and can help maintain proper tooth and gum hygiene.[10]

In addition to monitoring food intake, providing daily exercise to adult dogs maintains body condition and promotes health. Exercise can be in the form of daily walks or runs or several sessions of vigorous games such as fetch or hide-and-seek. Swimming is also an excellent form of exercise for dogs. Most dogs enjoy swimming if introduced to water at an early age and in a gradual manner. Monitoring an adult dog's daily food intake is best accomplished through portion-controlled feeding, but free-choice feeding can be used if the dog is able to self-regulate and maintain normal body weight. Fresh water should be available at all times.

Feeding during Gestation and Lactation

Pregnancy and lactation are periods of high physiological stress for female dogs. Increased energy and nutrients are needed for fetal growth during gestation and for milk production during lactation. The first 5 weeks of the 9-week gestation period is a time of rapid fetal development without any substantial increase in fetal size. As a result, there is only a slight increase in the dam's weight and nutritional needs.[11] The fetuses begin to grow in size after the fifth week, resulting in increased energy and nutrient needs in the mother. After 5 weeks of gestation, the bitch's food intake should be increased gradually so that at the time of whelping her daily intake is approximately 25 percent to 50 percent more than her maintenance intake. The total increase necessary depends on the size of the litter, and the age, size, and condition of the mother. A good rule of thumb is that the bitch's body weight should increase by approximately 15 percent to 20 percent and no more than 25 percent at the time of whelping.

It is most advantageous to begin feeding a high-quality, highly digestible food suitable for gestation and lactation at the time of breeding. Dog foods that contain highly digestible ingredients and increased nutrient density are appropriate. These foods are capable of supplying the extra energy and nutrients needed during reproduction without excess food consumption. Changing to this diet early during a female's reproductive cycle allows her to be fully adjusted to the new food when breeding takes place and prevents the need to abruptly change diets during either gestation or lactation. Food should be provided in several small meals per day. This is especially important during the last 2 to 3 weeks of gestation because the developing puppies will be infringing on abdominal space, making it uncomfortable for the mother to consume large meals. Many females become anorexic during the last day prior to whelping. This is a normal occurrence and should not be of concern unless anorexia persists beyond 24 hours. After whelping, the mother should be provided with fresh water and food. Most bitches will begin eating within 24 hours after whelping. If necessary, the mother's appetite can be stimulated by moistening her food with warm water. This also ensures that adequate fluid is consumed, which will be important for normal milk production.

Energy and water are the two nutrients of greatest concern during lactation. Ample energy intake allows sufficient milk production and prevents drastic weight loss from occurring during peak lactation. Adequate water intake is necessary for the production of a sufficient volume of milk. The nutritional demands of lactation are influenced by the bitch's nutritional status and weight at the time of whelping and the size of the litter. Dogs with large litters and with minimal body energy stores at parturition are at greatest risk for excessive weight loss and malnourishment during lactation. Peak lactation occurs when the puppies are 3 to 4 weeks old and corresponds to the highest energy needs of the bitch. After this time, milk production begins to decline as the puppies are slowly weaned onto solid food.

Depending on the size of the litter, a bitch will require up to two to three times her maintenance energy requirement during lactation. A general guideline is to feed 1.5 times maintenance during the first week of lactation, two times maintenance during the second week, and 2.5 to three times maintenance during the third to fourth week of lactation.[12] Peak lactation at 3 to 4 weeks postpartum is followed by the introduction of solid or semisolid food to the puppies. After the fourth week, the amount of mother's milk consumed by the puppies will decrease as their solid food intake gradually increases.

If a highly digestible, nutrient-dense diet is fed during gestation, this diet should be continued throughout lactation. The energy density of the diet is an important consideration during lactation because of the high energy needs of the bitch during this time. A primary goal of feeding lactating females is to prevent excessive weight loss during peak lactation. Studies have shown that diets with low energy densities (3,200 kcal/kg) can result in excessive weight loss in females, even when they are allowed to consume the food on an ad libitum basis.[13] In addition to causing weight loss in the mother, energy deficiency during lactation may also affect the quantity of milk that is produced. Decreased milk quantity can lead to impaired puppy growth and development. Therefore, a diet with an energy density of 4,000 to 4,400 kcal/kg is recommended for this demanding stage of life. Several small meals should be provided each day, and the mother should be fed separately from the litter to ensure that she (and not her puppies) has access to adequate amounts of food. Fresh, clean water should be available at all times, as the bitch's water intake will be very high during lactation.

By 3 to 4 weeks of age, puppies begin to become interested in solid food. After 4 weeks, as the bitch's interest in nursing begins to naturally decline and as the puppies begin to consume semisolid then solid food, the mother's daily food intake should be slowly reduced. By the time the puppies are of weaning age (7 to 8 weeks), the dam's food consumption should be less than 50 percent above her normal maintenance needs. Complete weaning will take place around 6 to 8 weeks, and puppies usually are consuming the major portion of their diet from solid food by the time they are 6 weeks of age. If the mother continues to produce milk immediately before weaning, several days of limited feeding will aid in decreasing her production of milk.

Weaning Puppies

At birth, it is important that puppies suckle from their mother as soon as possible to ensure they consume an adequate quantity of **colostrum**. Colostrum is a special form of milk that contains immunoglobulins and other protective factors that provide passive immunity against infectious diseases to puppies. Most of the immune factors in colostrum are large, intact protein molecules. The intestinal mucosa of newborn puppies is capable of absorbing intact immunoglobulins for only the first 24 to 48 hours after birth. After this time period, normal digestive processes begin to cause the complete digestion of these compounds, making them unavailable to the body as immune mediators. Therefore, it is vitally important that newborn puppies receive adequate colostrum during the first 24 hours of life.

Like the milk of many mammalian species, the milk of dogs changes during lactation to effectively meet the needs of their developing young. Several days after parturition, the composition of milk changes from colostrum to mature milk. During the first two weeks of life, puppies will nurse at least four to six times per day and spend a great deal of their time sleeping. Puppies survive exclusively on their mother's milk for the first 3 to 4 weeks of life. After that time, bitch's milk can no longer supply enough energy or essential nutrients for the rapidly growing puppies. At this age, puppies should be gradually introduced to supplemental food. The food should be a thick gruel made by mixing a small amount of warm water with the bitch's food or with the chosen puppy food. Cow's milk should not be used to make the gruel because it has a high lactose content and may cause diarrhea. The semisolid gruel should be provided in a shallow dish and puppies allowed to feed several times per day. At first, little food will be consumed, and the puppies' major food source will still be their mother's milk. However, by 4 1/2 weeks of age, the puppies will be readily consuming semisolid food. By 5 to 6 weeks of age, puppies are able to chew and consume dry food. Nutritional weaning usually is complete by 6 weeks of age, although some bitches will continue to allow their puppies to nurse until they are 7 to 8 weeks of age or older. Complete weaning (behavioral weaning) is not complete until puppies are at least 7 to 8 weeks of age.

Feeding Working Dogs

Although the majority of dogs that live in the United States today are kept as house pets, a substantial number of dogs also work with their owners or handlers in a variety of professions. These include guide dogs for the blind, hearing ear dogs, service dogs, sled dogs, livestock-herding dogs, livestock-guarding dogs, protection dogs, and hunting dogs (see Chapter 2). The type of training, level of exercise, and daily routine a dog experiences will vary with the type of work. In general, all working dogs have higher energy requirements than adult dogs during periods of normal maintenance. Depending on the type and intensity of work, modifications in the nutrient composition of the diet and changes in the daily feeding regimen of the working dog may be necessary.

The major concern when feeding working dogs is their increased need for energy. The energy requirement of a working dog is dependent on the environment, the duration and intensity of the exercise, and the dog's body composition and temperament. A general guideline suggests that energy needs increase to between 1.5 and 2.5 times maintenance requirements in dogs that are working in ambient temperatures. Working in cold weather can further increase energy needs by an additional 50 percent or more. It is generally accepted that sled dogs training in cold environments have higher energy needs than any other type of working dog. In fact, recent data collected from sled dogs racing as a team in the Alaskan bush showed that a working sled dog consumed more than 9,000 kcal per day! It is important to realize that these are extreme working conditions, in which the dogs are well conditioned and are running hard in cold conditions for long periods of time. Other types of prolonged work such as guarding, herding, aiding the disabled, and scenting for drugs or explosives will not cause such enormous increases in energy requirement. When feeding working dogs, it is important that the precise level and frequency of the animal's work are accurately assessed. Commercial diets formulated for performance are invariably energy-dense and highly palatable. Overfeeding this type of ration or feeding it to a dog who is not working hard enough to need it can lead to a loss of condition and the development of obesity.

Although it is generally accepted that energy is the nutrient of most concern for working dogs, there has been much debate about the best way to provide energy in diets formulated for performance. Carbohydrate and fat are the major sources of energy in food. In the dog, approximately 70 percent to 90 percent of the energy for sustained work is derived from fat metabolism, and only a small amount of energy is derived from carbohydrate metabolism.[17,18] Although human athletic performance and stamina are related to muscle glycogen stores and the ability to mobilize glycogen for energy, this does not seem to be as important in dogs. Results of field studies with sled dogs and laboratory studies with beagles suggest that the ability to use fatty acids may be more important than the use of muscle glycogen during strenuous exercise in this species.[19,20] These studies also showed that performance level in dogs is positively correlated with intake of digestible fat.

A diet's energy density and digestibility appear to be the two most important nutritional factors affecting performance in working dogs. Fat contributes a readily available, important energy source for working muscles. Equally important are the quality and digestibility of the nutrients in the diet. A dog with increased energy needs must consume a great deal of food to meet those needs. If the diet is low in digestibility, a large amount of dry matter must be ingested to meet total energy needs. The amount of dry matter that can be consumed during a meal will be limited by a working dog's gastric capacity and ability to digest and assimilate a large volume of food. High digestibility is necessary to limit the total amount of food the dog must consume at each meal. Because of their lower energy densities, maintenance diets may become bulk limiting and limit performance. Highly digestible, high-fat diets can supply the extra energy needed by working dogs and contribute positively to endurance performance.

A source of starch is also beneficial in the diets of working dogs to maintain normal muscle and liver glycogen levels. However, the carbohydrate in these diets must also be highly digestible, and its concentration should not be high enough to limit the energy density of the ration by replacing fat.

Water consumption is extremely important for all working dogs. Dogs lose water primarily through respiration and, to a much lesser degree, through perspiration. These water losses can increase by 10- to 20-fold during exercise.[21] All working dogs should be provided with fresh water at frequent intervals throughout a session of work. Even mild dehydration can lead to reduced work capacity, decreased strength, and hyperthermia.[22] Cool water should be provided because it is more palatable to most dogs, and it is more effective in helping to cool the body.

Portion-controlled meal feeding should always be the method of feeding used with working dogs. This allows careful attention to the amount that is fed and to the dog's response to feeding. Several small meals should be provided each day to prevent the consumption of a large volume of food at one time. The majority of the dog's daily food intake should be consumed after the longest period of exercise during the day to allow adequate digestion of food. When dogs are working for long periods of time, such as endurance sledding or hunting, feeding small snacks during the event may be beneficial. If the dog is adapted to a high-fat endurance diet, feeding a high-fat/high-protein snack during endurance performance is recommended.

Feeding Geriatric Dogs

Improvements in the control of infectious diseases and in the nutrition and health care of the domestic dog have resulted in a gradual increase in the average life span of companion animals. The maximum life span of the dog is estimated to be about 27 years, and the current average life span is approximately 13 years.[14] In general, the large and giant breeds of dogs have a shorter life span than the small and toy breeds. Some of the giant breeds, such as Great Danes and Irish Wolfhounds may have life spans as short as 6 or 7 years. These differences, plus the variability of aging between individuals, require that older animals be assessed as individuals, using functional changes in body systems rather than chronological age to categorize them with the elderly population.

Providing optimal nutrition during the geriatric years is essential for preventing or minimizing effects of chronic disease, maintaining proper body weight, and supporting vitality and health. One of the primary changes that occur with aging is a decline in a dog's resting metabolic rate (RMR). This is caused primarily by the natural decrease in lean body tissue that occurs with age. In addition, most dogs voluntarily reduce their physical activity as they become older. As a result, total daily energy requirements of older dogs may decrease by as much as 30 percent to 40 percent.[15] In addition to normal metabolic changes with age, the presence of chronic disease can present an additional nutritional challenge to geriatric dogs. Chronic renal disease is a leading cause of death in old dogs and is a major cause of chronic illness. Heart disease, diabetes mellitus, and cancer are other diseases that are more common in older pets. Dietary changes often can be helpful in relieving symptoms or decreasing progression of some of these diseases (see Chapter 19).

Aging dogs have a need for the same nutrients that were required during earlier physiological states and do not have requirements for any unique nutrients that are not needed earlier in life. However, the quantities of nutrients and the energy required per unit of body weight may change, and the way in which nutrients are provided to the pet may require modification. Such changes often depend on the presence or degree of degenerative disease. Nutrients that may be of specific concern in aging dogs are energy, protein, and fat.

Elderly pets will vary greatly in their energy needs, depending on individual temperament, the presence of degenerative disease, and the amount of daily exercise the dog receives. Caloric intake should be carefully monitored in older dogs to ensure adequate intake of calories and nutrients, while preventing the development of obesity. Protein intake is also of concern. The decrease in lean body mass that occurs with aging results in a loss of the protein reserves that normally can be used by the body during reaction to stress and illness. Older animals are subject to a high incidence of disease and stress and are, therefore, especially vulnerable if their ability to react is compromised. It is important that geriatric dogs are provided with high-quality protein at a level sufficient to supply the essential amino acids needed for body maintenance and to minimize losses of lean body tissue. Aging dogs should be fed diets with a lower percentage of calories from protein than those used for growth but with higher than the minimum necessary for adult maintenance.[16] Contrary to popular belief, dietary protein should not be restricted for healthy older dogs. It also has been theorized that the increase in the percentage of body fat that occurs with aging is partially a result of an increasing inability to metabolize lipids.[17] Slightly decreasing the amount of fat in the diet may benefit geriatric dogs, provided that the fat that remains in the diet is both highly digestible and rich in essential fatty acids.

The primary goals of feeding and care of geriatric dogs are to promote health, maintain normal body weight, slow or prevent the development of chronic disease, and minimize or improve clinical signs of diseases that may already be present. A diet that is moderate to low in energy density, but which still contains high-quality ingredients, especially high-quality, highly digestible protein should be selected. Generally, a dry dog food with 3,500 to

3,800 kcal/kg, 24 percent to 28 percent high-quality protein, and 10 percent to 12 percent fat is recommended. Optimal body weight can be maintained and obesity prevented through the judicious control of intake using portion-controlled meal feeding. A regular exercise schedule is also very important because it helps older pets maintain body weight, muscle tone, and vitality. Fresh water should be available at all times to older dogs. Proper care of the teeth and gums is also important for the geriatric pet. If an owner is unable or unwilling to regularly examine and brush the pet's teeth, yearly descaling by a veterinarian is necessary to prevent buildup of dental calculus and the development of periodontal disease. Dental problems can lead to decreased food intake, anorexia, and systemic disease if not treated promptly in older animals.

General Feeding Guidelines

The most important guideline for feeding dogs is that every dog should be evaluated and fed as an individual. Selecting a food based on the dog's age, life stage, living environment, and level of activity aids in providing optimal nutrition throughout life. Overall, a dog's response to a food in terms of vitality, health, body composition, and skin and coat condition provide the best assessment of a diet (Table 18.4). In addition to their dog's food, many owners enjoy feeding their dogs additional foods and treats. If table scraps and treats constitute only a small portion of the dog's daily diet, they will not imbalance the diet or cause harm. However, in some cases, ideas about what a dog needs or enjoys in its diet lead owners to provide food that may imbalance the diet or is harmful to the dog's health. A set of general guidelines are helpful in advising owners and professionals about what may or may not be healthy food for their dog.

Should table scraps be fed to dogs? Some owners enjoy feeding their dogs table scraps and other "people food" for the same reasons they like to

TABLE 18.4 General Guidelines for Feeding Dogs

✓ Avoid rapid changes in diet

✓ When the diet must be changed, the new diet should be introduced gradually by mixing it with the old diet in 25-percent increments each day

✓ Limit table scraps and human food to less than 10 percent of the dog's daily ration

✓ A dog should be fed as an individual: Select a food that promotes vitality, health, and optimal skin and coat condition, and results in the formation of well-formed stools and normal defecation frequency

✓ Feed amounts of food that support correct body condition and weight

✓ Select a diet that has been proved to provide optimal nutrition through AAFCO feeding trials

✓ Do not add nutritional supplements to a balanced diet

give them treats and snacks. Providing a special food is a way of showing affection and love. Adding table scraps and other choice food items to a pet's diet is believed to enhance the pet's enjoyment of the meal. However, it is important to realize that although the owner may eat a very nutritious and well-balanced diet, the nutritional requirements of dogs are not the same as a human's. Although some human food is unsuitable for companion animals and should not be fed at all, most only pose a danger to health if they make up a high proportion of the pet's diet. If table scraps are fed, a few guidelines should be followed to ensure that the dog's diet is not imbalanced or too many calories are not provided (Table 18.5).

TABLE 18.5   Recommendations on Table Scraps as Treats

✓ Table scraps and human food should never make up more than 5 to 10 percent of the dog's daily intake (calories)

✓ If meat, poultry, or fish is fed, it should be thoroughly cooked (never raw)

✓ All bones should be removed from meat, poultry, or fish

✓ Only small amounts of dairy products should be fed to dogs

✓ To prevent behavior problems such as begging or stealing food, all treats should be given away from the dinner table, preferably in the dog's food bowl

✓ No single type of food should be fed exclusively

✓ In all cases, the best type of treat to give a dog is a biscuit or dog snack formulated and sold as a dog treat (i.e., avoid giving "people food" if possible)

Several foods, however, are of special concern. These include dairy products, chocolate, and onions. Almost all dogs love the taste of dairy products, and many owners will treat their dog to a taste of ice cream or milk, now and then. Although dairy products are excellent sources of calcium, protein, phosphorus, and several vitamins, the consumption of high amounts of milk or milk products can cause digestive upsets and diarrhea in dogs. This occurs because the lactose present in milk requires the intestinal enzyme, lactase, for digestion. As in most mammals, the dog's intestinal mucosa has decreased lactase activity as the dog reaches maturity. The change results in lactose maldigestion. Undigested lactose travels to the large intestine where it is fermented by bacteria, resulting in the production of gas, loose stools, and possibly diarrhea. While some dogs continue to tolerate dairy products as adults, others do not. Most dogs can be fed and enjoy an occasional spoonful of ice cream or small bowl of milk, but, overall, the practice of feeding dairy products should be strictly limited.

Most dogs enjoy sweet flavors, including the taste of chocolate. Chocolate contains **theobromine**, a compound similar in structure and physiological action to caffeine. Theobromine is toxic to dogs when consumed in large quantities. This occurs because dogs have an unusually low rate of theobromine metabolism, resulting in a longer half-life of the chemical in the bloodstream and tissues. Following a single dose, the half-life of theobromine in the plasma of adult dogs is approximately 17.5 hours.[23] In humans, the half-life is less than 6 hours.[24] It appears that this extended half-life is responsible for dogs' sensitivity to theobromine.

Theobromine affects the dog's central nervous system, the cardiovascular system, the kidneys, and smooth muscle. Clinical signs of theobromine toxicity are increased heart rate, muscle tremors, increased urination and water consumption, vomiting, diarrhea, panting, and hyperactivity. Although it is not a common clinical problem, theobromine toxicity in dogs can be life threatening when it occurs. Signs usually occur about 4 to 5 hours after the dog has consumed chocolate. The onset of generalized motor seizures signifies severe toxicity in most cases and often results in death.[25,26] The only treatment for theobromine toxicity is to induce vomiting as soon as possible. Unfortunately, there is no specific systemic antidote for theobromine poisoning once the compound has been absorbed into the body.

Chocolate products differ greatly in their theobromine content and, therefore, in their ability to produce theobromine poisoning. Chocolate liquor, commonly called baking or cooking chocolate, is the base substance from which all other chocolate products are produced, so it contains the highest concentration of theobromine. Because of its theobromine content, as little as 3 ounces of baking chocolate could be fatal to a 25-pound dog. Fortunately, it is unusual for dogs to consume baking cocoa or baking chocolate because of the bitter taste of this product. The concentration of theobromine in chocolate candy and other chocolate products is much lower because of its dilution with milk solids, sugar, and other ingredients. For example, a 25-pound dog would have to consume approximately 1/2 pound of semisweet chocolate or 1 1/2 pounds of milk chocolate to reach a seriously toxic level. Despite the relatively low toxicity level of chocolate, dogs generally love the taste of chocolate, and many will gorge themselves on this treat if given the opportunity. Although it is not harmful to give a dog an occasional chocolate treat, the amount should be strictly limited and, more important, all chocolate foods should be stored in areas that are inaccessible to dogs.

A final people food that may pose a risk to dogs is onions. Like chocolate, a small amount of onion in a dog's diet is not harmful. However, the consumption of large amounts of onion, especially by small and toy breeds of dogs, can be highly toxic. The consumption of a high concentration of onion results in the formation of Heinz bodies on the dog's circulating red blood cells. Ultimately, this leads to a form of hemolytic anemia, which can be fatal in severe cases.[27,28] The reaction is caused by a toxic compound in onions called n-propyl disulfide. Signs of the hemolytic anemia that is produced by onion toxicity include diarrhea, vomiting, depression, elevated temperature, and production of a dark-colored urine. Although vomiting and diarrhea may be immediate, the remaining signs usually appear 1 to 4 days following the ingestion of onion. Overall, only limited amounts of onion should be given to dogs, and food containing high amounts of onion should not be fed to dogs at all.

Should mineral or vitamin supplements be given to dogs? Supplementing a pet's diet during growth or other periods of physiological stress is a common practice among breeders, trainers, and some owners. The most common mineral supplemented is calcium, and a commonly supplemented vitamin is vitamin C (ascorbic acid). Contrary to popular belief, there is no health benefit to supplementing a dog's diet with either of these nutrients, and, when supplementation is excessive, there may be some harm.

The reason most often cited for calcium supplementation relates to its essential role in normal skeletal growth and development. Supplements such as dicalcium phosphate and bone meal or calcium-containing foods such as cottage cheese or milk are added to a growing dog's diet with the intent of improving skeletal growth or preventing developmental skeletal disease. Regardless of good intentions, there are potential risks when excessively high levels of calcium are added to an adequate, balanced diet. Excess calcium in the diet can produce deficiencies in other nutrients and may contribute to abnormal bone development.[29] Studies indicate that a high level of calcium in the diet is associated with the occurrence of osteochondrosis, enlarged joints, limb deformities, and impaired growth.

The mechanism through which calcium exerts these effects relates to the homeostatic control of blood calcium and phosphorus levels. Excessive calcium intake in young dogs results in a transient hypercalcemia (elevated calcium) and hypophosphatemia (decreased serum phosphorus). This imbalance leads to chronically elevated levels of the hormone calcitonin, which is involved in calcium homeostasis. The ultimate effect of these changes are alterations in the rate and form of bone remodeling and retarded cartilage maturation in developing bone. Ironically, adding excessive amounts of calcium or calcium-containing foods to a balanced diet actually can contribute to the development of the very skeletal disorders owners are attempting to prevent. Also, adding excess calcium to a balanced diet can interfere with the absorption of other minerals such as zinc, iron, and copper. If a growing dog is fed an appropriate amount of a high-quality pet food formulated for growth, supplementation with calcium is unnecessary and contraindicated. If a pet owner is feeding his or her pet a food that appears to contain inadequate or unavailable levels of calcium, switching the dog to an adequate commercial diet is safer than attempting to correct the imbalance in the poor diet through supplementation.

Vitamin C (ascorbic acid) also is added to the diets of growing dogs because of the belief that this vitamin will promote healthy bone growth. Ascorbic acid is needed for the hydroxylation of the amino acids proline and lysine in the formation of the structural protein collagen. Collagen is the primary constituent of the protein matrix upon which bone is built. Interestingly, dogs do not have a requirement for dietary ascorbic acid. Like most species, they produce this vitamin in the liver from either glucose or galactose. Therefore, unless there is a high metabolic need or inadequate amounts are being synthesized by the body, a dietary source of ascorbic acid is unnecessary for the domestic dog. More importantly, controlled studies with growing dogs have shown that vitamin C supplementation does not benefit skeletal growth or prevent skeletal disease.[30,31] In addition to being unjustified, ascorbic acid supplementation in dogs may be detrimental. Excess ascorbic acid is excreted in the urine as oxalate, and high concentrations of oxalate have the potential to contribute to the formation of calcium oxalate uroliths in the urinary tract, leading to lower-urinary-tract disease.

Conclusions

Feeding dogs properly involves first evaluating and selecting a pet food that will provide optimal nutrition and support vitality and health. A method of feeding should be used that is suitable for the dog's age, lifestyle, and temperament and that fits with the owner's daily schedule. An amount of food that supports optimal growth and body condition, but which does not lead to rapid weight gain or obesity, should be provided. Also, general guidelines that allow regular feeding patterns to develop and limit the feeding of table scraps and treats should be followed. The following chapter examines one additional way in which diet can contribute to a dog's health and quality of life. Dietary management is an important component in the treatment or management of some types of chronic diseases.

Cited References

1. Allard, R.L., Douglass, G.M., and Kerr, W.W. **The effects of breed and sex on dog growth.** Companion Animal Practice, 2:9-12. (1988)

2. Sheffy, B.E. **Meeting energy-protein needs of dogs.** Compendium of Continuing Education for Small Animal Practitioners, 1:345-354. (1979)

3. Earle, K.E. **Calculations of energy requirements of dogs, cats and small psittacine birds.** Journal of Small Animal Practice, 34:163-183. (1993)

4. AAFCO. **AAFCO pet food regulatory update**. Proceedings of the Petfood Forum, Watts Publishing, Chicago, Illinois, pp. 141-147. (1998)

5. Hazewinkel, H.A.W., Goedegebuure, S.A., and Poulos, P.W. **Influences of chronic calcium excess on the skeletal development of growing Great Danes.** Journal of the American Animal Hospital Association, 21:377–391. (1985)

6. Kallfelz, F.A. and Dzanis, D.A. **Over nutrition: an epidemic problem in pet practice?** Veterinary Clinics of North America: Small Animal Practice, 19:433–466. (1989)

7. Hazewinkel, H.A.W. **Calcium metabolism and skeletal development of dogs.** In: Nutrition of the Dog and Cat (I.H. Burger. J.P.W. Rivers, editors), Cambridge University Press, Cambridge, United Kingdom, pp. 293–302. (1989)

8. Faust, I.M., Johnson, P.R., and Hirsch, J. **Long-term effects of early nutritional experience on the development of obesity in the rat.** Journal of Nutrition, 110:2027–2034. (1980)

9. Kulhman, G. and Biourge, V. **Nutrition of the large and giant breed dog with emphasis on skeletal development.** Veterinary Clinical Nutrition, 4:89-95. (1997)

10. Gorrel, C. and Rawlings, J.M. **The role of tooth brushing and diet in the maintenance of periodontal health in dogs.** Journal of Veterinary Dentistry, 13:139-143. (1996)

11. Moser, D. **Feeding to optimize canine reproductive efficiency.** Problems in Veterinary Medicine, 4:545–550. (1992)

12. Mosier, J.E. **Nutritional recommendations for gestation and lactation in the dog.** Veterinary Clinics of North America: Small Animal Practice, 7:683–692. (1977)

13. Ontko, J.A. and Phillips, P.H. **Reproduction and lactation studies with bitches fed semi-purified diets.** Journal of Nutrition, 65:211–218. (1958)

14. Brace, J.J. **Theories of aging.** Veterinary Clinics of North America: Small Animal Practice, 11:811–814. (1981)

15. Mosier, J.E. **Effect of aging on body systems of the dog.** Veterinary Clinics of North America: Small Animal Practice, 19:1–13. (1989)

16. Sheffy, B.E. and William, A.J. **Nutrition and the aging animal.** Veterinary Clinics of North America: Small Animal Practice, 11:669–675. (1981)

17. Therriault, D.G., Beller, G.A., and Smoake, J.A. **Intramuscular energy sources in dogs during physical work.** Journal of Lipid Research, 14:54–61. (1973)

18. Paul, P. and Issekutz, B. **Role of extramuscular energy sources in the metabolism of the exercising dog.** American Journal of Physiology, 22:615–622. (1976)

19. Downey, R.L., Kronfeld, D.S., and Banta, C.A. **Diet of beagles affects stamina.** Journal of the American Animal Hospital Association, 16:273–277. (1980)

20. Reynolds, A.J. **The effect of diet and training on energy substrate storage and utilization in trained and untrained sled dogs.** In: Nutrition and Physiology of Alaskan Sled Dogs, abstracts of a symposium held at the College of Veterinary Medicine, Ohio State University, Columbus, Ohio, September 5. (1992)

21. Hinchcliff, K.W. **Energy and water expenditure.** In: Proceedings of the Performance Dog Nutrition Symposium, Colorado State University, Fort Collins, Colorado, April 18, pp.4-9. (1995)

22. Gannon, J.R. **Nutritional requirements of the working dog.** Veterinary Annual, 21:161–166. (1981)

23. Gans, J.H., Korson, R., and Cater, M.R. **Effects of short-term and long-term theobromine administration to male dogs.** Toxicology and Applied Pharmacology, 53:481–496. (1980)

24. Drouillard, D.D., Vesell, E.S., and Dvorchick, B.N. **Studies on theobromine disposition in normal subjects.** Clinical Pharmacology Therapy, 23:296–302. (1978)

25. Decker, R.A. and Meyers, G.H. **Theobromine poisoning in a dog.** Journal of the American Veterinary Medical Association, 161:198–199. (1972)

26. Glauberg, A. and Blumenthal, P.H. **Chocolate poisoning in the dog.** Journal of the American Animal Hospital Association, 19:246–248. (1983)

27. Spice, R.N. **Hemolytic anemia associated with ingestion of onions in a dog.** Canadian Veterinary Journal, 17:181–183. (1976)

28. Kay, J.M. **Onion toxicity in a dog.** Modern Veterinary Practice, 6:477–478. (1983)

29. Hazewinkel, H.A. **Calcium metabolism and skeletal development of dogs.** In: Nutrition of the Dog and Cat (I.H. Burger and J.P.W. Rivers, editors), Cambridge University Press, Cambridge, United Kingdom, pp. 293–302. (1989)

30. Grondalen, J. **Metaphyseal osteopathy (hypertrophic osteodystrophy) in growing dogs: A clinical study.** Journal of Small Animal Practice, 17:721–735. (1976)[6]

31. Teare, J.A., Krook, L., and Kallfelz, A. **Ascorbic acid deficiency and hypertrophic osteodystrophy in the dog: A rebuttal.** Cornell Veterinarian, 69:384–401. (1979)

19   Common Nutrition Problems in Dogs

OPTIMAL NUTRITION IS ESSENTIAL for normal growth and the maintenance of health and vitality throughout life. As discussed in Chapter 18, supplementation, overfeeding, or providing inappropriate food items can lead to nutritional disorders or illness. In addition, there are several health problems in dogs that can be treated or managed through diet. Dietary therapy often plays an important role, even though the underlying cause of the disease may not be related to diet. Examples reviewed in this chapter include obesity, diabetes mellitus, chronic kidney disease, and food hypersensitivity.

Obesity

Obesity is the most common form of malnutrition in dogs in the United States, with an estimated rate of occurrence of between 24 percent and 34 percent.[1] The number of obese dogs has appeared to steadily increase as the dog has evolved from a working partner to a more sedentary house pet. These changes in lifestyle, coupled with the increase in highly palatable and energy-dense pet foods have contributed to the increased incidence of obesity in adult dogs. Regardless of predisposing factors, however, the underlying cause of obesity in any animal is a surplus of energy. Simply put, obesity occurs when a dog repeatedly consumes more energy than he or she expends.

Definition and diagnosis: A dog whose body weight is 20 percent or more above normal generally is considered to be obese. However, health problems associated with an overweight condition can arise when dogs are 10 percent to 15 percent above their ideal weight. For example, a Golden Retriever whose ideal body weight is determined to be 60 pounds is considered overweight at 66 to 69 pounds, and obese when his or her weight is greater than 72 pounds. Overweight dogs have decreased exercise tolerance and increased incidence of chronic illnesses such as diabetes mellitus, pulmonary and cardiovascular disease, and degenerative joint disease (arthritis). They are also at an increased surgical risk and have higher morbidity and mortality rates following surgical procedures.[2] Invariably, these problems contribute to a decreased quality of life for overweight dogs.

The diagnosis of obesity in companion animals should always include an examination by a veterinarian for the presence of underlying disease. Common disorders that may contribute to weight gain include hypothyroidism, hyperadrenocorticism, and diabetes mellitus. After these diseases have been ruled out, a comparison of the pet's current weight with previous weight measurements or with its weight shortly after reaching adulthood may indicate abnormal weight gain. In some cases involving purebred dogs, a comparison of the pet's body weight with the weights suggested by the breed's standard may also be a useful guideline for determining ideal body weight. Overall, visual assessment of the pet is the best method for diagnosing obesity. A dog at her ideal body weight should have an hourglass shape when viewed from above (Figure 19.1).[3] If the dog is heavily coated, the hourglass shape should be easily palpated beneath the dog's coat. The loss of a waist and the presence of a pendulous abdomen are both indicative of excess body fat. Subjective evaluation of the animal's gait, degree of exercise tolerance, and overall appearance also are used to support a diagnosis of obesity.

FIGURE 19.1   Visual assessment of the dog's body condition

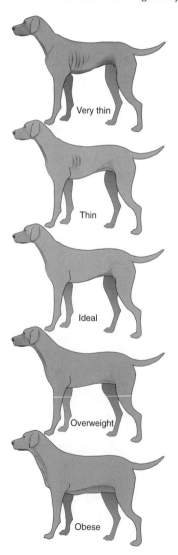

Contributing factors: The fundamental underlying cause in all cases of obesity is an energy surplus that arises because of an imbalance between energy intake and energy expenditure. Excess energy is stored primarily as fat, resulting in weight gain and an increased ratio of fat-to-lean tissue. Although the problem of obesity appears simple in terms of energy, several underlying factors can contribute to energy imbalances in dogs. Characteristics that may affect a predisposition for obesity include the dog's age, reproductive status, breed, level of activity, and health. Factors of the dog's lifestyle that may be important include the type of diet that is fed and the feeding regimen used.

Obesity is more prevalent in neutered than in intact companion animals. However, contrary to popular belief, spaying a female or castrating a male dog does not invariably lead to weight gain. Veterinarians often encourage clients to castrate or spay their pets before they become sexually mature, usually between 6 months and 1 year of age. This time period corresponds to a natural decrease in a dog's growth rate, level of activity, and energy needs (see Chapter 18). If owners are not aware of this change and continue to feed their dog the same amount of food, excess weight gain will result. Because spaying and neutering often occur just before maturity, neutering may erroneously be blamed for a weight gain that was actually the result of diminished energy needs and excess food intake. Although certain reproductive hormones do moderately affect food intake and activity, the absence of these hormones is not singularly responsible for the development of obesity.[4] Energy needs further decrease as dogs age and become elderly (see Chapter 18). Again, if energy intake is not decreased accordingly, older dogs may gain excess weight.

Breed and individual temperament may influence a dog's tendency to become overweight. Certain breeds of dogs have a disproportionately high incidence of obesity compared with the general population of dogs. Cocker Spaniels, Labrador Retrievers, Shetland Sheepdogs, and several of the small terrier breeds have a higher incidence of obesity than the general population of dogs.[5] In contrast, Boxers, German Shepherd Dogs, large terrier breeds, and the sight hound breeds have a comparatively low incidence of obesity. Even within breeds and breed types, a dog's natural activity level and response to exercise will affect energy expenditure. Similarly, some dogs behave as though they are perpetually hungry and will readily overeat if given the opportunity, while others can effectively self-regulate intake. These individual differences ultimately affect a dog's energy balance and tendency to maintain, gain, or lose weight.

The type of diet that is fed will affect food intake. The most important of these factors is feeding highly palatable diets that may induce some dogs to overconsume. Palatability is an important diet characteristic that is heavily promoted in the marketing of commercial pet foods. Semimoist foods contain variable amounts of simple sugars, while canned foods and some premium dry foods are very high in fat content. Fat contributes both to palatability and the food's caloric density. Feeding highly palatable foods on an ad libitum basis may contribute to both the development and the maintenance of obesity because many dogs will overconsume these foods. Therefore, portion-controlled meal feeding is recommended whenever a highly palatable food is fed.

The food's caloric distribution is also an important factor. Feeding dog foods that contain a relatively high proportion of fat can promote weight gain because they are usually more energy-dense and are always highly palatable to dogs. As the percentage of metabolizable energy (ME) calories from fat increases in a pet food, the ability of the diet to meet the energy demands of a working dog also increases (see Chapter 18). However, if this diet is fed to a dog that does not need it, weight gain may occur if intake is not strictly monitored. A diet that contains a low percentage of ME from fat will aid in weight loss and/or the maintenance of normal body weight in a sedentary adult animal.

Treatment: Dogs who are 10 percent to 15 percent or more above their ideal body weight should be placed on a weight-loss program. Short-term goals are to reduce body fat stores and decrease weight. Long-term goals are to attain ideal body weight and maintain this weight for the remainder of the dog's life. A weight-loss program should be designed to ensure a noticeable change in weight and body condition within several weeks, yet moderate enough to minimize excessive hunger and excessive losses of lean body tissue. Depending on the degree of obesity and the age and health of the dog, a weight loss of 1 percent to 2 percent of the animal's total body weight per week is recommended.[3] For example, the Golden Retriever whose ideal body weight is 60 pounds but actually weighs 75 pounds should lose between 3/4 pound (12 ounces) and 1 1/2 pounds per week.

Weight loss is best accomplished using a combination of caloric restriction and an exercise program to increase daily energy expenditure. This often requires changes in the way in which the owner lives with the dog in terms of eliminating extra treats, limiting table foods, and instituting a daily routine of walks or other type of exercise. For dogs that are less than 10 percent overweight, a normal maintenance diet can be fed but in restricted amounts. Dogs that are more than 10 percent overweight should be fed a dog food formulated for weight loss.

The inclusion of moderate, regular exercise in the treatment of obese pets increases daily energy expenditure and causes desired changes in body composition. In all animals, regular and continued exercise results in a higher proportion of lean-to-fat tissue. Because an animal's resting metabolic rate (RMR) is directly related to the amount of lean body tissue it has, increasing lean tissue contributes to the maintenance of a normal RMR during weight loss. This is important because, as weight decreases, the energy expenditure of voluntary activity also decreases. Maintaining a normal RMR helps offset this change and raises energy expenditure. If a dog is accustomed to a completely sedentary lifestyle, exercise should be initiated gradually. Twenty minutes of legitimate exercise three to five times per week is a good start. The duration and intensity can be increased as the dog begins to lose weight and becomes more athletically fit. Daily walking, running, swimming, or playing fetch and other games are recommended forms of exercise for dogs.

Caloric restriction is the second component of weight loss. As a rule of thumb, an amount of food that provides 60 percent to 70 percent of the calories necessary to maintain the dog's current body weight results in adequate weight loss. For example, the estimated daily caloric requirement of an inactive, overweight 75-pound Golden Retriever is approximately 1,400 kcal/day. Caloric restriction to 60 percent of this requirement equals 840 kcal/day. If a maintenance dog food that contains 350 kcal per 8-ounce cup is fed, this dog should receive only 2 1/2 cups of food per day. If the dog remained sedentary, a daily caloric deficit of 560 kcal per day would occur. A caloric deficit of 3,500 kcal is necessary to lose 1 pound of body fat. Therefore, the dog would lose about 1 pound per week on this dietary regimen. If exercise is included in the program, the additional energy deficit would be accounted for through increased energy expenditure, and a slightly greater weight loss will be seen (Table 19.1).

The example above illustrates the need to feed dogs who are obese commercial dog foods formulated for weight loss. Commercial pet foods formulated for adult maintenance contain adequate amounts of protein, fat, vitamins, and minerals to meet the needs of an animal at normal weight who is consuming adequate calories. If the volume of a maintenance diet is reduced too drastically in an effort to limit calories, nutrient deficiencies may develop.[6] Feeding a 75-pound dog only 2 1/2 cups of an adult maintenance diet per day may result in a nutrient deficiency because of the low volume of food that is fed. Diets designed for weight loss in dogs are formulated to contain adequate levels of nutrients while supplying fewer calories. Therefore, in cases of moderate to severe obesity, a change of diet to a commercially prepared food with a low energy density is recommended for weight reduction.

Several commercial pet foods that meet total nutrient requirements and are formulated to provide fewer calories than other adult maintenance foods are available. Some of these can be purchased through pet stores or grocery stores, while others are prescription diets and available only from veterinarians. These products all contain reduced levels of fat, and some may contain high amounts of indigestible fiber. Decreasing the fat content of a pet food results in the desired decrease in caloric density. Commercial, low-fat diets contain between 8 percent and 11 percent fat on a dry-matter basis. This per-

---

TABLE 19.1   Calculating Daily Intake for Weight Loss

(Golden Retriever: 75 lb; Ideal Weight Is 60 lb)

ME Requirement = $132 \times (34 \text{ kg})^{0.67}$ = **1,400 kcal/day**

60 Percent Restriction = $0.6 \times 1,400$ = **840 kcal/day**

Feeding: Adult Maintenance Diet **(ME = 3,800 kcal/kg; 350 kcal/cup)**
Cups per Day: 840/350 = **2½ cups of food**

Feeding: Reducing Diet **(ME = 3,400 kcal/kg; 300 kcal/cup)**
Cups per Day: 840/300 = **~ 3 cups of food**

centage is equivalent to 18 percent to 26 percent of the calories in a diet with an energy density of 3,500 kcal/kg. This decreased proportion of fat is low enough to reduce the caloric density of the food but high enough to still make the food palatable and acceptable to most dogs.

Complex carbohydrates (starch) provide an excellent source of energy for dogs because they are lower in energy than fat and are highly digestible. Adult maintenance diets for pets with normal activity levels contain between 30 percent and 50 percent of their calories from digestible carbohydrates. Diets formulated for the weight reduction of overweight dogs contain levels that are between 50 percent and 60 percent. Pet foods that replace fat with complex carbohydrates without adding additional fiber retain the level of digestibility of the higher fat products, but they contain fewer total calories. An added advantage to a low-fat diet high in complex carbohydrates is that, unlike reducing diets that are high in dietary fiber, this type of reducing diet does not cause increased fecal volume or defecation frequency.

Some pet foods formulated for weight reduction dilute calories through the addition of indigestible fiber. The rationale behind these products is that the increased bulk and decreased digestibility of the diet will cause a decrease in voluntary energy consumption by the dog. However, there are limited data to support this theory in companion animals, and some studies have shown that dogs consuming high-fiber diets did not lower their energy intakes.[7] Diets that dilute calories with indigestible fiber also result in increased defecation frequency and fecal volume, a side effect that is undesirable to most owners. For these reasons, a diet formulated for weight loss in dogs should contain reduced amounts of fat, increased amounts of digestible complex carbohydrates, and normal levels of indigestible fiber.

When reduced-calorie foods are fed, portion-controlled feeding should always be used. Most dogs, if given the opportunity, will merely increase the volume of food they eat in an effort to keep energy intake the same. The advantage of feeding a reducing diet is that lower calories can be consumed in a larger volume of food, and there is less risk of causing a nutrient imbalance during restricted feeding. For example, if a reducing pet food that contains 300 kcal/cup is fed, the Golden Retriever used in the previous example would receive 3 cups of food a day rather than 2 1/2 cups. This larger volume of food may result in a greater feeling of satiety and less tendency to beg or steal food. Moreover, these pet foods are specifically formulated by pet food manufacturers to provide balanced nutrition while lowering the amount of calories consumed.

The dietary and exercise habits that were established during the treatment of obesity must be maintained for dogs even after caloric restriction for weight loss has ended. Once the dog has attained his ideal weight, he should be fed a well-balanced, complete food designed for adult maintenance. In some cases, a diet formulated for adults with low levels of activity is appropriate. Owners should avoid reverting to old habits such as feeding table scraps, providing a large number of treats, or allowing begging behaviors. In all cases, portion-controlled feeding, twice daily, is the feeding schedule that should be used.

Diabetes Mellitus

Diabetes mellitus is a chronic endocrine disorder caused by the relative or absolute deficiency of the hormone insulin. Insulin is produced by the pancreas and is necessary for the transport of glucose and other nutrients into cells. A lack of insulin leads to elevated blood glucose levels, or **hyperglycemia**, and prevents tissues from receiving the nutrients they need. It is estimated that 0.5 percent of dogs in the United States are diabetic, the vast majority of which are either overweight or obese.[8] Other factors that appear to be related to the development of diabetes in dogs are hormonal abnormalities such as hypothyroidism and Cushing's syndrome, and genetic predispositions in some breeds.[9]

Clinical signs: The most common form of diabetes mellitus in dogs is insulin-dependent diabetes mellitus, or Type I diabetes, which occurs when the pancreas is incapable of producing or secreting insulin.[10] As a result, dogs with Type I diabetes require daily injections of insulin to maintain normal blood glucose levels and to promote normal nutrient metabolism. Noninsulin-dependent diabetes mellitus, or Type II diabetes, occurs when there is a relative deficiency of insulin. In this case, the pancreas still produces insulin, but cells and tissues of the body are insensitive to the effects of the hormone. This form of diabetes is seen in about 10 to 20 percent of the cases that are diagnosed in dogs, and is almost always associated with obesity.[10] Weight loss often results in a return to normal or near-normal insulin responsiveness in dogs with Type II diabetes.

All of the clinical symptoms observed in pets with diabetes mellitus are related to the short- or long-term effects of hyperglycemia. Signs that owners usually first notice are an increase in water consumption (polydypsia), an increase in urination (polyuria), and, occasionally, weight loss. If uncorrected, diabetes leads to serious chronic problems such as renal disease, neurological disorders, and the development of cataracts.

Dietary management: The therapeutic goal when treating diabetes is to maintain blood glucose levels within a normal range and to minimize **postprandial** (after-meal) fluctuations. This usually is achieved through exogenous insulin administration, oral hypoglycemic agents, controlled amounts of exercise, and diet. Therapy also may be aimed at controlling related illnesses that may be present, such as renal or neurological disease. Although diabetes cannot be cured, many dogs with this disorder can lead healthy and happy lives if the disease is properly managed. Providing an appropriate diet and feeding regimen are important components of treatment regimens because they affect fluctuations in blood glucose levels.

Dogs with insulin-dependent diabetes receive one or more insulin injections per day. The dietary goals for these dogs are to improve regulation of blood glucose concentrations by delivering nutrients to the body during periods when insulin is active and to prevent or minimize wide fluctuations in blood glucose levels. Dietary therapy will not eliminate the need for insulin replacement therapy, but it can be used to improve glycemic control. Dietary treatment for dogs who are not insulin-dependent is also aimed at improving glycemic control and toward prolonging or even preventing the need for insulin therapy. Weight reduction and control are important aspects of the dietary management of all diabetic animals who are overweight. In these cases, caloric intake should be designed for weight loss and the eventual maintenance of ideal body weight. Important dietary factors to consider when feeding diabetic dogs are the food's ingredients, its nutrient composition, and the schedule of feeding used.

Dogs who are insulin-dependent rely upon the delivery of insulin to the body to transport available nutrients into cells. Therefore, the presence of nutrients in the bloodstream should coincide as closely as possible with periods of peak insulin action. Supplying the same amount and type of nutrients each day facilitates this balance. Therefore, a diet that is consistent in the type and quantity of nutrients it contains should be selected. The proportions of calories supplied by carbohydrate, protein, and fat should be constant, and these nutrients should always be supplied by the same ingredients. Changes in the diet's ingredients or caloric distribution can disrupt the tight coupling of blood glucose levels with insulin activity needed for proper glycemic control. Manufacturers of premium-quality pet food use fixed formulations in their products. This means that the ingredients do not vary according to market prices, and the consumer is guaranteed that the food is consistent from batch to batch. In contrast, most grocery store products and private label brands use variable formulations. The ingredients in these products may change between batches depending upon ingredient availability and market prices. These differences are significant when selecting a pet food for a diabetic animal. Only foods guaranteed to use a fixed formulation should be considered.

The form and quality of ingredients are also important. Because the digestion of complex carbohydrates provides glucose to the bloodstream at a slower rate than simple carbohydrates, complex carbohydrates should supply most of the diet's carbohydrates. As a general rule, complex carbohydrates should make up 40 percent or more of the calories in diets for diabetic pets. The level of fat in the diet should be moderately restricted, especially if the pet is overweight. This decreases the food's caloric density and contributes to the control of hypercholesterolemia and hepatic lipidosis (fatty liver) that may occur as a complication of diabetes. As a general rule, the fat content of pet food for diabetic pets should not exceed 18 percent to 20 percent of the ME calories in the diet. Dietary protein in the diet should be of high quality and included in quantities that meet but do not greatly exceed the dog's requirement. If chronic kidney disease is present as a complication of diabetes, protein must be restricted to a level that is effective in controlling clinical signs. In most cases, a dry-type, premium dog food formulated for maintenance or for less active adults is appropriate for diabetic pets. Semimoist pet food is not a good choice because much of it contains high amounts of simple sugars. Simple sugars are quickly digested and absorbed following a meal, leading to rapid elevations of blood glucose.

The feeding schedule of pets with diabetes should be planned so nutrients are delivered to the body during peak periods of insulin activity.[11] This span will be determined by the type of insulin used and the time of day it is administered. The owner's veterinarian can provide a feeding schedule appropriate for the type and level of insulin being used. In most situations, several small meals are fed throughout the period of insulin activity, as opposed to feeding a single meal. This procedure helps minimize postprandial fluctuations in blood glucose levels. A small meal should always be given before insulin injections. This is recommended because if the dog refuses to eat on any occasion, the insulin injection can be withheld, thereby preventing the subsequent onset of hypoglycemia. The remaining meals in the day are then spaced at 4- to 6-hour intervals, depending on the action of the insulin that is used.[12] Once an appropriate diet and feeding schedule have been selected, the program should be strictly adhered to. Supplemental foods should not be given, and feeding times should vary as little as possible. Periodic monitoring of blood glucose levels is used to adjust the diet as the pet loses weight, to change the amount of exercise it receives, or to make adjustments in insulin dosage (Table 19.2).

Chronic Kidney Disease

The kidney has many regulatory and excretory functions and is essential for normal homeostasis and health. The functional units of the kidney are called nephrons. Each nephron consists of a glomerulus and a system of tubules within which reabsorption and excretion occur. The glomerulus is a tuft of capillaries where waste products and electrolytes from the blood are filtered. The tubules originate at the base of the glomerulus and selectively reabsorb many of the blood components present in the filtrate. When the filtrate reaches the final portion of the tubule, it contains only those compounds

---

TABLE 19.2   Nutritional Management of Diabetes Mellitus

✓ Feed a premium dog food that has a fixed formulation, with high-quality ingredients and a consistent caloric distribution of carbohydrate, fat, and protein

✓ Complex carbohydrates (starch) should make up more than 40 percent of the calories

✓ Fat should be moderately restricted (18 percent to 20 percent of calories)

✓ Portion-controlled meal feeding should be used

✓ Feeding times should be strictly regulated to coincide with peak insulin action (Insulin-dependent diabetes)

✓ A meal should always be offered prior to administering insulin. If the dog does not eat, insulin can be withheld until food is consumed

that are going to be excreted as waste in the urine. These include the waste products of protein catabolism, such as urea, creatinine, uric acid, and ammonia. In addition, the urine contains electrolytes, trace minerals, and metabolites of certain vitamins. The kidney is also important in the normal regulation of fluid balance, pH, and blood pressure, and for the production of two hormones.

Dogs with chronic kidney (renal) disease have experienced a progressive loss of functioning nephrons. The kidney has a significant reserve capacity and ability to compensate for damage or disease. As a result, clinical signs of kidney disease will be observed only after a loss of 70 percent to 85 percent of functioning nephrons has occurred.[13] There are many potential underlying causes for the initial kidney damage. These causes include, but are not limited to, trauma, infection, immunological disease, tumors, renal ischemia (decreased blood flow to the kidney), and exposure to toxins. In most cases, the initial underlying cause is no longer present and may not even be known when the pet develops signs of chronic kidney failure. The onset of chronic kidney disease occurs when the kidney's compensatory mechanisms break down and lead to progressive loss of kidney function and signs of chronic disease.

Clinical signs: One of the first signs owners notice in their dog is increased water consumption and increased urination. This effect is caused by a reduced capacity to concentrate the urine, resulting in an increased volume of urine and increased frequency of urination. Polydypsia accompanies the increased urination as the dog consumes more water in an effort to maintain fluid balance. Other clinical signs that are seen are associated with the degree of **azotemia** and **uremia** that is present. Azotemia refers to the accumulation of nitrogenous waste products, such as creatinine, in the blood. Urea is a major by-product of the metabolism of amino acids and is normally excreted in the urine. The term uremia technically means elevated concentrations of urea in the blood, but it commonly refers to the collection of clinical signs associated with renal failure.[14] Plasma creatinine levels of between 1.5 and 4 milligrams per deciliter (mg/dl) are indicative of mild to moderate renal disease, while levels higher than 4 mg/dl indicate end-stage renal disease.[15] Fasting blood urea nitrogen (BUN) levels that are greater than 35 mg/dl indicate some level of kidney dysfunction. Clinical signs of uremia in dogs include decreased appetite or anorexia, vomiting, depression, electrolyte and pH disturbances, mucosal ulcers, and weight loss. Some dogs also develop chronic diarrhea and neurological signs such as staggering or disorientation. Calcium and phosphorus homeostasis are negatively affected in dogs with renal disease. Over time, these changes lead to bone demineralization. The inability of the kidney to produce the hormone erythropoietin, which is necessary for the production of red blood cells, can lead to anemia in some dogs.

Dietary management: Dietary management is provided to dogs with chronic kidney disease as a method for minimizing the clinical signs associated with uremia, azotemia, and alterations in calcium and phosphorus homeostasis. Although dietary therapy does not provide a cure for renal disease, it can minimize the clinical signs and contribute to the pet's health, well-being, and longevity. Dietary protein is of primary concern because it is the breakdown products of protein metabolism that are responsible for uremia. The diet used should minimize the accumulation of protein end products in the blood while still providing adequate protein for the dog's maintenance needs. Contrary to popular belief, restricting dietary protein does not halt the progression of renal disease, nor is there any evidence that high-protein diets are an underlying cause of renal disease in dogs.[16, 17, 18] The restriction of dietary protein in dogs with renal disease is instituted primarily as a means of controlling the clinical signs associated with uremia and azotemia. Adequate calories from carbohydrate and fat must be provided in these diets to prevent the use of either body tissues or dietary protein for energy.

The generation of urea is directly proportional to the daily turnover of dietary and body protein. Protein ingested in excess of the animal's requirement is metabolized, producing urea and other end products that must then be excreted by the kidneys. Similarly, when inadequate calories are ingested, some body protein will be used for energy, again resulting in the synthesis of urea. Dogs with chronic kidney disease have a reduced ability to excrete these compounds efficiently, so they accumulate to abnormal levels in the bloodstream. Elevated plasma levels of urea and other waste products cause nausea, vomiting, and anorexia. Normalizing the levels of these waste products through restriction of dietary protein contributes to a return of appetite, weight gain, and a lessening of other clinical signs.[19]

The level of protein restriction is completely dependent on the severity of the dog's clinical signs and the degree of impaired renal function. Protein restriction is recommended only when the dog's BUN is greater than 80 mg/dl and when serum creatinine is greater than 2.5 mg per 100 milliliters (ml). This recommendation is a result of studies showing that dogs with lower levels of dysfunction do not benefit from dietary protein restriction.[20] The goal of dietary protein restriction is to maintain the dog's BUN below a level of 60 mg/dl, while still providing adequate amounts of protein essential for tissue maintenance and health.

The potential to cause protein deficiency requires conservative restriction of dietary protein in dogs with renal disease. Protein nutrition is particularly of concern because some dogs may be losing protein in their urine (proteinuria) and so may require more dietary protein than dogs without this symptom. The basic rule of thumb when managing renal disease in dogs is to feed a level of dietary protein that will improve clinical signs and promote well-being but not compromise the dog's nutritional status. A diet containing between 12 percent and 28 percent protein on a dry-matter basis is recommended for dogs with mild to moderate renal disease. Only protein sources that are highly digestible and of high biological value should be included in the diet. The exact level of protein can be adjusted relative to the dog's clinical and biochemical (i.e. BUN levels) response to the diet.[21] In severe and end-stage disease, protein must be progressively restricted to approach a level that is close to the pet's minimum daily requirement. If protein restriction is adequate, decreased BUN occurs rapidly, and improvement in clinical signs generally is seen within 3 to 4 weeks. Most dogs will show a reduction in vomiting, improved appetite, weight gain, and improved physical activity. Consistent monitoring of BUN levels and of clinical response to the diet should be used to indicate the need to either increase or decrease protein level.

Other nutrients of concern for dogs with renal disease are energy, phosphorus, sodium, potassium, and water-soluble vitamins. The diet fed to dogs with renal disease should supply adequate calories from carbohydrate and fat to minimize the catabolism of protein for energy. Dietary fat has the added advantages of increasing the energy density of the diet and contributing to the diet's palatability and acceptability. Most dogs who are uremic have a decreased appetite, and enticing them to eat is a major challenge of dietary therapy. The fat in the prescribed diet makes the diet more palatable and may stimulate increased consumption in sick pets.

The phosphorus content of the diet is important because dogs with chronic kidney disease have a decreased ability to excrete this mineral. This results in chronically elevated serum phosphorus levels, which leads to aberrations in calcium and phosphorus metabolism, bone demineralization, and the formation of calcium phosphate crystals in the kidney and other soft tissues. These changes appear to cause further loss of nephrons and can contribute to the progression of renal disease.[22] Dietary restriction of phosphorus is helpful in the early stages of renal disease. In more severe cases, phosphate-binding agents such as aluminum hydroxide and aluminum carbonate must be used in conjunction with reduced dietary phosphorus to normalize serum phosphorus concentration.

Additional nutrients that are of concern in the diets of dogs and cats with renal disease include sodium, potassium, the water-soluble vitamins, and, possibly, bicarbonate. Dietary sodium should be restricted in dogs that develop systemic hypertension as a complication of renal disease. In these cases, the concentration of sodium should be adjusted to meet the needs of the individual animal, with the goal of controlling hypertension while still providing adequate sodium. Diets for pets with renal disease also should contain adequate levels of potassium, and, if polyuria is present, supplementation with water-soluble vitamins is advisable because of excessive losses of these vitamins in the urine.

The therapeutic diet used for dogs with chronic kidney disease can be either a commercially prepared product or a homemade diet. Commercially prepared prescription diets usually are preferable because of their convenience and the assurance of consistency in the formulation. In addition, these products are always sold through veterinarians, so the dog's clinical response can be carefully monitored and evaluated by the attending veterinarian. An advantage to using a homemade diet is that these diets allow greater flexibility in the level of protein and other nutrients that are included, thus providing a diet specifically formulated to meet an individual dog's needs. Homemade diets may also be more palatable for some pets than commercially prepared products. Decisions regarding the type of diet to use can be made based on the veterinarian's recommendations, the pet's response to treatment, and the capabilities and preferences of the owner (Table 19.3).

TABLE 19.3   Nutritional Management of Chronic Kidney Disease

✓ Restrict dietary protein when there are clinical signs of uremia and BUN is greater than 60 mg/dl

✓ A diet that contains high-quality protein and adequate levels of nonprotein calories from fat and carbohydrate should be selected

✓ The protein level of the diet should be low enough to decrease BUN and clinical signs but still high enough to provide optimal protein nutrition

✓ Dietary phosphorus should be restricted, and, if necessary, phosphate-binding agents should be used to further moderate serum phosphorus levels

✓ Adjustments in dietary sodium may be necessary if secondary hypertension develops

✓ Provide supplemental water-soluble vitamins if polyuria leads to excessive losses

---

Food Hypersensitivity (Allergy)

Dietary hypersensitivity occurs when an animal develops an allergic reaction to one or more dietary components. In dogs, the body's hypersensitivity reaction to a food component usually is in the form of an allergic reaction in the skin. Allergic skin diseases are very common in dogs. Flea bite hypersensitivity accounts for the largest number of inflammatory skin disease cases reported, with atopic disease (allergic inhalant dermatitis) ranking second.[23] Although food hypersensitivity is probably less common than flea bite allergy or atopy, its actual incidence rate is difficult to determine because dogs who are allergic to food components also are often allergic to other substances.[24] Regardless, dietary hypersensitivity is of concern to owners because of the severity of symptoms involved, and because it is one type of hypersensitivity response over which owners and veterinarians can have a significant measure of control. This fact is important because when food hypersensitivities are correctly diagnosed, treatment can mean the difference between a dog that is chronically uncomfortable and one that is healthy and free from skin lesions and pruritus (itchiness).

Clinical signs and occurrence: Food allergies can be manifested in several ways in dogs. Survey studies have reported that 97 percent of allergic dogs show only dermatological signs, while between 10 percent and 15 percent also develop gastrointestinal disease.[25,26] When gastrointestinal signs occur, vomiting and the development of chronic diarrhea are typically reported. However, the most common signs are a severe and persistent pruritus and skin injury and lesions that are associated with scratching and self trauma.[27] Initially, this usually occurs between 4 and 24 hours after consuming the offending antigen. However, chronic cases of food allergy show constant pruritus, with no evident association between eating a meal and the onset of pruritus.

The behavior of dogs with allergic skin disease indicates that the pruritus is intense and the dog is very uncomfortable. Over time, the dog's scratching, biting, and digging at affected areas of skin lead to hair loss, damaged skin, and the development of lesions. Secondary bacterial infections of the skin often develop as well as chronic inflammation, crusting, seborrhea, and regional hyperpigmentation. Areas of the body most intensely affected are the bottom side of the dog's feet, the inside of the front legs where the leg meets the body, and around the region of the groin.[28] In severe cases, owners report that the dog seems to itch incessantly over the entire body. In some cases, a persistent inflammation of the outer ear, called "otitis externa," is observed. This may or may not be associated with bacterial or fungal infections and, in a small number of cases, is the only presenting sign of food hypersensitivity. Some dogs also have been reported to show only a recurrent pyoderma that was not associated with pruritus. The pyoderma subsided with antibacterial therapy but continued to recur until food hypersensitivity was diagnosed and the diet was changed.[29]

Dietary hypersensitivity can develop at any age and, unlike other forms of allergic skin disease, commonly is seen in dogs that are less than 1 year of age.[28] A recent study of 25 dogs diagnosed with food allergy found that the average age dogs began to show clinical signs was 1 year.[29] A second difference between food allergies and flea bite allergy and atopy is that food allergies are not typically seasonal. However, if multiple sensitivities are present (for example, dietary allergy plus atopy or flea bite allergy), the food allergy may not cause clinical signs until other allergic reactions also are triggered. This refers to the dog's pruritic threshold. The presence of several types of allergies at the same time can make a food allergy appear to be seasonal in nature.[30]

An unexpected finding and one that is counter to most pet owners' intuitions is that the onset of signs usually is not associated with a recent change in diet. It is not unusual for the dog to be consuming the same diet for 2 years or more before clinical signs of food hypersensitivity develop.[31] No gender predilections for food allergies have been reported. However some breeds of dogs seem to be more often diagnosed with this problem. Breeds that have been identified as being at greater risk are German Shepherd Dogs, Golden Retrievers, Labrador Retrievers, Dalmatians, Cocker Spaniels, English Springer Spaniels, Collies, and some terrier breeds.[29,32]

Common food allergens: Food antigens are generally large proteins, most commonly proteins associated with one or more of the protein sources in a commercial pet food. Dogs with food hypersensitivity usually have an allergic response to only one or, occasionally, two specific ingredients in the diet. The most common food allergens are beef and dairy proteins. Though less common, other allergens include pork, cereal grains, chicken, eggs, and fish.[27,29] It is relatively rare for a dog to develop sensitivities to several ingredients at the same time. However, dogs can develop sequential hypersensitivities, sometimes over a time span of several years, as their diet is changed in attempts to avoid offending ingredients.[26] Luckily, these cases are relatively rare, as they present a particularly difficult challenge for dietary management. It has been suggested that some of the cooking and processing procedures used to produce commercial pet foods increase the antigenicity of proteins.[27,33] As a result, some dogs with food allergies seem to be able to tolerate homemade diets but develop an allergic response to commercial diets that contain the same ingredients.

Diagnosis: Diagnosis of food hypersensitivity involves first ruling out other causes of the allergic disease, especially flea bite allergy and atopy (see chapters 12 and 14). Obtaining a full diet history is equally important. When food allergy is suspected in a dog, the standard method of diagnosis involves three steps: (1) feeding an elimination diet and demonstrating a decrease or elimination of clinical signs, (2) "challenging" the dog with the original diet and observing a return of clinical signs, and (3) feeding select ingredients to identify the specific dietary component to which the dog is allergic. The use of a feeding program is necessary because both skin tests and blood tests for allergens have been shown to be unreliable in diagnosing food allergies in dogs.[33,34]

An elimination diet refers to a diet that contains protein and carbohydrate sources to which the dog has not previously been exposed. In the past, lamb and rice were appropriate for this usage. However, an increase in the inclusion of lamb meat in commercial pet food in recent years has made these ingredients unacceptable for elimination diets in many cases. The use of fish and potatoes in some commercially available prescription diets are suitable for most dogs. If possible, a homemade pet food should be used for the elimination phase of diagnosis because some dogs with food hypersensitivity react to any type of commercial diet.[25,33] It is thought that the processing of commercial pet foods may enhance the antigenicity of some food components. In cases in which the preparation of a homemade elimination diet is cost-prohibitive or in which there is poor owner compliance, a commercially prepared prescription diet should be used. These foods are sold through veterinarians and have the benefits of economy, convenience, and assurance of consistency and nutritional adequacy.

The elimination diet should then be fed exclusively, with no additional treats, table scraps, or chew toys for the dog during this phase of the diagnostic program. The elimination diet should be fed for a minimum of 8 to 10 weeks. If food allergy is the cause of the dog's symptoms, some dogs will begin to show a decrease in clinical signs, primarily pruritus, within 2 to 3 weeks. However, a substantial proportion of dogs take a longer period of time to respond.[32] For this reason, the diet should be fed exclusively for the entire 8- to 10-week period before making any conclusions. Owners should be aware that not all dogs with food allergy will show a complete termination of skin inflammation and pruritus when fed an elimination diet. This occurs because some dogs are allergic to other substances in the environment. Therefore, a reduction in pruritus of 50 percent or more generally is considered to be a positive diagnosis for food allergy.[24]

The challenge portion of the diagnostic program is used to make a conclusive diagnosis of food allergy. This is conducted by reintroducing the dog's original diet and observing the dog for a return of clinical signs. If signs of pruritus recur within 4 hours and 14 days of the start of the challenge, this is indicative of food allergy. In contrast, if no change is seen, the dog probably is not food allergic or is allergic to other compounds in its environment.

The final phase, identification of specific antigens, is accomplished by adding single food items to the elimination diet and observing the dog for a return of pruritus. Beef and dairy products usually are tested first, as these are the most common food allergens in dogs. The owner adds a few teaspoons of ground beef or powdered milk to the dog's elimination diet at each meal. Only one ingredient should be added and tested at a time, and if an ingredient causes an allergic reaction, the elimination diet should be refed until all signs are resolved before proceeding with another item. If no clinical signs are observed within 14 days of adding a test ingredient, the pet probably is not allergic to that food.

Treatment: Treatment of food hypersensitivity involves lifetime nutritional management in which the dog is fed a diet that is acceptable, palatable, nutritionally complete, and does not contain any ingredients to which the dog is allergic. This can be either a homemade diet that has been determined to be complete and balanced or a commercial product that contains a protein and carbohydrate source the dog tolerates. Lamb traditionally has been used as the protein source in diets for dogs with food allergies. However, the ubiquitous use of lamb in commercial pet food now precludes its use for most dogs with diagnosed food allergy. Other protein sources that may be acceptable are fish, venison, or rabbit. Possible novel carbohydrate sources include potato, barley, and oats.

In many cases, owners will proceed through the elimination and challenge phases of diagnosis but refrain from the identification phase. This phase can be very time-consuming and tedious, and many owners are reluctant to conduct this phase because it involves exposing their dog to potential allergens and causing a return of the allergic signs. Therefore, after completing the elimination and challenge phases and arriving at a diagnosis of food allergy, some owners choose to simply find a diet their dog will tolerate and do not attempt to identify the specific ingredients to which the dog is allergic. In these cases, a diet that contains protein and carbohydrate sources new to the dog should be selected. Feeding the elimination diet as the dog's long-term maintenance diet is acceptable if the food has been determined to be complete and balanced. Most commercially available prescription diets formulated as elimination diets meet these criteria.

Some dogs with diagnosed food hypersensitivities may eventually develop additional sensitivities to ingredients in the new diet.[30] This may take several years to occur and can develop even when the owner diligently feeds the dog only one type of diet. In these cases, the identification phase must be repeated and another suitable diet must be found. Occasionally, the dog loses her original sensitivity and can once again consume a diet containing the original ingredients.[30] Overall, the underlying goal of dietary management of food hypersensitivity is to avoid feeding any food that contains ingredients to which the dog is allergic. This includes treats, human food, and even chew toys (Table 19.4). In cases in which the dog is fed only an appropriate diet, the elimination of pruritus and skin infections can be long term and can lead to a long, healthful life for the dog.

TABLE 19.4   Diagnosis and Management of Food Hypersensitivity

✓ Select an elimination diet containing novel protein and carbohydrate sources (example: fish and potato)

✓ Feed the elimination diet for 8 to 10 weeks and observe for diminishing clinical signs of hypersensitivity

✓ If the elimination diet causes a decrease in clinical signs, refeed the original diet and observe for a return of pruritus. If signs reappear, this is a definitive diagnosis of food hypersensitivity

✓ Food allergens can be identified by adding a small amount of a single suspected allergen (example: beef or milk) to the elimination diet and observing for a return of signs

✓ For lifelong management, a diet that is nutritionally complete and balanced and does not contain the food allergens to which the dog reacts must be fed exclusively

✓ Any dog treats, human food, and other snacks should not be fed unless they are known to be free of the allergen

Conclusions

Providing a complete and balanced diet throughout a dog's life is an important contributor to health and vitality. In addition, new knowledge and recent advances in the understanding of canine health and disease have allowed the development of dietary management and treatment programs that effectively manage or treat certain types of disease. The use of dietary management to treat obesity and to manage diabetes mellitus, chronic kidney disease, and food hypersensitivity are some examples. The growing body of knowledge and understanding of the needs of healthy and ill dogs will lead to additional dietary prescriptions that aid in the prevention, management, and treatment of disease.

Cited References

1. Markwell, P.J., Erk, W., and Parkin, G.D. **Obesity in the dog.** Journal of Small Animal Practice, 31:533–537. (1990)

2. Sloth, C. **Practical management of obesity in dogs and cats.** Journal of Small Animal Practice, 33:178–182. (1992)

3. Branam, J.E. **Dietary management of obese dogs and cats.** Veterinary Technician, 9:490–493. (1988)

4. Houpt, K.A., Coren, B., and Hintz, H.F. **Effect of sex and reproductive status on sucrose preference, food intake, and body weight of dogs.** Journal of the American Veterinary Medical Association, 174:1083–1085. (1979)

5. Edney, A.T.B. and Smith, A.M. **Study of obesity in dogs visiting veterinary**

practices in the United Kingdom. Veterinary Record, 118:391–396. (1986)

6. Sibley, K.W. **Diagnosis and management of the overweight dog.** British Veterinary Journal, 140:124–131. (1984)

7. Butterwick, R.F. and Markwell, P.J. **Effect of level and source of dietary fibre on food intake in the dog.** In: *Waltham Symposium on the Nutrition of Companion Animals,* September 23–25, 1993 (abstract).

8. Stogdale, L. **Definition of diabetes mellitus.** Cornell Veterinarian, 76:156–174. (1985)

9. Williams, L. **Canine diabetes mellitus.** Veterinary Technician, 9:168–170. (1988)

10. Robertson, K.A., Feldman, E.C., and Polonsky, K. **Spontaneous diabetes mellitus in 24 dogs: incidence of type I versus type II disease.** Proceedings of the American College of Veterinary Internal Medicine, pp. 1036-1040. (1989)

11. Nelson, R.W. **Nutritional management of diabetes mellitus.** Seminars in Veterinary Medicine and Surgery, Small Animal, 5:178–186. (1990)

12. Ferguson, D. C., Hoenig, M., and Cornelius, L. M. **Diabetes mellitus in dogs and cats.** In: *Small Animal Medical Therapeutics* (M.D. Lorenz, L.M. Cornelius, and D.C. Ferguson, editors), Lippincott Co., Philadelphia, Pennsylvania, pp. 85-96. (1992)

13. Bovee, K.C. **Diet and kidney failure.** In: *Kal Kan Symposium for the Treatment of Dog and Cat Disease,* Kal Kan Foods, Inc., Vernon, California, pp. 25–28. (1977)

14. Bovee, K.C. **The uremic syndrome: Patient evaluation and treatment.** Compendium of Continuing Education of the Practicing Veterinarian, 1:279–283. (1979)

15. Cowgill, L.D. and Spangler, W.L. **Renal insufficiency in geriatric dogs.** Veterinary Clinics of North America: Small Animal Practice, 11:727–749. (1981)

16. Finco, D.R., Crowell, W.A., and Barsanti, J.A. **Effects of three diets on dogs with induced chronic renal failure.** American Journal of Veterinary Research, 46:646–653. (1985)

17. Bovee, K.C. **Influence of dietary protein on renal function in dogs.** Journal of Nutrition, 121:S128–S139. (1991)

18. Robertson, J.L., Goldschmidt, M., and Kronfeld, D.S. **Long-term renal responses to high dietary protein in dogs with 75 percent nephrectomy.** Kidney International, 29:511–519. (1986)

19. Polzin, D.J., Osborne, C.A., and Lulich, J.P. **Effects of dietary protein/phosphate restriction in normal dogs and dogs with chronic renal failure.** Journal of Small Animal Practice, 32:289–295. (1991)

20. Hansen. B., DiBartola, S.P., and Chew, D.J. **Clinical and metabolic findings in dogs with chronic renal failure fed two diets.** American Journal of Veterinary Research, 53:326–334. (1992)

21. Kronfeld, D.S. **Dietary management of chronic renal disease in dogs: a critical appraisal.** Journal of Small Animal Practice, 34:211–219. (1993)

22. Finco, D.R., Brown, S.A., and Crowell, W.A. **Effect of phosphorus/calcium-restricted and phosphorus/calcium-replete 32 percent diets in dogs with chronic renal failure.** American Journal of Veterinary Research, 53:157–163. (1992)

23. Scott, D.W., Miller, W.H., and Griffin, C.E. In: *Muller and Kirk's Small Animal Dermatology,* fifth edition, W.B. Saunders, Philadelphia, Pennsylvania, pp. 500-520. (1995)

24. Scott, D.W. **Immunologic skin disorders in the dog and cat.** Veterinary Clinics of North America: Small Animal Practice, 8:641–664. (1978)

25. White, S.D. **Food hypersensitivity in 30 dogs.** Journal of the American Veterinary Medical Association, 188:695–698. (1986)

26. August, J.R. **Dietary hypersensitivity in dogs: cutaneous manifestations, diagnosis and management.** Compendium of Continuing Education for the Practicing Veterinarian, 7:469–477. (1985)

27. Doering, G.G.. **Food allergy: where does it fit as a cause of canine pruritus**? Pet Veterinarian, May/June, pp 10-16. (1991)

28. Leib, M.S. and August, J.R. **Food hypersensitivity.** In: *Textbook of Veterinary Internal Medicine,* third edition (S.J. Ettinger, editor), W.B. Saunders, Philadelphia, Pennsylvania, pp. 194–197. (1989)

29. Harvey, R.G. **Food allergy and dietary intolerance in dogs: a report of 25 cases.** Journal of Small Animal Practice, 34:175–179. (1993)

30. Halliwell, R.E.W. **Management of dietary hypersensitivity in the dog.** Journal of Small Animal Practice, 33:156–160. (1992)

31. Walton, G.S. **Skin responses in the dog and cat due to ingested allergens: observations on one hundred confirmed cases.** Veterinary Record, 81:709–713. (1967)

32. Rosser, E.J. **Diagnosis of food allergy in dogs.** Journal of the American Veterinary Medical Association, 203:259–262. (1993)

33. Jeffers, J.G., Shanley, K.J., and Meyer, E.K. **Diagnostic testing of dogs for food hypersensitivity.** Journal of the American Veterinary Medical Association, 198:245–250. (1991)

34. Kunkle, G. and Horner, S. **Validity of skin testing for diagnosis of food allergy in dogs.** Journal of the American Veterinary Medical Association, 200:677–680. (1992)

References and
Recommended Reading

PART 1
Books

Ackerman, L. *Healthy Dog!* Doarl Publishing, Wilsonville, Oregon, 126 pp. (1993)

American Kennel Club. *The Complete Dog Book.* Howell Book House, Inc., New York, New York, 724 pp. (1995)

American Kennel Club. *Obedience Regulations.* American Kennel Club, New York, New York, 2 pp. (1990)

Anderson, R.K., Hart, B.L., and Hart, L.A. *The Pet Connection: Its Influence on Our Health and Quality of Life.* Center to Study Human-Animal Relationships and Environments, Minneapolis, Minnesota, 455 pp. (1984)

Beck, A.M. and Katcher, A.A. *Between Pets and People.* G.P. Putman's Sons, New York, New York. (1983)

Fogle, B. *The Dog's Mind.* Howell Book House, New York, New York, 201 pp. (1990)

Fox, M.W. *Behaviour of Wolves, Dogs and Related Canids.* Harper and Row, New York, New York. (1971)

Fox, M.W. *The Dog: Its Domestication and Behavior.* Garland STPM Press, New York, New York. (1978)

Genoways, H.H. and Burgwin, M.A. (editors). *Natural History of the Dog.* Carnegie Museum of Natural History, Washington, DC. 65 pp. (1984)

Gibbs, M. *Leader Dogs for the Blind.* Denlinger's Publishers Ltd., Fairfax, Virginia. (1982)

Gilbert, E.M. and Brown, T.R. *K-9 Structure and Terminology.* Howell Book House, New York, New York, 233 pp. (1995)

Hall, R.L. and Sharp, H.S. (editors). *Wolf and Man: Evolution in Parallel.* Academic Press, New York, New York, 210 pp. (1978)

Hoage, R.J. (editor). *Perceptions of Animals in American Culture.* Smithsonian Institution Press, Washington, D.C., 151 pp. (1989)

Holst, P.A. *Canine Reproduction: A Breeder's Guide.* Alpine Publications, Inc., Loveland, Colorado, 223 pp. (1985)

James, R.B. *The Dog Repair Book.* Alpine Press, Mills, Wyoming, 242 pp. (1990)

Kay, W.J. and Randolph, E. (editors). *The Complete Book of Dog Health.* Macmillan Publishing Company, New York, New York, 253 pp. (1985)

Lopez, Barry Holstun. *Of Wolves and Men.* Charles Scribner's Sons, New York, New York, 308 pp. (1978)

Lorenz, Konrad. *Man Meets Dog.* Kodansha International, New York, New York, 211 pp. First printed in 1953. (1994)

Manning, A. and Serpell, J. *Animals and Human Society: Changing Perspectives.* Routledge, London, United Kingdom. (1994)

Marder, A. *Your Healthy Pet: A Practical Guide to Choosing and Raising Happier, Healthier Dogs and Cats.* Rodale Press, Emmaus, Pennsylvania, 216 pp. (1994)

O'Farrell, V. *Dog's Best Friend.* Methuen, London, United Kingdom. (1994)

Olsen, S.J. *Origins of the Domestic Dog.* University of Arizona Press, Tucson, Arizona. (1985)

Ritchie, C.I.A. *The British Dog: Its History from Earliest Times.* Robert Hale, London, United Kingdom. (1981)

Robinson, I. *The Waltham Book of Human-Animal Interaction: Benefits and Responsibilities of Pet Ownership.* Pergamon Press, Oxford, United Kingdom, 148 pp. (1995)

Scott, J.P and Fuller, J.L. *Genetics and the Social Behavior of the Dog.* University of Chicago Press, Chicago, Illinois. (1965)

Seigal, M. (editor). *UC Davis School of Veterinary Medicine Book of Dogs.* HarperCollins Publishers, Inc., New York, New York, 538 pp. (1995)

Serpell, J.A. (editor). *The Domestic Dog: Its Evolution, Behavior, and Interactions with People.*, Cambridge, United Kingdom, 268 pp. (1995)

Serpell, J.A. *In the Company of Animals.* Blackwell, Oxford, United Kingdom. (1986)

Thorne, C. (editor). *The Waltham Book of Dog and Cat Behaviour.* Pergamon Press, Oxford, England, 158 pp. (1992)

Willis, M.B. *Genetics of the Dog,* Howell Book House, New York, New York, 417 pp. (1989)

Zeuner, F.E. *A History of Domesticated Animals.* Harper and Row, New York, New York. (1963)

Articles

Abrantes, R. **The expression of emotions in man and canid.** In: *Canine Development Throughout Life,* Waltham Symposium, No. 8, (A.T.B. Edney, editor), Journal of Small Animal Practice, 28:1030-1036. (1987)

Albert, A. and Bulcroft, K. **Pets and urban life.** Anthrozoos, 1:9-23. (1987)

Albert, A. and Bulcroft, K. **Pets, families and the life**

course. Journal of Marriage and the Family, 50:543-552. (1988)

Anderson, W., Reid, P., and Jennings, G.L. **Pet ownership and risk factors for cardiovascular disease.** Medical Journal of Australia, 157:298-301. (1992)

Arkow, P. **A new look at overpopulation.** Anthrozoos, 3:202-205. (1994)

Arkow, P.S. and Dow, S. **The ties that do not bind: A study of the human-animal bonds that fail.** In: *The Pet Connection,* (R.K. Anderson, B.L. Hart, and L.A. Hart, editors), Center to Study Human-Animal Relationships and Environments, University of Minnesota, Minneapolis, Minnesota, pp. 348-354. (1984)

Barker, S.B. and Barker, R.T. **The human-canine bond: closer than family ties?** Journal of Mental Health Counseling, 10:46-56. (1988)

Bassing, J. **Companion animals for the blind.** In: *The Loving Bond: Companion Animals in the Helping Professions* (P. Arkow, editor), R & E Publishers, Inc., Saratoga, California, pp. 171-189. (1987)

Baun, M., Bergstrom, N., Langston, N., and Thoma, I. **Physiological effects of petting dogs: Influences of attachment.** In: *The Pet Connection: Its Influence on Our Health and Quality of Life* (R. Anderson, B. Hart, and L. Hart, editors), Grove Publishing, St. Paul, Minnesota, pp. 162-170. (1984)

Birney, B.A. **Children, animals and leisure settings.** Animals and Society, 3:171-187. (1995)

Bradshaw, J.W.S. and Brown, S.L. **Behavioural adaptations of dogs to domestication.** In: *Pets: Benefits and Practice* (I.H. Burger, editor), BVA Publications, London, United Kingdom, pp. 18-24. (1990)

Brown, L.T., Shaw, T.G., and Kirland, K.D. **Affection for people as a function of affection for dogs.** Psychological Reports, 31:957-958. (1972)

Bulcroft, K. **Pets in the American family.** People, Animals, Environment, 8:13-15. (1990)

Bustad, L.K. and Hines, L.H. **Historical perspectives of the human-animal bond.** In: *The Pet Connection* (R.K. Anderson, B.L. Hart, and L.A. Hart, editors), Center to Study Human-Animal Relationships and Environments, University of Minnesota, Minneapolis, Minnesota, pp. 15-29. (1984)

Cain, A.O. **Pets as family members.** Marriage, Family Review, 8:5-10. (1985)

Cain, A.O. **A study of pets in the family system.** In: *New Perspectives on Our Lives with Companion Animals* (A.H. Katcher and A.M. Beck, editors), University of Philadelphia Press, Philadelphia, Pennsylvania, pp. 72-81. (1983)

Clutton-Brock, J. **Dog.** In: *Evolution of Domesticated Animals* (I.L. Mason, editor), Longman Press, London, United Kingdom, pp. 198-211. (1984)

Clutton-Brock, J. **Man-made dogs.** Science, 197:1340-1342. (1977)

Clutton-Brock, J. **A review of the family Canidae with a classification by numerical methods.** Bulletin of the British Museum of Natural History, Zoology, 29:117-199. (1976)

Clutton-Brock, J. and Jewell, P. **Origin and domestication of the dog.** In: *Miller's Anatomy of the Dog,* third edition (H.E. Evans, editor), W.B. Saunders, Philadelphia, Pennsylvania, pp. 21-31. (1993)

Concannon, P.W. **Canine pregnancy and parturition.** Veterinary Clinics of North America: Small Animal Practice, 16:453-475. (1986)

Concannon, P.W., Hansel, W., and McEntee, K. **Changes in LH, progesterone and sexual behavior associated with preovulatory lutenization in the bitch.** Biology and Reproduction, 17:604-615. (1977)

Coppinger, R.P. and Feinstein, M. **Why dogs bark.** Smithsonian Magazine, January:119-129. (1991)

Coppinger, R.P. and Schnieder, R. **Evolution of working dogs.** In: *The Domestic Dog: Its Evolution, Behavior and Interactions with People* (J.A. Serpell, editor), Cambridge University Press, Cambridge, United Kingdom, pp. 21-47. (1995)

Coppinger, R.P. and Smith, C.K. **A model for understanding the evolution of mammalian behavior.** In: *Current Mammalogy,* volume 2 (H. Genoways, editor), Plenum Press, New York, New York, pp. 33-74. (1989)

Currier, R.W., Raithel, W.F., Martin, R.J., and Potter, M.E. **Canine brucellosis.** Journal of the American Veterinary Medical Association, 180:187-198. (1982)

Davis, S.J. and Valls, F.R. **Evidence for domestication of the dog 12,000 years ago in the natufian of Israel.** Nature, 276:608-610. (1978)

Dodd, G.H. and Squirrel, D.J. **Structure and mechanism in the mammalian olfactory system.** Symposia of the Zoological Society of London, 45:35-36. (1980)

Dodds, W.J. **Further studies of canine Von Willebrands disease.** Journal of Laboratory and Clinical Medicine, 76:713-721. (1970)

Dodds, W.J. **Inherited bleeding disorders.** Canine Practice, 5:49-58. (1978)

Endenburg, N., Hart, H., and de Vries, H.W. **Differences between owners and non-owners of companion animals.** Anthrozoos, 4:120-126. (1990)

Fletch, S.M., Pinkerton, P.H., and Brueckner, P.J. **The Alaskan Malamute chondrodysplasia (dwarfism-anemia) syndrome—a review.** Journal of the American Animal Hospital Association, 11:353-361. (1975)

Fogle, B. **The bond between people and pets—a**

review. Veterinary Annual, 26:361-365. (1986)

Fox, M.W. **Origin and history of the dog.** In: *Understanding Your Dog,* Coward, McCann and Geoghegan, New York, New York, pp. 1-17. (1974)

Fox, M.W. **Socio-ecological implications of individual differences in wolf litters: a developmental and evolutionary perspective.** Behaviour, 41:298-313. (1972)

Frank, H. and Frank, M.G. **On the effects of domestication on canine social development and behavior.** Applied Animal Ethology, 8:507-525. (1982)

Freedman, D.G., King, J.A., and Elliot, O. **Critical period in the social development of dogs.** Science, 133:1016-1017. (1961)

Friedmann, E., Katcher, A.H., Thomas, S.A., Lynch, J.J., and Messent, P.R. **Social interaction and blood pressure: Influence of animal companions.** Journal of Nervous and Mental Disease, 171:461-465. (1983)

Grossberg, J.M. and Alf, E.F., Jr. **Interactions with pet dogs: Effects on human cardiovascular response.** Journal of the Delta Society, 2:20-27. (1986)

Grossberg, J.M., Alf, E.F. Jr., and Vormbrock, J.K. **Does pet dog presence reduce human cardiovascular responses to stress?** Anthrozoos, 2:38-44. (1988)

Harcourt, R.A. **The dog in prehistoric and early historic Britain.** Journal of Archeological Science, 1:151-175. (1974)

Hart, L., Hart, B.L., and Bergin, B. **Socializing effects of service dogs for people with disabilities.** Anthrozoos, 1:41-44. (1987)

Heffner, H.E. **Hearing in large and small dogs: absolute thresholds and size of the tympanic membrane.** Behavioral Neuroscience, 97:310-318. (1983)

Hodgeman, S.F.J., Parr, H.B., Rasbridge, W.J., and Steel, J.D. **Progressive retinal atrophy in dogs. 1. The disease in Irish Setters (red).** Veterinary Record, 61:185-190. (1949)

Johnson, G.F., Sternlieb, I., Twedt, D.C., Grushoff, P.S., and Scheinberg, I.H. **Inheritance of copper toxicosis in Bedlington Terriers.** American Journal of Veterinary Research, 41:1865-1866. (1980)

Kaimus, H. **The discrimination by the nose of the dog of individual human odours and in particular of the odours of twins.** Animal Behaviour, 3:25-31. (1955)

Katcher, A.H. **Interactions between people and their pets: Form and function.** In: *Interrelationships Between People and Pets* (B. Fogle, editor), Charles C. Thomas, Springfield, Illinois, pp. 41-67. (1981)

Katcher, A.H. and Beck, A.M. **Health and caring for living things.** In: *Animals and People Sharing the World* (A.R. Rowan, editor), University Press of New England, Hanover, New Hampshire, pp. 53-73. (1988)

Katcher, A.H. and Friedmann, E. **Potential health value of pet ownership.** Compendium on Continuing Education for the Practicing Veterinarian, 2:117-122. (1980)

Katcher, A.H., Friedmann, E., Goodman, M., and Goodman, L. **Men, women and dogs.** California Veterinarian, 2:14-16. (1983)

Kidd, A.H. and Kidd, R.M. **Factors in adults' attitudes toward pets.** Psychological Reports, 65:903-910. (1989)

Kidd, A.H. and Kidd, R.M. **Personality characteristics and preferences in pet ownership.** Psychological Reports, 46:939-949. (1980)

Kretchmer, K.R. and Fox, M.W. **Effects of domestication on animal behavior.** Veterinary Record, 96:102-108. (1975)

Marx, M.B., Stalones, L., Garrity, T.F., and Johnson, T.P. **Demographics of pet ownership among U.S. adults 21 to 64 years of age.** Anthrozoos, 2:33-37. (1988)

Messent, P.R. **Facilitation of social interaction by companion animals.** In: *New Perspective on our Lives with Companion Animals* (A.H. Katcher and A.M. Beck, editors), University of Pennsylvania Press, Philadelphia, Pennsylvania, pp. 37-46. (1983)

Messent, P.R. **Pets as social facilitators.** Veterinary Clinics of North America: Small Animal Practice, 15:387-397. (1985)

Miller, M. and Lage, D. **Observed pet-owner in-home interactions: species differences and association with the pet relationship scale.** Anthrozoos, 4:49-54. (1990)

Morey, D.F. **The early evolution of the domestic dog.** American Scientist, 82:336-347. (1994)

Morey, D.F. **Size, shape and development in the evolution of the domestic dog.** Journal of Archaeological Science, 19:181-204. (1992)

Moulton, D.G., Ashton, E.H., and Eayrs, J.T. **Studies in olfactory acuity. 4. Relative detectability of n-aliphatic acids by the dog.** Animal Behaviour, 8:117-128. (1960)

Mugford, R.A. **The social significance of pet ownership.** In: *Ethology and Nonverbal Communication in Mental Health* (S.A. Corson and E.O. Corson, editors), Pergamon Press, Oxford, England, pp. 111-122. (1980)

Myers, O.E., Jr. **Child-animal interaction: Nonverbal dimensions.** Society and Animals, 4:19-35. (1996)

Neitz, J., Geist, T., and Jacobs, J.H. **Color vision in the**

dog. Visual Neuroscience, 3:119-125. (1989)

Ory, M., and Goldberg, E. **Pet possession and life satisfaction.** In: *New Perspectives on Our Lives With Companion Animals* (A.H. Katcher and A.M. Beck, editors), University of Pennsylvania Press, Philadelphia, Pennsylvania. (1983)

Paul, E.S. and Serpell, J.A. **Why children keep pets: The influence of child and family characteristics.** Anthrozoos, 5:231-244. (1992)

Podberscek, A.L. and Serpell, J.A. **The English Cocker Spaniel: Preliminary findings on aggressive behavior.** Applied Animal Behaviour Science, 47:750-89. (1996)

Purswell, B.J. and Freeman, L.E. **Reproduction in the canine male: Anatomy, endocrinology, and spermatogenesis.** Canine Practice, 18(3):8-13. (1993)

Ritvo, H. **The emergence of modern pet-keeping.** In: *Animals and People Sharing the World* (A.R. Rowan, editor), University Press of New England, Hanover, New Hampshire, pp. 13-31. (1988)

Schenkel, R. **Submission: its features and functions in the wolf and dog.** American Zoologist, 7:319-330. (1967)

Serpell, J.A. **Beneficial effects of pet ownership on some aspects of human health.** Journal of the Royal Society of Medicine, 84:717-720. (1991)

Serpell, J. A. **Childhood pets and their influence on adults' attitudes.** Psychological Reports, 49:651-654. (1981)

Serpell, J.A. **Evidence for an association between pet behavior and owner attachment levels.** Applied Animal Behavior Science, 47:49-60. (1996)

Serpell, J.A. **The personality of the dog and its influence on the pet-owner bond.** In: *New Perspectives on Our Lives with Companion Animals* (A.H. Katcher and A.M. Beck, editors), University of Philadelphia Press, Philadelphia, Pennsylvania, pp. 57-63. (1983)

Serpell, J.A. and Paul, E. **Pets and the development of positive attitudes to animals.** In: *Animals and Human Society: Changing Perspectives* (Manning, A. and Serpell, J. editors), Routledge, London, United Kingdom, pp. 127-144. (1994)

Sokolowski, J.H. **Prostaglandin-F2-alpha-THAM for medical treatment of endometriosis, metritis, and pyometra in the bitch.** Journal of the American Animal Hospital Association, 16:119-122. (1980)

Thorne, C. **Feeding behaviour of domestic dogs and the role of experience.** In: *The Domestic Dog: Its Evolution, Behavior and Interactions with People* (J.A. Serpell, editor), Cambridge University Press, Cambridge, United Kingdom, pp. 103-114. (1995)

Voith, V. **Attachment of people to companion an-**

imals. Veterinary Clinics of North America: Small Animal Practice, 15:289-295. (1985)

Watson, N.L. and Weinstein, M. **Pet ownership in relation to depression, anxiety, and anger in working women.** Anthrozoos, 6:135-138. (1993)

Wayne, R.K. **Molecular evolution of the dog family.** Trends in Genetics, 9:218-224. (1993)

Wayne, R.K. **Phylogenetic relationships of canids to other carnivores.** In: *Miller's Anatomy of the Dog,* third edition (H.E. Evans, editor), W.B. Saunders Company, Philadelphia, Pennsylvania, pp. 15-21. (1993)

Willis, M.B. **Breeding dogs for desirable traits.** Journal of Small Animal Practice, 28:965-983. (1987)

Young, M.S. **The evolution of domestic pets and companion animals.** Veterinary Clinics of North America: Small Animal Practice, 15:297-309. (1985)

PART 2
Books

Beck, A.M. *The Ecology of Stray Dogs: A Study of Free-Ranging Urban Animals.* York Press, Baltimore, Maryland. (1973)

Beck, A.M., Overall, K.L., and McKeown, D.B. *Behavioural Problems in Small Animals.* Ralston Purina, St. Louis, Missouri. (1992)

Burns, M. and Fraser, M.N. *Genetics of the Dog: The Basis of Successful Breeding.* Oliver and Boyd, Edinburgh, Scotland. (1966)

Campbell, W.E. *Behavior Problems in Dogs.* American Veterinary Publications, Santa Barbara, California. (1992)

Donaldson, J. *Culture Clash: A Revolutionary New Way of Understanding the Relationship between Humans and Domestic Dogs.* James and Kenneth Publishers, Oakland, California, 221 pp. (1996)

Fisher, J. *Dogwise; The Natural Way to Train Your Dog.* Souvenir Press, London, United Kingdom. (1992)

Fisher, John (editor). *The Behaviour of Dogs and Cats.* Stanley Paul and Co., London, United Kingdom, 164 pp. (1993)

Fox, M.W. *Behavior of Wolves, Dogs and Related Canids.* Harper and Row, New York, New York. (1971)

Fox, M.W. *The Dog: Its Domestication and Behavior.* Garland STPM Press, New York, New York. 1978

Hart, B.L. *The Behavior of Domestic Animals.* W.H. Freeman Company, New York, New York. (1985)

Hart, B.L. and Hart L.A. *Canine and Feline Behavioral Therapy.* Lea and Febiger, Philadelphia, Pennsylvania, 275 pp. (1985)

Hart, B.L. and Hart, L.A. *The Perfect Puppy: How to Choose Your Dog by Its Behavior.* W.H. Freeman and

Company, New York, New York. (1988)

Johnston, B. *The Skillful Mind of the Guide Dog: Towards a Cognitive and Holistic Model of Training.* Guide Dogs for the Blind Association, Reading, United Kingdom. (1990)

Koehler, W. *The Koehler Method of Dog Training.* Howell Book House, New York, New York, 208 pp. (1962)

Landsberg, G., Hunthausen, W., and Ackerman, L. *Handbook of Behaviour Problems in the Dog and Cat.* Butterworth-Heinemann, Oxford, United Kingdom, 211 pp. (1997)

Lorenz, K. *Man Meets Dog.* Penguin Books, Harmondsworth, Middlesex, United Kingdom. (1953)

Mech, L.D. *The Wolf: The Ecology and Behaviour of an Endangered Species.* Natural History Press, New York, New York. (1970)

Neville, P. *Do Dogs Need Shrinks?* Carol Publishing Group, New York, New York. (1992)

O'Farrell, V. *Dog's Best Friend: How Not to Be a Problem Owner.* Methuen Press, London, United Kingdom. (1994)

O'Farrell, V. *Manual of Canine Behavior.* BSAVA Publications, Cheltenham, United Kingdom. (1986)

Pfaffenberger, C.J. Scott, J.P., and Fuller, J.L. *Guide Dogs for the Blind: Their Selection, Development and Training.* Elsevier, Amsterdam, Netherlands. (1976)

Polsky, R.H. *User's Guide to the Scientific Literature on Dog and Cat Behavior.* Animal Behavior Counseling Services, Inc., Los Angeles. California. (1991)

Pryor, K. *Don't Shoot the Dog.* Bantam Books, New York, New York, 187 pp. (1984)

Pryor, K. *Karen Pryor on Behavior.* Sunshine Books, North Bend, Washington. (1995)

Reid, P. *Excel-Erated Learning: Explaining How Dogs Learn and How Best to Teach Them.* James and Kenneth Publishing, Oakland, California, 172 pp. (1996)

Robinson, I. *The Waltham Book of Human-Animal Interaction: Benefits and Responsibilities of Pet Ownership.* Pergamon Press, Oxford, United Kingdom, 148 pp. (1995)

Rogerson, J. *Your Dog: Its Development, Behaviour, and Training.* Popular Dogs Publishing Company, London, United Kingdom, 174 pp. (1990)

Saunders, B. *The Complete Book of Dog Obedience: A Guide for Trainers.* Howell Book House, New York, New York, 261 pp. (1976)

Scott, J.P and Fuller, J.L. *Genetics and the Social Behavior of the Dog.* University of Chicago Press, Chicago, Illinois. (1965)

Serpell, J.A. (editor). *The Domestic Dog: Its Evolution, Behavior, and Interactions with People.* Cambridge University Press, Cambridge, United Kingdom, 268 pp. (1995)

Skinner, B.F. *The Behavior of Organisms: An Experimental Approach.* Appleton-Century, New York, New York. (1938)

Thorne, C. (editor). *The Waltham Book of Dog and Cat Behaviour.* Pergamon Press, Oxford, England, 158 pp. (1992)

Tortora, D.L. *The Right Dog for You.* Simon and Schuster, New York, New York. (1986)

Voith, V.L. and Borchelt, P.L. (editors). *Readings in Companion Animal Behavior.* Veterinary Learning Systems, Trenton, New Jersey, 276 pp. (1996)

Walkowicz, C. *The Perfect Match: A Dog Buyer's Guide.* Howell Book House, New York, New York. (1996)

Wilkes, G. *A Behavior Sampler.* Sunshine Books, North Bend, Washington, 237 pp. (1994)

Articles

Abrantes, R. **The expression of emotions in man and canid.** In: *Canine Development Throughout Life,* Waltham Symposium, No. 8 (A.T.B. Edney, editor), Journal of Small Animal Practice, 28:1030-1036. (1987)

Arons, C.D., Shoemaker, W.J. **The distribution of catecholamines and beta-endorphin in the brain of three behaviorally distinct breeds of dogs and their F1 hybrids.** Brain Research, 594:31-39. (1992)

Barrette, C. **The 'inheritance of dominance,' or an aptitude to dominate.** Animal Behaviour, 46:591-593. (1993)

Bartlett, C.R. **Heritabilities and genetic correlations between hip dysplasia and temperament traits of seeing-eye dogs.** Master's Thesis, Rutgers University, New Brunswick, New Jersey. (1976)

Bateson, P. **How do sensitive periods arise and what are they for?** Animal Behaviour, 27:470-486. (1979)

Beaver, B.V. **Clinical classification of canine aggression.** Applied Animal Ethology, 10:35-43. (1983)

Beaver, B.V. **Distance-increasing postures of dogs.** Veterinary Medicine: Small Animal Clinician, 77:1023-1024. (1982)

Beaver, B.V. **Friendly communications by the dog.** Veterinary Medicine: Small Animal Clinician, 76:647-649. (1981)

Beaver, B.V. **Profiles of dogs presented for aggression.** Journal of the American Animal Hospital Association, 29:564-569. (1993)

Bekoff, M. **Scent-marking by free ranging domestic dogs: Olfactory and visual components.** Biology of Behaviour, 4:123-139. (1979)

Bekoff, M. **Social play and play-soliciting by infant canids.** American Zoologist, 14:323-340. (1974)

Blackshaw, J.K. **Human and animal inter-relationships. Review series 3: Normal behaviour patterns of dogs. Part 1.** Australian Veterinary

Practitioner, 15:110-112. (1985)

Bolles, R.C. **Species-specific defense reactions and avoidance learning.** Psychology Review, 77:32-48. (1970)

Borchelt, P.L. **Aggressive behavior of dogs kept as companion animals: Classification and influence of sex, reproduction status and breed.** Applied Animal Ethology, 10:45-61. (1983)

Borchelt, P.L. **Behavioral development of the puppy.** In: *Nutrition and Behavior in Dogs and Cats* (R.S. Anderson, editor), Pergamon Press, Oxford, United Kingdom, pp. 165-174. (1984)

Borchelt, P.L. **Separation-elicited behavior problems in dogs.** In: *New Perspectives on Our Lives with Companion Animals,* (A.H. Katcher and A.M. Beck, editors), University of Pennsylvania Press, Philadelphia, Pennsylvania, pp. 187-196. (1983)

Borchelt, P.L. and Coppola, M.C. **Characteristics of dominance aggression in dogs.** Paper presented at annual meeting of the Animal Behavior Society, North Carolina, June. (1985)

Borchelt, P.L. and Voith, V.L. **Classification of animal behavior problems.** Veterinary Clinics of North America: Small Animal Practice, 12:571-585. (1982)

Borchelt, P.L. and Voith, V.L. **Diagnosis and treatment of separation-related behavior problems in dogs.** Veterinary Clinics of North America: Small Animal Practice, 12:625-635. (1982)

Borchelt, P.L. and Voith, V.L. **Dominance aggression in dogs.** In: *Readings in Companion Animal Behavior* (V.L. Voith and P.L. Borchelt, editors), Veterinary Learning Systems, Trenton, New Jersey, pp. 230-239. (1996)

Bradshaw, J.W.S. and Brown, S.L. **Behavioral adaptations of dogs to domestication.** In: *Pets: Benefits and Practice* (I.H. Burger, editor), BVA Publications, London, United Kingdom, pp. 18-24. (1990)

Bradshaw, J.W.S., Natynczuk, S.E., and Macdonald, D.W. **Potential applications of anal sac volatiles from domestic dogs.** In: *Chemical Signals in Vertebrates,* fifth edition (D.W. Macdonald, D. Muller-Schwarze, and S.E. Natynczuk, editors), Oxford University Press, Oxford, United Kingdom, pp. 640-644. (1990)

Bradshaw, J.W.S., Wickens, S.M., and Goodwin, D. **Dogs and wolves: Do they really speak the same language?** Association of Pet Behaviour Counsellors' Newsletter. (1994)

Clark, R.S., Heron, W., Fetherstonhaugh, M.L., Forgays, D.G., and Hebb, D.O. **Individual differences in dogs: preliminary report on the effects of early experience.** Canadian Journal of Psychology, 5:150-156. (1951)

Coppinger, R. and Coppinger, L. **Biological basis of behavior of domestic dog breeds.** From: *Readings in Companion Animal Behavior* (V.L. Voith and P.L. Borchelt, editors), Veterinary Learning Systems, Trenton, New Jersey, pp. 9-18. (1996)

Coppinger, R.P. and Feinstein, M. **Why dogs bark.** Smithsonian Magazine, January:119-129. (1991)

Coppinger, R., Coppinger, L., Langeloh, G., Gettler, L., and Lorenz, J. **A decade of use of livestock guarding dogs.** In: *Proceedings of the Vertebrate Pest Conference,* Vol. 13 (A.C. Crabb and R.E. Marsh, editors), University of California at Davis, pp. 209-214. (1988)

Crowell-Davis, S.L. **Identifying and correcting human-directed dominance aggression of dogs.** Veterinary Medicine, October:990-998. (1991)

Denenberg, V.H. **A consideration of the usefulness of the critical period hypothesis as applied to the stimulation of rodents in infancy.** In: *Early Experience and Behaviour* (G. Newton and S. Levine, editors), Charles Thomas, Springfield, Illinois, pp. 142-167. (1968)

Doty, R.L. and Dunbar, I.F. **Attraction of beagles to conspecific urine, vaginal and anal sac secretion odours.** Physiology and Behaviour, 12:325-333. (1974)

Dykman, R.A., Murphree, O.D., and Ackerman, P.T. **Litter patterns in the offspring of nervous and stable dogs. II. Autonomic and motor conditioning.** Journal of Nervous and Mental Disease, 141:419-431. (1966)

Dykman, R.A., Murphree, O.D., and Reese, W.G. **Familial anthropophobia in Pointer dogs?** Archives of Genetics and Psychiatry, 36:988-993. (1979)

Elliot, O. and Scott, P. **The development of emotional distress reactions to separation in puppies.** Journal of Genetic Psychology, 99:3-22. (1961)

Estep, D.Q. **The ontogeny of behavior.** In: *Readings in Companion Animal Behavior* (V.L. Voith and P.L. Borchelt, editors), Veterinary Learning Systems, Trenton, New Jersey, pp. 19-31. (1996)

Falt, L. **Inheritance of behaviour in the dog.** In: *Nutrition and Behaviour in Dogs and Cats* (R.S. Anderson, editor), Pergamon Press, Oxford, United Kingdom, pp. 183-187. (1984)

Fox, M.W. **Behavioral effects of rearing dogs with cats during the "critical period of socialization."** Behaviour, 35:273-280. (1969)

Fox, M.W. **The behaviour of dogs.** In: *The Behaviour of Domestic Animals,* third edition (E.S.E. Hafez, editor), Bailliere Tindall Press, London, United Kingdom, pp. 370-409. (1975)

Fox, M.W. **Socialization, environmental factors, and abnormal behavioral development in animals.** In: *Abnormal Behavior in Animals* (M.W.

Fox, editor), W.E. Saunders, Philadelphia, Pennsylvania, pp. 332-355. (1968)

Fox, M.W. and Stelzner, D. **Behavioural effects of differential early experience in the dog.** Animal Behaviour, 14:273-281. (1966)

Freedman, D.G., King, J.A., and Elliot, O. **Critical periods in the social development of dogs.** Science, 133:1016-1017. (1961)

Ginsberg, B.E. and Hiestrand, L. **Humanity's "best friend": The origins of our inevitable bond with dogs.** In: *The Inevitable Bond: Examining Scientist-Animal Interactions* (A. Davis and D. Balfour, editors), Cambridge University Press, Cambridge, United Kingdom, pp. 93-108. (1992)

Goddard, M.E. and Beilharz, R.G. **Factor analysis of fearfulness in potential guide dogs.** Applied Animal Behaviour Science, 12:253-265. (1984)

Goddard, M.E. and Beilharz, R.G. **Genetic and environmental factors affecting the suitability of dogs as guide dogs for the blind.** Theoretical and Applied Genetics, 62:97-102. (1982)

Hart, B.L. and Hart, L.A. **Selecting pet dogs on the basis of cluster analysis of breed behavior profiles and gender.** Journal of the American Veterinary Medical Association, 186:1181-1195. (1985)

Hetts, S. and Estep, D.Q. **Behavior management: Preventing elimination and destructive behavior problems.** Veterinary Forum, November:60-61. (1994)

Jagoe, J.A. **Behaviour problems in the domestic dog: A retrospective study to identify factors influencing their development.** Unpublished Ph.D. Thesis, Cambridge University Press, Cambridge, United Kingdom. (1994)

Landsberg, G. **The distribution of canine behavior cases at three behavior referral practices.** Veterinary Medicine, 86:1011-1018. (1991)

Landsberg, G., Hunthausen, W., and Ackerman, L. **Drugs used in behavioral therapy.** In: *Handbook of Behaviour Problems of the Dog and Cat,* Butterworth/Heinemann, Oxford, United Kingdom, pp.47-64. (1997)

Landsberg, G., Hunthausen, W., and Ackerman, L. **Fears and phobias.** In: *Handbook of Behaviour Problems of the Dog and Cat,* Butterworth/Heinemann, Oxford, United Kingdom, pp.119-128. (1997)

Levine, S. **Maternal and environmental influences on the adrenal cortical response to stress in weanling rats.** Science, 135:795-796. (1962)

Line, S. and Voith, V.L. **Dominance aggression of dogs toward people: Behavior profile and response to treatment.** Applied Animal Behavior Science, 16:77-83. (1986)

Markwell, P.J. and Thorne, C.J. **Early behavioral development of dogs.** Journal of Small Animal Practice, 28:984-991. (1987)

McCrave, E.A. **Diagnostic criteria for separation anxiety in the dog.** Veterinary Clinics of North America: Small Animal Practice, 21:247-255. (1991)

Miller, D.D., Staats, S.R., and Partlo, C. **Factors associated with the decision to surrender a pet to an animal shelter.** Journal of the American Animal Hospital Association, 209:738-742. (1996)

Mugford, R.A. **Aggressive behaviour in the English Cocker Spaniel.** The Veterinary Annual, 24:310-314. (1984)

Mugford, R.A. **Attachment versus dominance: an alternate view of the man-dog relationship.** In: *The Human-Pet Relationship,* Proceedings of the Institute for Interdisciplinary Research on the Human-Pet Relationship, Vienna, Austria, pp. 157-165. (1985)

Mugford, R.A. **Behavior problems in the dog.** In: *Nutrition and Behavior in Dogs and Cats* (R.S. Anderson, editor), Pergamon Press, Oxford, United Kingdom, pp. 207-215. (1984)

Murphree, O.D. and Dykman, R.A. **Litter patterns in the offspring of nervous and stable dogs. I. Behavioral tests.** Journal of Nervous and Mental Disease, 141:321-332. (1965)

Murphree, O.D., Angel, C., DeLuca, D.C., and Newton, J.E.O. **Longitudinal studies of genetically nervous dogs.** Biological Psychiatry, 12:573-576. (1977)

Natynczuk, S., Bradshaw, J.W.S., and Macdonald, D.W. **Chemical constituents of the anal sacs of domestic dogs.** Biochemical Systematics and Ecology, 17:83-87. (1989)

Nott, H.M.R. **Behavioural development in the dog.** In: *The Waltham Book of Dog and Cat Behaviour* (C. Thorne, editor), Pergamon Press, Oxford, United Kingdom, pp. 65-78. (1992)

Nott, H.M.R. **Social behaviour of the dog.** In: *The Waltham Book of Dog and Cat Behaviour* (C. Thorne, editor), Pergamon Press, Oxford, United Kingdom, pp. 97-114. (1992)

O'Farrell, V. and Peachey, E. **Behavioral effects of ovariohysterectomy on bitches.** Journal of Small Animal Practice, 31:595-598. (1990)

Peters, R.P. and Mech, L.D. **Scent marking in wolves.** American Scientist, 63:628-637. (1975)

Polsky, R.H. **Factors influencing aggressive behavior in dogs.** California Veterinarian, 37:12-15. (1983)

Reid, P.J. and Borchelt, P.L. **Learning.** In: *Readings in Companion Animal Behavior* (V.L. Voith and P.L. Borchelt, editors), Veterinary Learning Systems, Trenton, New Jersey, pp. 62-71 (1996)

Sacks, J.J., Sattin, R.W., and Bonzo, S.E. **Dog bite: Related fatalities from 1979 through 1988.** Journal of the American Medical Association, 262:1489-1492. (1989)

Schenkel, R. **Submission: its features and function in the wolf and dog.** American Zoologist, 7:319-329. (1967)

Scott, J.P. **Critical periods in behavioral development.** Science, 138:949-958. (1962)

Scott, J.P. **The evolution of social behaviour in dogs and wolves.** American Zoologist, 7:373-381. (1967)

Scott, J.P. and Marston, M.V. **Critical periods affecting the development of normal and maladjustive social behaviour of puppies.** The Journal of Genetic Psychology, 77:25-60. (1950)

Serpell, J.A. **The influence of inheritance and environment on canine behaviour: myth and fact.** Journal of Small Animal Practice, 28:949-956. (1987)

Serpell, J.A. and Jagoe, J.A. **Early experience and the development of behaviour.** In: *The Domestic Dog: Its Evolution, Behavior, and Interactions with People* (J.A. Serpell, editor), Cambridge University Press, Cambridge, United Kingdom, pp. 80-102. (1995)

Shull-Selcer, E.A. and Stagg, W. **Advances in the understanding and treatment of noise phobias.** Veterinary Clinics of North America: Small Animal Practice, 21:353-367. (1991)

Simpson, B.S. and Simpson, D.M. **Behavioral pharmacotherapy.** In: *Readings in Companion Animal Behavior* (V.L. Voith and P.L. Borchelt, editors), Veterinary Learning Systems, Trenton, New Jersey, pp. 100-115. (1996)

Slabbert, J.M. and Rasa, O.A. **The effect of early separation from the mother on pups in bonding to humans and pup health.** Journal of the South African Veterinary Association, 64:4-8. (1993)

Stanley, W.C. and Elliot, O. **Differential human handling as reinforcing events and as treatment influencing later social behavior in Basenji puppies.** Psychology Reports, 10:775-788. (1962)

Stead, S.C. **Euthanasia in the dog and cat.** Journal of Small Animal Practice, 23:37-43. (1982)

Stur, I. **Genetic aspects of temperament and behavior in dogs.** Journal of Small Animal Practice, 28:957-964. (1987)

Thompson, W.R. and Heron, W. **The effects of restricting early experience on the problem-solving capacity of dogs.** Canadian Journal of Psychology, 8:17-31. (1954)

Thorne, F.C. **The inheritance of shyness in dogs.** Journal of Genetic Psychology, 65:275-279. (1944)

Tryon, R.C. **Genetic differences in maze-learning ability in rats.** In: *39th Yearbook of the National Society for the Study of Education,* Public School Publishing Company, Bloomington, Indiana, pp. 111-119. (1940)

Tuber, D.S., Hothersall, D., and Peters, M.F. **Treatment of fears and phobias in dogs.** Veterinary Clinics of North America: Small Animal Practice, 12:607-623. (1982)

Vangen, O. and Klemetsdal, G. **Genetic studies of Finnish and Norwegian test results in two breeds of hunting dog.** VI World Conference on Animal Production, Helsinki, Finland. Paper 4.25. (1988)

Vila, C., Savolainen, P., Maldonado, J.E., Amorim, I.R., Rice, J.E., Honeycutt, R.L., Crandall, K.A., Lundeburg, J., and Wayne, R.K. **Multiple and ancient origins of the domestic dog.** Science, 276:1687-1689. (1997)

Voith, V.L. **Human/animal relationships.** In: *Nutrition and Behaviour in Dogs and Cats* (R.S. Anderson, editor), Pergamon Press, Oxford, United Kingdom, pp. 147-156. (1984)

Voith, V.L. and Borchelt, P.L. **Elimination behavior and related problems in dogs.** In: *Readings in Companion Animal Behavior* (V.L. Voith and P.L. Borchelt, editors), Veterinary Learning Systems, Trenton, New Jersey, pp. 168-178. (1996)

Voith, V.L. and Borchelt, P.L. **History taking and interviewing.** In: *Readings in Companion Animal Behavior* (V.L. Voith and P.L. Borchelt, editors), Veterinary Learning Systems, Trenton, New Jersey, pp. 42-47. (1996)

Voith, V.L. and Borchelt, P.L. **Separation anxiety in dogs.** In: *The Domestic Dog: Its Evolution, Behavior, and Interactions with People,* Cambridge University Press, Cambridge, United Kingdom, pp. 124-139. (1995)

Voith, V.L. and Ganster, D. **Separation anxiety: Review of 42 cases—an abstract.** Applied Animal Behavior Science, 37:84-85. (1993)

Voith, V.L., Goodloe, L., Chapman, B., and Marder, A.R. **Comparison of dogs presented for behavior problems by source of dog.** Paper presented at AVMA annual meeting, Seattle, Washington, July 18. (1993)

Wilsson, E. **The social interaction between mother and offspring during weaning in German Shepherd Dogs: individual differences between mothers and their effects on offspring.** Applied Animal Behaviour Science, 13:101-112. (1984)

Wright, J.C. **The development of social structure during the primary socialization period in German shepherds.** Developmental Psychobiology, 13:17-24. (1980)

Wright, J.C. **Early development of exploratory behavior and dominance in three litters of German Shepherds.** In: *Early Experiences and Early Behavior: Implications for Social Development* (E.C. Simmes, editor), Academic Press, New York, New York, pp. 181-206. (1980)

Wright, J.C. and Nesselrote, M.S. **Classification of behavior problems in dogs: Distributions of age, breed, sex and reproductive status.** Applied Animal Behaviour Science, 19:169-178. (1987)

Young, M.S. **Treatment of fear-induced aggression in dogs.** Veterinary Clinics of North America: Small Animal Practice, 12: 645-653. (1982)

PART 3
Books

Ackerman, L. *Healthy Dog!* Doarl Publishing, Wilsonville, Oregon, 126 pp. (1993)

Aeolic, A.L., Weisiger, R., Siegel, A.M., Campbell, K.L., Krawiec, D.R., and McKiernan, B.C. **Trends of bacterial infections in dogs: Characterization of *Staphylococcus intermedius* isolages (1990-1992).** Canine Practice, 21:12-19. (1996)

Allen, D., Pringle, J.K., Smith, D., and Conlon, P.D. *Handbook of Veterinary Drugs.* J.B. Lippincott Company, Philadelphia, Pennsylvania. (1993)

Bamberger, M. *The Quick Guide to First Aid for Your Dog.* Howell Book House, New York, New York, 147 pp. (1993)

Foster, R. and Smith, M. *Just What the Doctor Ordered: A Complete Guide to Drugs and Medications for Your Dog.* Howell Book House, New York, New York, 248 pp. (1996)

Fowler, M.E. *Plant Poisoning in Small Companion Animals.* Ralston Purina Company, St. Louis, Missouri. (1980)

Greene, C.E. *Infectious Diseases of the Dog and Cat.* W.B. Saunders Company, Philadelphia, Pennsylvania. (1990)

James, R.B. *The Dog Repair Book.* Alpine Press, Mills, Wyoming, 242 pp. (1990)

Kay, W.J. and Randolph, E. (editors). *The Complete Book of Dog Health.* Macmillan Publishing Company, New York, New York, 253 pp. (1985)

Lane, D.R. *Jone's Animal Nursing,* fifth edition. Pergamon Press, Oxford, United Kingdom, 821 pp. (1989)

McCurnin, D.M. *Clinical Textbook for Veterinary Technicians,* third edition. W.B. Saunders Company, Philadelphia, Pennsylvania, 655 pp. (1994)

Morgan, R.V. (editor). *Handbook of Small Animal Practice,* second edition. W.B. Saunders Company, Philadelphia, Pennsylvania. (1992)

Seigal, M. (editor). *UC Davis School of Veterinary Medicine Book of Dogs.* Harper Collins Publishers, Inc., New York, New York, 538 pp. (1995)

Articles

Alexander, J.W., Richardson, J.W., and Selcer, B.A. **Osteochondritis dissecans of the elbow, stifle and hock: A review.** Journal of the American Animal Hospital Association, 17:51-56. (1981)

American Heartworm Society. **American Heartworm Society recommended procedures for the diagnosis, prevention, and management of Heartworm (*Dirofilaria immitis*) infection in dogs.** Canine Practice, 22:8-15. (1997)

Appel, M.J. **Canine infectious tracheobronchitis (kennel cough): A status report.** Compendium on Continuing Education for the Practicing Veterinarian, 3:70-79. (1981)

Appel, M.J.G. **Lyme disease in dogs and cats.** Compendium on Continuing Education for the Practicing Veterinarian, 5:617-624. (1990)

Baker, R.F. and Huebner, R.B. **Ampicillin as therapy in canine upper respiratory disease.** Veterinary Medicine: Small Animal Clinician, 65:855-857. (1970)

Bardens, J.W. and Hardwick, H. **New observations on the diagnosis and cause of hip dysplasia.** Veterinary Medicine: Small Animal Clinician, 63:238-245. (1968)

Becker, M. **New weapons in the battle against fleas.** Compendium on Continuing Education for the Practicing Veterinarian, Supplement, 19:41-47. (1997)

Blagburn, B.L., Hendrix, C.M., Vaughan, J.L. **Efficacy of lufenuron against developmental stages of fleas (*Ctenocephalides felis felis*) in dogs housed in simulated home environments.** American Journal of Veterinary Research, 56:464-470. (1995)

Blake, S. and Lapinski, A. **Hypothyroidism in different breeds.** Canine Practice, 7:48-51. (1980)

Brunner, C.J. and Swango, L.J. **Canine parvovirus infection: Effects on the immune system and factors that predispose to severe disease.** Compendium on Continuing Education for the Practicing Veterinarian, 7:979-989. (1985)

Calvert, C.A. and Rawlings, C.A. **Treatment of heartworm disease in dogs.** Canine Practice, 18:13-28. (1993)

Canine Practice. **Canine respiratory disease.** 20:27-29. (1995)

Corley, E.A. **Hip dysplasia: A report from the Orthopedic Foundation for Animals.** Seminars in Veterinary Medicine and Surgery (Small Animal), 2:141-151. (1987)

Corley, E.A. **Role of the Orthopedic Foundation for Animals in the control of canine hip dysplasia.** Veterinary Clinics of North America: Small Animal Practice, 22:579-593. (1992)

Courtney, C.H. and Zeng, Q.Y. **The structure of heartworm populations in dogs and cats in Florida.** In: *Proceedings of the Heartworm Symposium of the American Heartworm Society,* Washington, D.C., pp. 1-6. (1989)

Cox, U.H., Hoskins, J.D., and Newman, S.S. **Temporal study of Staphylococcal species on healthy dogs.** American Journal of Veterinary Research, 49:747-751. (1988)

Cunningham, J.G. and Farnbach, G.C. **Inheritance of idiopathic canine epilepsy.** Journal of the American Animal Hospital Association, 24:421-424. (1988)

Dillon, A.R., Brawner, W.R., and Hanrahan, L. **Influence of number of parasites and exercise on the severity of heartworm disease in dogs.** In: *Proceedings of the Heartworm Symposium of the American Heartworm Society,* Washington, D.C., p.113. (1995)

Dworkin, N. **Hornets, spiders and snakes.** American Kennel Club Purebred Dog Gazette, April:46-52. (1996)

Everann, J.F., McKeirman, A.J., Eugster, A.K., Sosozano, R.F., Collins, J.K., Black, J.W., and Kim, J.S. **Update on canine coronavirus infections and interactions with other enteric pathogens of the dog.** Companion Animal Practice, 18:6-12. (1989)

Font, A., Closa, J.M., and Mascort, J. **Tick-transmitted diseases: A comparative study of Lyme disease, canine ehrlichiosis and rickettsiosis in the dog.** Veterinary International, 3:3-14. (1992)

Ford, R.B. **Canine infectious tracheobronchitis.** Veterinary Technician, 13:660-664. (1992)

Ford, R.B. **Canine vaccination protocols.** Veterinary Technician, 13:475-482. (1992)

Fox, S.M. and Walker, A.M. **The etiopathogenesis of osteochondrosis.** Veterinary Medicine, February:116-122. (1993)

Glickman, L.T. and Appel, M.J. **Intranasal vaccine trial for canine infectious tracheobronchitis (kennel cough).** Laboratory Animal Science, 31:397-399. (1981)

Glickman, L.T., Domanski, L.M., Patronek, G.J., and Visintainer, F. **Breed-related risk factors for canine parvovirus enteritis.** Journal of the American Veterinary Medical Association, 187:589-594. (1985)

Greene, R.T. and Lammler, C.H. *Staphylococcus intermedius:* **Current knowledge of a pathogen of veterinary importance.** Journal of Veterinary Medicine, 40:206-214. (1993)

Haan, J.J., Beale, B.S., and Parker, R.B. **Diagnosis and treatment of canine hip dysplasia.** Canine Practice, 18:24-28. (1993)

Harari. J. **Identifying and managing osteochondrosis in dogs.** Veterinary Medicine, June, pp. 508-509. (1997)

Hedhammer, A., Olssom, S.E., and Anderson, S.A. **Canine hip dysplasia: Study of heritability in 401 litters of German Shepherd Dogs.** Journal of the American Veterinary Medical Association, 174:1012-1019. (1979)

Hedhammer, A., Wu, F., Krook, L.. et al. **Over nutrition and skeletal disease: An experimental study in growing Great Dane dogs.** Cornell Veterinarian, Supplement 5, 64:1-59. (1974)

Heyman, S.J., Smith, G.K., and Cofone, M.A. **Biomechanical study of the effect of coxofemoral positioning on passive hip joint laxity in the dog.** American Journal of Veterinary Research, 54:210-215. (1993)

Heynold, Y., Faissler, D., Steffen, F., and Jaggy, A. **Clinical, epidemiological and treatment results of idiopathic epilepsy in 54 Labrador Retrievers: A long-term study.** Journal of Small Animal Practice, 38:7-14. (1997)

Hoover, J.P., Campbell, G.A., and Fox, J.C. **Comparison of eight diagnostic blood tests for Heartworm infection in dogs.** Canine Practice, 21:11-19. (1996)

Hoover, J.P., Fox, J.C., Claypool, P.L., Campbell, G.A., and Mullins, S.B. **Comparison of visual interpretations and optical density measurements of two antigen tests for Heartworm infections in dogs.** Canine Practice, 21:12-20. (1996)

Hopkins, T.J., Woodley, I., and Gyr, P. **Imidacloprid topical formulation: Larvicidal effect against** *Ctenocephalides felis* **in the surroundings of treated dogs.** Compendium on Continuing Education for the Practicing Veterinarian, Supplement, 19:4-10. (1997)

Hutt, F.B. **Genetic selection to reduce the incidence of hip dysplasia in dogs.** Journal of the American Veterinary Medical Association, 151:1041-1048. (1967)

Jaggy, A. **Neurological manifestations of hypothyroidism: A retrospective study of 29 dogs.** Journal of Veterinary Internal Medicine, 8:328-336. (1994)

Jenkins, S.R., Clark, K.A., Leslie, M.J., Martin, R.J., Miller, G.B., Satalowich, F.T., and Sorhage, F.E. **Compendium of animal rabies control, 1997.** Journal of the American Veterinary Medical Association, 210:33-37. (1997)

Jensen, A.L., Iveersen, L., Koch, J., Hoier, R., and Petersen, T.K. **Evaluation of the urinary corti-sol:creatinine ratio in the diagnosis of hyperadrenocorticism in dogs.** Journal of Small Animal Practice, 38:99-102. (1997)

Kaman, C.H. and Grossling, H.R. **A breeding program to reduce hip dysplasia in German Shepherd Dogs.** Journal of the American Veterinary Medical Association, 151:562-571. (1967)

Kealy, R.D., Olsson, S.E., and Monti, K.L. **Effects of limited food consumption on the incidence of hip dysplasia in growing dogs.** Journal of the American Veterinary Medical Association, 201:857-863. (1992)

Keister, D.M., Meo, N.J., and Tanner, P.A. **A comparison of flea control efficacy of Frontline™ Spray Treatment against the flea infestation prevention pack (Vet-Kem) in the dog and cat.** Proceedings of the American Association of Veterinary Parasitologists, July 20-23, Louisville, Kentucky. (1996)

Kennedy, M.A., Mellon, V.S., Caldwell, G., and Potgieter, L.N.D. **Virucidal efficacy of the newer quaternary ammonium compounds.** Journal of the American Animal Hospital Association, 31:254-258. (1995)

Kern, M.S. **Deworming your dogs.** American Kennel Club Purebred Dog Gazette, July:77-80. (1992)

Knight, M.W. and Dorman, D. **Selected poisonous plant concerns in small animals.** Veterinary Medicine, March:260-272. (1997)

Krebs, J.W., Strine, T.W., Smith, J.S., Noah, D.L., Rupprecht, C.E., and Childs, J.E. **Rabies surveillance in the United States during 1995.** Journal of the American Veterinary Medical Association, 209:2031-2044. (1996)

Larson, L.J. and Schultz, R.D. **High titer canine parvovirus vaccine: Serologic response and challenge of immunity study.** Veterinary Medicine, 91:210-218. (1996)

Leib, M.S., Wingfield, W.E., and Twedt, D.C. **Plasma gastrin immunoreactivity in dogs with acute gastric dilatation-volvulus.** Journal of the American Veterinary Medical Association, 185:205-208. (1984)

Leighton, E.A., Lin, J.M., and Willham, R.F. **A genetic study of canine hip dysplasia.** American Journal of Veterinary Research, 38:241-244. (1977)

Levy, S.A. and Dreesen, D.W. **Lyme borreliosis in dogs.** Canine Practice, 17:5-17. (1992)

Lippincott, C.L. **Femoral head and neck excision in the management of canine hip dysplasia.** Veterinary Clinics of North America: Small Animal Practice, 22:721-737. (1992)

Lorenz, M.D. **What is canine Cushing's Syndrome?** American Kennel Club Purebred Dog Gazette, April:42-46. (1985)

Lust, G., Williams, A.J., and Burton-Wurster, N. **Effects**

of intramuscular administration of glycosaminoglycan polysulfates on signs of incipient hip dysplasia in growing pups. American Journal of Veterinary Research, 53:1836-1843. (1992)

Lust, G., Williams, A.J., and Burton-Wurster, N. **Joint laxity and its association with hip dysplasia in Labrador Retrievers.** American Journal of Veterinary Research, 54:1990-1999. (1993)

MacDonald, J.M. **Flea control in animals with flea allergy dermatitis.** Compendium on Continuing Education for the Practicing Veterinarian, Supplement, 19:38-40. (1997)

MacDonald, J.M. **Flea control: An overview of treatment concepts for North America.** Veterinary Dermatology, 6:121-129. (1995)

Macintire, D.K. and Smith-Carr, S. **Canine parvovirus. Part II: Clinical signs, diagnosis, and treatment.** Compendium on Continuing Education for the Practicing Veterinarian, 19:291-300. (1997)

Magnarelli, L.A., Anderson, J.F., and Schreider, A.B. **Clinical and serologic studies of canine Borreliosis.** Journal of the American Veterinary Medical Association, 191:1089-1094. (1987)

Martini, M., Capellie, G., Poglayen, G., Bertotti, F., and Turilli, C. **The validity of some hematological and ELISA methods for the diagnosis of canine heartworm disease.** Veterinary Research Communications, 20:331-339. (1996)

Maupin, G. **Comparative susceptibility of nymphal *Ixodes scapularis*, the principal vector of Lyme disease, to Fipronil and Permethrin.** Fourth International Symposium on Ectoparasites of Pets, April 6-8, Riverside, California. (1977)

McCall, J.W., McTier, T.L., Ryan, W.G., Gross, S.J., and Soll, M.D. **Evaluation of ivermectin and milbemycin oxime efficacy against *Dirofilaria immitis* infections of three and four months duration in dogs.** American Journal of Veterinary Research, 57:1189-1192. (1996)

McCandlish, I.A.P., Thompson, H., and Fisher, E.W. **Canine parvovirus infection.** In Practice, 3:14. (1981)

McTier, T.L. **A guide to selecting adult heartworm antigen test kits.** Veterinary Medicine, 89:528-544. (1994)

Milton, J.L. **Osteochondritis dissecans in the dog.** Veterinary Clinics of North America: Small Animal Practice, 13:117-133. (1983)

Moore, M.G. **Promising responses to a new oral treatment for degenerative joint disorders.** Canine Practice, 21:7-11. (1996)

Nesbitt, G.H., Izzo, J., Peterson, L., and Wilkins, R.J. **Canine hypothyroidism: A retrospective study of 108 cases.** Journal of the American Veterinary Medical Association, 177:1117-1122. (1980)

Nettifee, A. **Canine heartworm antigen testing: current concepts in selecting a screening program.** Veterinary Technician, 13:674-677. (1992)

O'Brien, S.E. **Serologic response of pups to the low-passage, modified-live canine parvovirus-2 component in a combinaton vaccine.** Journal of the American Veterinary Medical Association, 204:1207-1209. (1994)

Olmstead, M.L. **Total hip replacement in the dog.** Seminars in Veterinary Medical Surgery, Small Animal, 2:131-140. (1987)

Owens, J.G. and Dorman, D.C. **Common household hazards for small animals.** Veterinary Medicine, February:140-148. (1997)

Panciera, D. **Clinical manifestations of canine hypothyroidism.** Veterinary Medicine, January:44-49. (1997)

Parrish, C.R. **Emergence, natural history and variation of canine, mink, and feline parvoviruses.** Advances in Virus Research, 38:403-450. (1990)

Parrish, C.R., Aquadrom, C.F., and Strassheim, M.L. **Rapid antigenic-type replacement and DNA sequence evolution on canine parvovirus.** Journal of Virology, 65:6544-6552. (1991)

Paul, A.J. **Evaluation of the safety of administering high doses of a chewable Ivermectin tablet to Collies.** Veterinary Medicine, 86:623-625. (1991)

Pollock, R.V.H. and Carmichael, L.E. **Maternally derived immunity to canine parvovirus infection: Transfer, decline, and interference with vaccination.** Journal of the American Veterinary Medical Association, 180:37-42. (1982)

Pulliam, J.D. **Investigating Ivermectin toxicity in Collies.** Veterinary Medicine, 80:36-40. (1985)

Rawlings, C.A. **Post-adulticide changes in *Dirofilaria immitis*-infected Beagles.** American Journal of Veterinary Research, 44:8-15. (1983)

Rawlings, C.A. and McCall, J.W. **Melarsomine: A new heartworm adulticide.** Compendium on Continuing Education for the Practicing Veterinarian, 10:373-379. (1996)

Richardson, D.C. **The role of nutrition in canine hip dysplasia.** Veterinary Clinics of North America: Small Animal Practice, 22:529-540. (1992)

Riser, W.H. and Shirer, J.F. **Correlation between canine hip dysplasia and pelvic muscle mass: A study of 95 dogs.** American Journal of Veterinary Research, 28:769-777. (1967)

Schlotthauer, J.C. **Safety and acceptability of Ivermectin in dogs with naturally acquired patent infection of *Dirofilaria immitis*.** In: *Proceedings of the Heartworm Symposium of the American Heartworm Society,* Washington, D.C., pp. 45-97. (1989)

Schwartz-Porsche, D. **Seizures.** In: *Clinical Syndromes in Veterinary Neurology,* second edition, (K.G. Braund, editor), Mosby-Year Book, Inc., St. Louis, Missouri, pp. 234-251. (1994)

Smith, C.S. **Seizures.** American Kennel Club Purebred Dog Gazette, December:54-57. (1996)

Smith, G.K., Biery, D.N., and Gregor, T.P. **New concepts of coxofemoral joint stability and the development of a clinical stress-radiographic method for quantitating hip joint laxity in the dog.** Journal of the American Veterinary Medical Association, 196:59-70. (1990)

Smith, G.K., Gregor, T.P., and Rhodes, W.H. **Coxofemoral joint laxity from distraction radiography and its contemporaneous and prospective correlation with laxity, subjective score, and evidence of degenerative joint disease from conventional hip-extended radiography in dogs.** American Journal of Veterinary Research, 54:1021-1042. (1993)

Smith, G.K., Popovitch, C.A., and Gregor, T.P. **Evaluation of risk factors for degenerative joint disease associated with hip dysplasia in dogs.** Journal of the American Veterinary Medical Association, 206:642-647. (1995)

Smith-Carr, S., MacIntie, D.K., and Swango, L.J. **Canine parvovirus. Part I: Pathogenesis and vaccination.** Compendium on Continuing Education for the Practicing Veterinarian, 19:125-133. (1997)

Swango, L. **Choosing a canine vaccine regimen, Part 1.** Canine Practice, 20:10-14. (1995)

Swango, L., Barta, R., Fortney, W., Garnett, P., Leedy, D., and Stevenson, J. **Choosing a canine vaccine regimen. Part 3.** Canine Practice, 20:21-26. (1995)

Swift, W.B. **Getting hip to hip dysplasia.** Animals, May/June:29-31. (1995)

Talcott, P.A. and Dorman, D.C. **Pesticide exposures in companion animals.** Veterinary Medicine, February:167-181. (1997)

Tanner, P.A., Meo, N.J., Sparer, D., Butler, S., Romano, M.N., and Keister, D.M. **Advances in the treatment of heartworm, fleas and ticks.** Canine Practice, 22:40-47. (1997)

Theis, J.H. **Occult rate of heartworm infected dogs in California appears to be significantly lower than that of infected dogs from Florida and Texas.** Canine Practice, 22:5-7. (1997)

Thrushfield, M.V. **Canine kennel cough: A review.** Veterinary Annual, 32:1-12. (1992)

Thrushfield, M.V., Aitken, C.G.C., and Muirhead, R.H.

A field investigation of kennel cough: Efficacy of vaccination. Journal of Small Animal Practice, 30:550-560. (1989)

Thrushfield, M.V., Aitken, C.G.C., and Muirhead, R.H. **A field investigation of kennel cough: Efficacy of different treatments.** Journal of Small Animal Practice, 32:455-459. (1991)

Thrushfield, M.V., Aitken, C.G.C., and Muirhead, R.H. **A field investigation of kennel cough: Incubation period and clinical signs.** Journal of Small Animal Practice, 32:215-220. (1991)

Todhunter, R.J. and Lust, G. **Polysulfated glycosamioglycan in the treatment of osteoarthritis.** Journal of the American Veterinary Medical Association, 204:1245-1251. (1994)

Tomlinson, J. and McLaughlin, R. **Canine hip dysplasia: Development factors, clinical signs and initial examination steps.** Veterinary Medicine, 91:26-33. (1996)

Turner, J.L. **Canine coronavirus.** Canine Practice, 18:13-15. (1989)

Ueland, K. **Serological, bacteriological and clinical observations on an outbreak of canine infectious tracheobronchitis in Norway.** Veterinary Record, 126:481-483. (1990)

Wallace, L.J. **A half century of canine hip dysplasia: perspectives of the eighties.** Seminars in Veterinary Medicine and Surgery (Small Animal), 2:97-98. (1987)

Wease, G.N. and Corley, E.A. **Control of canine hip dysplasia: Current status.** KalKan Forum, 4:80–88. (1985)

Wilford, C. *Ehrlichia:* **A poorly understood organism, uses ticks to spread it dangerous infection nationwide.** American Kennel Club Purebred Dog Gazette, June, pp. 48-52. (1994)

Wilford, C. **Treating shifting leg lameness.** American Kennel Club Purebred Dog Gazette, December:58-62. (1994)

P A R T   4
Books

Association of American Feed Control Officials: *Official Publication.* AAFCO, Atlanta, Georgia. (1998)

Carey, D.P., Norton, S.A., and Bolser, S.M. (editors) *Recent Advances in Canine and Feline Nutritional Research: Proceedings of the Iams International Nutrition Symposium.* Orange Frazer Press, Wilmington, Ohio, 284 pp. (1996)

Case, L.P., Carey, D.P, and Hirakawa, D.A. *Canine and Feline Nutrition: A Resource for Companion Animal Professionals.* Mosby-Year Book, Inc., St. Louis, Missouri, 455 pp. (1995)

Edney, A.T.B. (editor). *Dog and Cat Nutrition.* Pergamon Press, Oxford, United Kingdom, 143 pp. (1988)

Irlbeck, N.A. *Nutrition and Care of Companion Animals.* Kendall/Hunt Publishing Company, Dubuque, Iowa, 369 pp. (1996)

Lewis, L.D., Morris, M.L., and Hand, M.S. *Small Animal Clinical Nutrition,* third edition. Mark Morris Associates, Topeka, Kansas. (1987)

National Research Council: *Nutrient Requirements of Dogs.* National Academy of Sciences, National Academy Press, Washington, D.C. (1985)

Wang, X. *Effect of Processing Methods and Raw Material Sources on Protein Quality of Animal Protein Meals.* Ph.D. Thesis, University of Illinois, Urbana. (1996)

Articles

AAFCO. **AAFCO pet food regulatory update.** Proceedings of the Petfood Forum, Watts Publishing, Chicago, Illinois, pp. 141-147. (1998)

Alexander, J.E. and Wood, L.L.H. **Growth studies in Labrador Retrievers fed a calorie-dense diet: time-restricted versus free choice feeding.** Canine Practice, 14:41–47. (1987)

Allard, R.L., Douglass, G.M., and Kerr, W.W. **The effects of breed and sex on dog growth.** Companion Animal Practice, 2:9-12. (1988)

Anderson, R.S. **Water balance in the dog and cat.** Journal of Small Animal Practice, 23:588–598. (1982)

Anderson, R.S. **Water content in the diet of the dog.** Veterinary Annual, 21:171–178. (1981)

August, J.R. **Dietary hypersensitivity in dogs: cutaneous manifestations, diagnosis and management.** Compendium of Continuing Education for the Practicing Veterinarian, 7:469–477. (1985)

Bartges, J. and Anderson, W.H. **Dietary fiber.** Veterinary Clinical Nutrition, 4:25-28, (1997)

Bisset, S.A., Guilford, W.G., Lawoko, C.R., and Sunvold, G.D. **Effect of food particle size on carbohydrate assimilation assessed by breath hydrogen testing in dogs.** Veterinary Clinical Nutrition, 4:82-88. (1997)

Blaxter, A.C., Cripps, R.J., and Gruffyd-Jones, T.J. **Dietary fibre and postprandial hyperglycemia in normal and diabetic dogs.** Journal of Small Animal Practice, 31:229-233. (1990)

Blaza, S.E. and Burger, I.H. **Is carbohydrate essential for pregnancy and lactation in dogs?** In: *Nutrition of the Dog and Cat* (I.H. Burger and J.P.W. Rivers, editors), Cambridge University Press, Cambridge, United Kingdom, pp. 229–242. (1989)

Bovee, K.C. **Diet and kidney failure.** In: *Kal Kan Symposium for the Treatment of Dog and Cat Disease,* Kal Kan Foods, Inc., Vernon, California, pp. 25–28. (1977)

Bovee, K.C. **Influence of dietary protein on renal**

function in dogs. Journal of Nutrition, 121:S128–S139. (1991)

Bovee, K.C. **The uremic syndrome: patient evaluation and treatment.** Compendium of Continuing Education of the Practicing Veterinarian, 1:279–283. (1979)

Brace, J.J. **Theories of aging.** Veterinary Clinics of North America: Small Animal Practice, 11:811–814. (1981)

Branam, J.E. **Dietary management of obese dogs and cats.** Veterinary Technician, 9:490–493. (1988)

Brown, R.G. **Protein in dog foods.** Canadian Veterinary Journal, 30:528–531. (1989)

Butterwick, R.F. and Markwell, P.J. **Effect of level and source of dietary fibre on food intake in the dog.** *Waltham Symposium on the Nutrition of Companion Animals* (abstract), September 23–25, (1993)

Case, L.P. and Czarnecki-Maulden, G.L. **Protein requirements of growing pups fed practical dry-type diets containing mixed-protein sources.** American Journal of Veterinary Research, 51:808–812. (1990)

Codner, E.C. and Thatcher, C.D. **The role of nutrition in the management of dermatoses.** Seminars in Veterinary Medicine and Surgery (Small Animal), 5:167–177. (1990)

Cowgill, L.D. and Spangler, W.L. **Renal insufficiency in geriatric dogs.** Veterinary Clinics of North America: Small Animal Practice, 11:727–749. (1981)

Dammrich, K. **Relationship between nutrition and bone growth in large and giant dogs.** Journal of Nutrition, 121:114S-121S. (1991)

Danforth, E. and Landsberg L. **Energy expenditure and its regulation.** In: *Obesity—Contemporary Issues in Clinical Nutrition* (M.R.C. Greenwood, editor), Churchill Livingstone, New York, New York, pp. 103–121. (1983)

Decker, R.A. and Meyers, G.H. **Theobromine poisoning in a dog.** Journal of the American Veterinary Medical Association, 161:198–199. (1972)

Deshmukh, A.R. **Regulatory aspects of pet foods.** Veterinary Clinical Nutrition, 3:4-9. (1996)

Doering, G.G. **Food allergy: where does it fit as a cause of canine pruritus?** Pet Veterinarian, May/June:10–16. (1991)

Downey, R.L., Kronfeld, D.S., and Banta, C.A. **Diet of Beagles affects stamina.** Journal of the American Animal Hospital Association, 16:273–277. (1980)

Drouillard, D.D., Vesell, E.S., and Dvorchick, B.N. **Studies on theobromine disposition in normal subjects.** Clinical Pharmacology Therapy, 23:296–302. (1978)

Durrer, J.L. and Hannon, J.P. **Seasonal variations in caloric intake of dogs living in an arctic environment.** American Journal of Physiology, 202:375–384. (1962)

Dzanis, D.A. **Complete and balanced? Substantiating the nutritional adequacy of pet foods: Past, present and future.** Petfood Industry, July/August:22-27. (1997)

Dzanis, D.A. **Regulatory update.** In: *Proceedings of the Petfood Forum,* Watts Publishing, Chicago, Illinois, pp. 106-111. (1996)

Dzanis, D.A. **Safety of ethoxyquin in dog foods.** Journal of Nutrition, 121:S163–S164. (1991)

Earle, K.E. **Calculations of energy requirements of dogs, cats and small psittacine birds.** Journal of Small Animal Practice, 34:163-183. (1993)

Fahey, G. and Hussein, S.H. **The nutritional value of alternative raw materials used in pet foods.** *Proceedings of the Pet Food Forum,* Watts Publishing, Chicago, Illinois, pp. 12-24. (1997)

Faust, I.M., Johnson, P.R. and Hirsch, J. **Long-term effects of early nutritional experience on the development of obesity in the rat.** Journal of Nutrition, 110:2027–2034. (1980)

Ferguson, D.C., Hoenig, M., and Cornelius, L. **Diabetes mellitus in dogs and cats.** In: *Small Animal Medical Therapeutics* (M.D. Lorenz, L. Cornelius, and D.C. Ferguson, editors), Lippincott Co., Philadelphia, Pennsylvania, pp. 85-96. (1992)

Finco, D.R., Brown, S.A., and Crowell, W.A. **Effect of phosphorus/calcium-restricted and phosphorus/calcium-replete 32% diets in dogs with chronic renal failure.** American Journal of Veterinary Research, 53:157–163. (1992)

Finco, D.R., Crowell, W.A., and Barsanti, J.A. **Effects of three diets on dogs with induced chronic renal failure.** American Journal of Veterinary Research, 46:646–653. (1985)

Finke, M.D. **Evaluation of the energy requirements of adult kennel dogs.** Journal of Nutrition, 121:S22–S28. (1991)

Gannon, J.R. **Nutritional requirements of the working dog.** Veterinary Annual, 21:161–166. (1981)

Gans, J.H., Korson, R., and Cater, M.R. **Effects of short-term and long-term theobromine administration to male dogs.** Toxicology and Applied Pharmacology, 53:481–496. (1980)

Glauberg, A. and Blumenthal, P.H. **Chocolate poisoning in the dog.** Journal of the American Animal Hospital Association, 19:246–248. (1983)

Gorrel, C. and Rawlings, J.M. **The role of tooth brushing and diet in the maintenance of periodontal health in dogs.** Journal of Veterinary Dentistry, 13:139-143. (1996)

Grondalen, J. **Metaphyseal osteopathy (hypertrophic osteodystrophy) in growing dogs. A clinical study.** Journal of Small Animal Practice, 17:721-735. (1976)

Halliwell, R.E.W. **Management of dietary hypersensitivity in the dog.** Journal of Small Animal Practice, 33:156-160. (1992)

Hansen, B., DiBartola, S.P., and Chew, D.J. **Clinical and metabolic findings in dogs with chronic renal failure fed two diets.** American Journal of Veterinary Research, 53:326-334. (1992)

Harlow, J. **U.S. pet food trends.** Proceedings of the Pet Food Forum, Watts Publishing, Chicago, Illinois, pp. 355-364. (1997)

Harvey, R.G. **Food allergy and dietary intolerance in dogs: a report of 25 cases.** Journal of Small Animal Practice, 34:175-179. (1993)

Hazewinkel, H.A. **Calcium metabolism and skeletal development of dogs.** In: *Nutrition of the Dog and Cat* (I.H. Burger and J.P.W. Rivers, editors), Cambridge University Press, Cambridge, England, pp. 293-302. (1989)

Hazewinkel, H.A.W., Goedegebuure, S.A., and Poulos, P.W. **Influences of chronic calcium excess on the skeletal development of growing Great Danes.** Journal of the American Animal Hospital Association, 21:377-391. (1985)

Hedhammer, A., Wu, F.M., and Krook, L. **Over nutrition and skeletal disease: an experimental study in growing Great Dane dogs.** Cornell Veterinarian, Supplement 5, 64:1-160. (1974)

Hill, R. **Soy in petfoods: myth vs. fact.** Proceedings of the Pet Food Forum, Watts Publishing, Chicago, Illinois, pp. 71-80. (1995)

Hilton, J.W. **Antioxidants: function, types and necessity of inclusion in pet foods.** Canadian Veterinary Journal, 30:682-684. (1989)

Hilton, J.W. and Atkinson, J.L. **High lipid and high protein dog foods.** Canadian Veterinary Journal, 29:76-78. (1988)

Hinchcliff, K.W. **Energy and water expenditure.** In: *Proceedings of the Performance Dog Nutrition Symposium,* Colorado State University, Fort Collins, Colorado, pp. 4-9. (1995)

Hinchcliff, K.W. and Reinhart, G.A. **Energy metabolism and water turnover in Alaskan sled dogs during running.** In: *Recent Advances in Canine and Feline Nutritional Research: Proceedings of the Iams International Nutrition Symposium,* Orange Frazer Press, Wilmington, Ohio, April 18-21, pp. 199-206. (1996)

Houpt, K.A. and Smith, S.L. **Taste preferences and their relation to obesity in dogs and cats.** Canadian Veterinary Journal, 22:77-81. (1981)

Houpt, K.A., Coren, B., and Hintz, H.F. **Effect of sex and reproductive status on sucrose preference, food intake and body weight of dogs.** Journal of the American Veterinary Medical Association, 174:1083-1085. (1979)

Huber, T.L., Wilson, R.C., and McGarity, S.A. **Variations in digestibility of dry dog foods with identical label guaranteed analysis.** Journal of the American Animal Hospital Association, 22:571-575, (1986)

Jeffers, J.G., Shanley, K.J., and Meyer, E.K. **Diagnostic testing of dogs for food hypersensitivity.** Journal of the American Veterinary Medical Association, 198:245-250. (1991)

Jensen, L., Logan, E., Finney, O., and Lowry, R. **Reduction in accumulation of plaque, stain, and calculus in dogs by dietary means.** Journal of Veterinary Dentistry, 12:161-163. (1996)

Kallfelz, F.A. **Evaluation and use of pet foods: general considerations in using pet foods for adult maintenance.** Veterinary Clinics of North America: Small Animal Practice, 19:387-403. (1989)

Kallfelz, F.A. and Dzanis, D.A. **Over nutrition: an epidemic problem in pet practice?**, Veterinary Clinics of North America: Small Animal Practice, 19:433-466. (1989)

Kaufman, E. **Obesity in dogs.** Veterinary Technician, 7:5-8. (1986)

Kay, J.M. **Onion toxicity in a dog.** Modern Veterinary Practice, 6:477-478. (1983)

Kealy, R.D., Olsson, S.E., and Monti, K.L. **Effects of limited food consumption on the incidence of hip dysplasia in growing dogs.** Journal of the American Veterinary Medical Association, 201:857-863. (1992)

Kendall, P.T. **Comparable evaluation of apparent digestibility in dogs and cats,** Proceedings of the Nutrition Society, 40:45a. (1981)

Kendall, P.T. and Holme, D.W. **Studies on the digestibility of soya bean products, cereal, cereal and plant by-products in diets of dogs.** Journal of Science and Food Agriculture, 33:813-820. (1982)

Kendall, P.T., Holme, D.W., and Smith, P.M. **Methods of prediction of the digestible energy content of dog foods from gross energy value, proximate analysis and digestible nutrient content.** Journal of Science and Food Agriculture, 3:823-828. (1982)

Kienzle, E. and Meyer, H. **The effects of carbohydrate-free diets containing different levels of protein on reproduction in the bitch.** In: *Nutrition of the Dog and Cat* (I.H. Burger and J.P.W. Rivers, editors), Cambridge University Press, New York, New York, pp. 113-132. (1989)

Kronfeld, D.S. **Dietary management of chronic re-**

nal disease in dogs: a critical appraisal. Journal of Small Animal Practice, 34:211–219. (1993)

Kulhman, G. and Biourge, V. **Nutrition of the large and giant breed dog with emphasis on skeletal development.** Veterinary Clinical Nutrition, 4:89-95. (1997)

Kunkle, G. and Horner, S. **Validity of skin testing for diagnosis of food allergy in dogs.** Journal of the American Veterinary Medical Association, 200:677–680. (1992)

Leib, M.S. and August, J.R. **Food hypersensitivity.** In: *Textbook of Veterinary Internal Medicine,* third edition (S.J. Ettinger, editor). W.B. Saunders, Philadelphia, Pennsylvania, pp. 194–197. (1989)

Markham, R.W. and Hodgkins, E.M. **Geriatric nutrition.** Veterinary Clinics of North America: Small Animal Practice, 19:165-185. (1989)

Markwell, P.J., Erk, W., and Parkin, G.D. **Obesity in the dog.** Journal of Small Animal Practice, 31:533–537. (1990)

McNamara, J.H. **Nutrition for military working dogs under stress.** Veterinary Medicine and Small Animal Surgery, 67:615–623. (1972)

Miller, W.H., Jr. **Nutritional considerations in small animal dermatology.** Veterinary Clinics of North America: Small Animal Practice, 19:497–511. (1989)

Morgan, T. **Treat trends.** Petfood Industry, September/October:32-37. (1997)

Morris, J.G. and Rogers, Q.R. **Comparative dog and cat nutrition.** In: *Nutrition of the Dog and Cat* (I.H. Burger and J.P.W. Rivers, editors), Cambridge University Press, Cambridge, England, pp. 35–66. (1989)

Morris, J.G. and Rogers, Q.R. **Evaluation of commercial pet foods.** Tijdschrehund Diergeneesk, 1:67S–70S. (1991)

Moser, D. **Feeding to optimize canine reproductive efficiency.** Problems in Veterinary Medicine, 4:545–550. (1992)

Mosier, J.E. **Effect of aging on body systems of the dog.** Veterinary Clinics of North America: Small Animal Practice, 19:1–13. (1989)

Mosier, J.E. **Nutritional recommendations for gestation and lactation in the dog.** Veterinary Clinics of North America: Small Animal Practice, 7:683–692. (1977)

Nap, R.C. and Hazewinkel, H.A.W. **Growth and skeletal development in the dog in relation to nutrition: A review.** Veterinary Quarterly, 1:50-59. (1994)

Nelson, R.W. **Nutritional management of diabetes mellitus.** Seminars in Veterinary Medicine and Surgery (Small Animal), 5:178-186. (1990)

Nelson, R.W., Ihle, S.L., and Lewis, L.D. **Effects of di-etary fiber supplementation on glycemic control in dogs with alloxan-induced diabetes mellitus.** American Journal of Veterinary Research, 52:2060–2066. (1991)

Newsholme, E.A. **Control of metabolism and the integration of fuel supply for the marathon runner.** In: *Biochemistry of Exercise.* (H.G. Knuttgen, J.A. Vogel, and J. Poortmans, editors), Human Kinetic Publishers, Champaign, Illinois, pp. 144–150. (1983)

Ontko, J.A. and Phillips, P.H. **Reproduction and lactation studies with bitches fed semi-purified diets.** Journal of Nutrition, 65:211–218. (1958)

Papas, A.M. **Antioxidants: which ones are best for your pet food products?** Pet Food Industry, May/June:8–16. (1991)

Paul, P. and Issekutz, B. **Role of extra muscular energy sources in the metabolism of the exercising dog.** American Journal of Physiology, 22:615–622. (1976)

Polzin, D.J. and Osborne, C.A. **Current progress in slowing progression of canine and feline chronic renal failure.** Companion Animal Practice, 3:52–62. (1988)

Polzin, D.J., Osborne, C.A., and Lulich, J.P. **Effects of dietary protein/phosphate restriction in normal dogs and dogs with chronic renal failure.** Journal of Small Animal Practice, 32:289–295. (1991)

Reinhart, G. **Fiber nutrition and intestinal function critical for recovery.** DVM News Magazine, 24: June. (1993)

Reynolds, A.J. **The effect of diet and training on energy substrate storage and utilization in trained and untrained sled dogs.** In: *Nutrition and Physiology of Alaskan Sled Dogs,* abstracts of a symposium held at the College of Veterinary Medicine, Ohio State University, September 5. (1992)

Reynolds, A.J., Fuhrer, H.L., and Dunlap, M.D. **Lipid metabolite responses to diet and training in sled dogs.** Journal of Nutrition, 124:2754S-2759S. (1994)

Richardson, D.C. **The role of nutrition in canine hip dysplasia.** Veterinary Clinics of North America: Small Animal Practice, 22:529-540. (1992)

Robertson, J.L., Goldschmidt, M., and Kronfeld, D.S. **Long term renal responses to high dietary protein in dogs with 75% nephrectomy.** Kidney International, 29:511–519. (1986)

Robertson, K.A., Feldman, E.C., and Polonsky, K. **Spontaneous diabetes mellitus in 24 dogs: incidence of type I versus type II disease.** Proceedings of the American College of Veterinary Internal Medicine, pp. 1036-1040. (1989)

Romsos, D.R., Hornshus, M.J., and Leveille, G.A. **Influence of dietary fat and carbohydrate on food intake, body weight and body fat of adult dogs.** Proceedings of the Society of Experimental Biology and Medicine, 157:278–281. (1978)

Rosser, E.J. **Diagnosis of food allergy in dogs.** Journal of the American Veterinary Medical Association, 203:259–262. (1993)

Samuelson, A.C. and Cutter, G.R. **Dog biscuits: an aid in canine tartar control.** Journal of Nutrition, 121:S162. (1991)

Scott, D.W. **Immunologic skin disorders in the dog and cat.** Veterinary Clinics of North America: Small Animal Practice, 8:641–664. (1978)

Sheffy, B.E. **Meeting energy-protein needs of dogs.** Compendium of Continuing Education for Small Animal Practitioners, 1:345-354. (1979)

Sheffy, B.E. and William, A.J. **Nutrition and the aging animal.** Veterinary Clinics of North America: Small Animal Practice, 11:669–675. (1981)

Shields, R.G., Kigin, P.D., and Izquierdo, J.A. **Counting calories: caloric claims—measuring digestibility and metabolizable energy.** Pet Food Industry, January/February:4–10. (1994)

Sibley, K.W. **Diagnosis and management of the overweight dog.** British Veterinary Journal, 140:124–131. (1984)

Sloth, C. **Practical management of obesity in dogs and cats.** Journal of Small Animal Practice, 33:178–182. (1992)

Sousa, C.A., Stannard, A.A., and Ihrke, P.J. **Dermatosis associated with feeding generic dog food: 13 cases (1981–1982).** Journal of the American Veterinary Medical Association, 192:676–680. (1988)

Spice, R.N. **Hemolytic anemia associated with ingestion of onions in a dog.** Canadian Veterinary Journal, 17:181–183 (1976)

Stogdale, L. **Definition of diabetes mellitus.** Cornell Veterinarian, 76:156–174. (1985)

Teare, J.A., Krook, L., and Kallfelz, A. **Ascorbic acid deficiency and hypertrophic osteodystrophy in the dog: a rebuttal.** Cornell Veterinarian, 69:384–401. (1979)

Thorne, C.J. **Understanding pet response: Behavioural aspects of palatability.** In: *Focus on Palatability*, Proceedings of the Petfood Industry, Watt Publishing, Chicago, Illinois, pp. 17-34. (1995)

Walton, G.S. **Skin responses in the dog and cat due to ingested allergens: observations on one hundred confirmed cases.** Veterinary Record, 81:709–713. (1967)

White, S.D. **Food hypersensitivity in 30 dogs.** Journal of the American Veterinary Medical Association, 188:695–698. (1986)

Wiernusz, C.J., Shields, R.G., Van Vlierbergen, D.J., Kigin, P.D., and Ballard, R. **Canine nutrient digestibility and stool quality evaluation of canned diets containing various soy protein supplements.** Veterinary Clinical Nutrition, 2:49-56. (1995)

Williams, L. **Canine diabetes mellitus.** Veterinary Technician, 9:168–170. (1988)

Glossary

acute—symptoms that are of short duration, relatively severe, and with a rapid onset

ad libitum—self-feeding; unlimited access to food and water

adipsia—absence of thirst; avoidance of drinking

agonistic—any behavior elicited during conflict; most commonly refers to aggressive behaviors but also can involve fear, flight, or pacifying behaviors

agoraphobia—fear of new or unfamiliar places

alleles—several expressions of a particular gene; for example, the gene for black/red coat color has two alleles: b (red coat) and B (black color)

allergy—hypersensitivity; enhanced state of the immune response in which exposure to a particular allergen causes a noxious or physically harmful immunologic reaction

alopecia—loss of hair coat

altricial—requiring parental care and feeding for survival at birth; refers to a species whose young is born at a relatively immature stage of development

anabolism—process of synthesizing or building complex compounds

androgenization—development of male characteristics in response to exposure to androgens

androgens—male sexual hormones: androsterone and testosterone

anemia—abnormally low red blood cell concentration or hemoglobin levels

anestrus—period of reproductive quiescence or rest in the bitch's reproductive cycle occurring between estrus periods

anorexia—loss of appetite for food

antibodies—proteins produced by the immune system in response to an antigen; functions to protect the animal from infection by destroying antigens

antigen—substance such as a virus, bacteria, or foreign microbe that stimulates an immune response and the production of antibodies

avascular—lacking a blood supply

azotemia—excess concentrations of nitrogenous wastewater products in the blood

bacteremia—presence of bacteria in the blood

basal cells—bottom cell layer of the epidermis

bloat—gastric dilatation volvulus; abnormal distension of the stomach

brachycephalic—canine head type that has a wide skull base and short muzzle; cephalic index of > 80

bradycardia—abnormally slow heart rate

bronchi—the two main branches of the trachea that lead to the bronchioles within the lungs

carnassial teeth—upper fourth premolar and lower first molar teeth in the dog's mouth

castration—surgical removal of the testes in the male

catabolism—breakdown of complex chemical compounds into simpler compounds; opposite of anabolism

caudal—anatomical term for "toward the tail" or relating to the tail

cervix—oval-shaped fibrous structure that serves as the opening between the vagina and the uterus in the female

chromosome—structures found in the nucleus of cells that carry genes responsible for inherited characteristics; dogs have 39 pairs (78 total) of chromosomes

chronic—occurring or persisting for a long duration

clitoris—female secondary sexual organ analogous to the penis

collagen—structural protein that forms the chief constituent of connective tissue, cartilage, tendon, bone, and skin

colostrum—milk produced by a lactating female immediately after birth; contains high levels of antibodies and immunoprotective compounds

conjunctiva—mucous membranes of the eye, covering the sclera of the eyeball

conspecific—belonging to the same species or social group

coprophagy—consumption of feces

cornified—converted to keratinized material

cranial—anatomical term denoting "toward the head"

degradation—metabolic breakdown or catabolism

diapedesis—seepage or leaking of red blood cells and serum out of capillary vessels

diaphysis—central shaft of long bones

digestible energy—energy in a food that is available for absorption; gross energy minus fecal energy

digigrade—walking on the toes (digits or phalanges)

dissacharide—simple carbohydrate consisting of two monosaccharides linked together; for example, sucrose and lactose

distal—anatomical term denoting "farther away; distant"

dolichocephalic—canine head type that has a narrow skull base and long muzzle; cephalic index of < 75

dysplasia—abnormal growth or development of cells

dystocia—difficulty with labor or parturition (birth)

ectoparasites—external parasites; for example, fleas and mites

endemic—constantly present to a greater or lesser extent in a particular region or environment

endogenous—synthesized or derived by the body; originating within

endoparasite—internal parasites; for example, heartworm and ascarids (roundworm)

energy density—concentration of energy, expressed as metabolizable energy per unit of weight; in dog food, typically expressed as kcal ME/kg

enteritis—inflammation of the small intestine, usually resulting in abdominal discomfort and diarrhea

eosinophil—a leukocyte (white blood cell) with a bilobate nucleus, which stains with eosin dye

epithelial cells—cells that cover a surface or cavity of the body and have protective and secreting functions

erythema—abnormal redness of the skin as a result of local congestion or inflammation

etiology—the underlying cause of a disease

exfoliation—scaling off or peeling in thin layers or fragments

extinction burst—a temporary increase in behavior in response to the removal of reinforcing stimuli; precedes extinction (termination) of the behavior

familial—observed within a family lineage

febrile—having a fever

gastric—pertaining to the stomach

genetic plasticity—existence of high degree of variation in the genetic material of a species, allowing for high degree of variability between individuals

genotype—genetic makeup of an individual

glycogen—animal starch; found in the liver and muscle and used as a source of glucose when needed by the body

gross energy—total chemical energy of a food; also called its potential energy

hematocrit—also called packed cell volume; represents the proportion of red blood cells in a volume of whole blood

hematoma—localized swelling filled with blood

hematuria—presence of blood in the urine

hemorrhagic diathesis—disease syndrome in which spontaneous bleeding or an enhanced tendency for bleeding occurs

hemorrhagic enteritis—gastrointestinal syndrome characterized by inflammation of the intestine and severe and bloody diarrhea

heterozygous—presence of dissimilar genes (alleles) at a given locus on homologous chromosomes for a hereditary characteristic

homeostasis—maintenance of chemical and physiological stability in the body's internal environment

homologous—matched pair of chromosomes; one of maternal origin, the other of paternal origin

homozygous—presence of identical genes (alleles) at a given locus on homologous chromosomes

hybrid—offspring from the breeding of two animals of different breeds, varieties, or lineages

hybrid vigor—enhanced health or vitality as a result of increased numbers of heterozygous gene pairs and decreased numbers of homozygous recessive gene pairs in an individual

hydrolysis—chemical reaction involving splitting of a compound through the addition of water

hyperglycemia—abnormally elevated blood glucose concentration

hyperkeratosis—abnormal thickening of the protective (horny) layer of the epidermis

hyperthermia—abnormally elevated body temperature; seen with fever or heatstroke

hypothermia—abnormally low body temperature; occurs with shock or overexposure to cold weather

iatrogenic—arising as a result of veterinary or medical treatment

idiopathic—of unknown causation

inguinal—pertaining to the groin region of the body

jaundice—yellowing of the mucous membranes or skin as a result of the accumulation of bile pigments in the blood; indicative of liver or bile duct disorders

keratin—structural protein found in skin, hair, and nails

kilocalorie—unit of energy defined by the amount of energy required to raise the temperature of 1 kilogram of water, 1 degree Celsius

labia-external folds of the vulva in the female

larvae—immature stage of life in life cycle of some insects and parasites

larynx—muscular, cartilage-containing organ located within the trachea that contains the vocal cords

locus—site on a chromosome where a specific gene is found

luxation—dislocation of a joint

meiosis—type of cellular division that produces reproductive cells (ova and sperm)

mesaticephalic—canine head type that has a moderate skull base and muzzle; a balanced head type

metabolism—life-sustaining chemical reactions and biochemical processes of the body; conversion of nutrients into energy

metabolizable energy—energy in a food that is available to tissues; gross energy minus fecal energy and urinary energy

mitochondria—cell organelle within which most energy transformation reactions occur

monosaccharide—single carbohydrate unit; for example, glucose and fructose

morphology—an organism's or organ's form and structure

myocarditis—inflammation of the myocardium (muscular tissue of the heart)

myoclonus—involuntary, rapid muscular tremors; seen as a complication of canine distemper

necrosis—cell death

neophobia—fear of the unknown or unfamiliar

neoplasm—abnormal growth of new tissue; tumor

neoteny—selection for infantile (neotenous) characteristics that persist into adulthood

nephritis—inflammation of the nephrons; kidney disease

occlude—to close off or obstruct

olfactory—involving the nose and sense of smell

ontogeny—development of an individual from birth to adulthood

oocyst—encapsulated ovum (egg)

ossification—process of bone formation

ovariohysterectomy—surgical removal of the female reproductive tract (ovaries, oviducts, and uterus); spaying

palliative—alleviation of pain or clinical signs without curing

palpate—examine through feel or touch

paresis—partial motor paralysis

pathogenic—capable of causing disease or infection

peracute—extremely rapid onset

perianal—in the region of the anus

periosteum—connective tissue covering all bones; contains blood supply and provides protection

phenotype—set of observable characteristics determined by genotype

pheromones—hormone-like substances secreted by an individual that affect the behavior of another individual of the same species; often related to reproductive behavior

piloerection—reflex in which the muscles at the base of the dog's hairs contract; causes the hairs on the dog's back to stand up

pituitary gland—endocrine gland located at the base of the brain

placenta—mammalian organ formed in the lining of the uterus with membranes of the fetuses; functions to supply nourishment to and remove wastes from the developing fetuses

pleomorphic—existing in two or more distinct forms during the life cycle

polysaccharide—complex carbohydrate consisting of many single monosaccharide units linked together; for example, starch and glycogen

postprandial—following a meal

proglottids—segments of the tapeworm, each of which contains complete male and female reproductive systems

prognosis—prediction of the probable course of a disease and possibility for recovery

prolapse—slipping or falling out of place of an organ

purulent—containing or discharging pus

relaxin—reproductive hormone that functions to relax the symphysis pubis and helps prepare the uterus for parturition

replication—duplication; production of a copy

resorption—biochemical dissolution of tissue; loss of tissue

scolex—anterior, headlike portion of the tapeworm that attaches to the lining of the intestine

sebaceous glands—glands located within the skin that produce sebum, a protective, waxy substance

sebum—oily secretion of the sebaceous glands that lubricates and protects the skin

septicemia—invasions and persistence of pathogenic microorganisms in the blood

sesamoid—small, nodular bones of the foot

shock—circulatory collapse occurring as a result of injury or disease

social facilitation—effect of group interactions upon individual behavior

stop—junction between the muzzle (maxilla bone) and the frontal bone of the skull

strobila—the entire body of a tapeworm

syndrome—a collection of symptoms that typify a particular disease state

tachycardia—abnormally fast heartbeat

talus—the uppermost, protruding tarsal bone of the hock

taxonomy—classification of organisms according to physical, genetic, and biochemical relationships and characteristics

teres ligament—major ligament connecting the femur to the acetabulum of the pelvis

theobromine—chemical compound structurally related to caffeine found in relatively high amounts in chocolate

thromboembolism—occlusion by an embolus that has broken away from a thrombus; fibrous clot obstructing a blood vessel

titer—strength of a solution as determined through titration with a standard substance; or, sequential dilutions

toxemia—presence of toxins in the blood and associated signs of disease

trachea—tubular airway leading from the larynx into the chest, branching into two bronchi that enter the lungs

trochlea—a smooth articular surface of bone upon which another bone glides

turgid—swollen, congested

uremia—abnormally elevated levels of urea in the blood and associated clinical signs

vascular—pertaining to blood vessels

viremia—presence of virus particles in the blood

volvulus—twisting of the stomach or intestine

xenophobia—fear of strangers; fear of the unfamiliar

zygote—fertilized ovum

Index